I0968939

dispatches

from the war zone of environmental health

What You Need to Know and What You Can Do

*Information from the Files
of a Medical Science Reporter*

Helke Ferrie

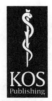

KOS
Publishing

BOOKS ON MEDICINE THAT WORKS

gmos • cancer • fluoride • government betrayal • pesticides • chlorine
multiple chemical sensitivity • toxic drugs • contaminated vaccines
•autism • antidepressants • asthma • gmos • cancer • fluoride • government
betrayal • pesticides • chlorine • multiple chemical sensitivity • toxic drugs
contaminated vaccines • autism • antidepressants • asthma • gmos

Copyright © 2004 Helke Ferrie and Robert K. Ferrie

All Rights reserved. No part of this book may be reproduced in any manner whatsoever without prior written permission from the publisher except in the case of brief quotations embodied in review.

National Library of Canada Cataloguing in Publication

Ferrie, Helke, 1948–
Ferrie, Robert K. 1937–

Dispatches from the war zone of environmental health

Includes bibliographical references

ISBN 0-9731945-3-7

1. Medical politics. 2. Environmental health
3. Environmental toxicology

Cover and text design/layout: Heidy Lawrance Associates

Published and distributed by
KOS Publishing Inc.
1997 Beechgrove Road
Alton, ON, Canada   L0N 1A0
Tel: 519-927-1049
Fax: 519-927-9542
www.kospublishing.com
Quantity discounts available

The nutritional, medical and health information presented in this book is based on the research and interviews conducted by the authors and are true to the best of their knowledge. The opinions are those expressed of the authors. This book is intended only as an informative guide for those who wish to know more about the subject matters covered therein. Every effort has been made to achieve accuracy. The authors and KOS Publishing Inc. shall have no liability or responsibility to any person or entity with respect to any loss, damage, or injury caused or alleged to be caused directly or indirectly by the information contained in this book. The information herein contained is in no way intended to replace supervision by a doctor for medical or health related problems.

For
Hilary Balmer
Director and Founder of RAINET*

because she continues to be outraged
at what deserves outrage
and does something about it,
especially for MCS (see Section 7)

*RESEARCH ADVOCACY & INFORMATION NETWORK
*Established as a volunteer, not-for-profit organization in 1997, RAINET provides services to
disabled individuals who have become financially disadvantaged*
P.O. Box 943 Uxbridge, ON, L9P 1N3
canrainet@sympatico.ca
905-852-2672

Contents

What You Need to Know and What You Can Do
Information from The Files of a Medical Science Reporter

Introduction

Reporting on Crime and Progress

The weapons of mass destruction have been found, at least in medicine, and only we—the people, the consumers, the patients—can stop their proliferation by rouge corporations and their buddies in government. We have known about them for a long time actually, but their origins have been attributed to different sources over time. In antiquity, malevolent deities were thought responsible for the plagues that wiped out city-states and later caused economic disaster for the Roman Empire. In the Middle Ages, God was believed to be angry with sinful humanity and therefore visited epidemics on them, as he was believed to have done in the biblical stories about the Egypt at the time of Moses. In the mid-19th century, the poor of the vast slums associated with Europe's great cities were blamed for spreading mysterious diseases whose bacterial and viral causes were not yet understood by science.

Today, we know that the weapons of mass destruction are human-made chemicals, causing our current plague of chronic and degenerative diseases, and they are found in those substances intended to kill bugs, slugs, dandelions as well as in most of the drugs manufactured to fight cancer, impotence, heart disease, arthritis and other illnesses. These chemicals are the basis of an amoral economic system that sells toxic chemicals in all their forms with the promise of perfect lawns, perfect agricultural produce, perfectly hygienic kitchens, perfect white laundry, and perfect magic-bullet drugs. In fact, they harm us and are guaranteed to harm coming generations as well. Marketing techniques ensure that the whole truth is as carefully disguised as possible. That truth being, that our chemically saturated food, air, water, and soil are the sources of all our diseases—either directly, or by compromising our immune responses, or by giving pathogens the evolutionary advantage.

These toxic chemicals create phantom needs and dependencies by which their manufacturers *enforce* profits. This has to do with power and is a political process. The famous Swiss psychotherapist, Marie-Louise von Franz used to say that the challenge posed by evil boiled down to understanding within oneself and others the nature of "PP and FF" which stands for "power, pride, fame and fortune". There is no essential difference between the claims of a lawn care product, a toxic pharmaceutical drug, and the invasion of Iraq, except the field of action: they share the aim of seeking to profit at somebody else's expense and covering up the deadly truth of long-term environmental and social destruction or deadly side-effects; advertising and present-day war propaganda are the same devil in two different disguises. One promises to free you from lawn pests (at best with temporary success and at the risk of cancer to your family and neighbor), the second promises symptom control (at the price of worse sickness or death), and the third touts political liberation—but all of it boils down to: just hand over your money or oil.

How This Book Came To Be

I am actually an anthropologist by training, not a journalist. I studied human evolution and had fun researching stone tools, the evolution of agriculture, and taking part in the amusing and arcane academic scuffles over whether the Neanderthals went extinct or evolved into us, *Homo sapiens*, and whether either or both are related or not to the oldest humans, *Homo erectus*. My main area of interest was the evolution of disease about which science knows surprisingly much. Most people don't know that every disease known to humanity has a history with a beginning and sometimes even an end—that is to say: the history of disease is the history of human behavior in a given environment.

Pandora's Box contains what our interactions with each other and our environment inadvertently promoted. Pathogens that were harmless for millions of years mutated and became harmful through close proximity with animals we domesticated, or as a function of our choice to live in more and more crowded villages and eventually cities. Chronic illnesses, such as arthritis, are known from Neanderthal skeletons and became a sign of deficiency when the wide variety of foods from hunting and gathering practiced for several million years was replaced by reliance on a comparatively monotonous diet of a few so-called staple foods. Indeed, with the increasing reliance on agriculture the archaeological record shows the simultaneous proliferation of diseases: with planting and domestication begin the diagnoses listed in *Harrison's Principles of Internal Medicine*.

Illness is the price of civilization. The variety of experience higher civilizations made possible resulted also in an unexpected variety of physical problems. Comparisons with modern hunter-gatherer societies have conclusively proven this observation to be true. They don't develop heart disease or cancer until they start eating and living like "civilized" people do. Their average daily intake of vitamin C would shock the historically and anthropologically naive scientists who determine the Recommended Daily

Allowances (RDAs) of vitamins, minerals and other nutrients: a !Kung hunter-gatherer gets about 60,000 mg of vitamin C in his *daily* diet, which is about the same amount a chimpanzee gets also. Our absurd RDAs suggest a maximum of 1,000 mg, and most doctors will actually tell you that 200 mg is all you need. Maybe to avoid something awful like scurvy, but certainly not if we want to be as healthy as those few remaining hunter-gatherer tribes and those equally threatened chimpanzees.

So, yes, polio has a beginning (Old Kingdom Egypt), as does tetanus, the flu, small pox, and the ability of the body to respond in a way we call cancer (all associated with the rise of the Neolithic). These illnesses all arose out of the environment, where they were dormant and harmless, in interaction with and as a response to human behavior. Today, science knows that even the mutations in our genes, that can give rise to disease, require enabling human-made conditions. As ecologist Sandra Steingraber puts it, "A cancer cell is made, not born."

When I became seriously ill in the early 1990s with what turned out to be a chronic illness called Myasthenia gravis and was told that the cause is unknown and no cure exists, the doctors were talking to an anthropologist who knew that every disease has a history and therefore had a cause that's knowable. That implies, in principle, the possibility of a cure. I did not accept this standard verdict, found the cause of my illness to be a combination of years of exposure to DDT, while living in India, and a mouth full of mercury amalgam fillings; their removal and a subsequent detoxification protocol restored my health.

This experience of disease and medical ignorance (medicine in general and the education of doctors sorely lack the historical perspective) and coming face to face with the criminal refusal by the majority of the dental community to take responsibility for their toxic treatments, led me to write an article for *The Medical Post* about me journey back to health. I was mad as hell and wanted everybody to know about this. It has been a matter of profound satisfaction to me that, as a result of my articles on my own experience, I have helped a great many myasthenics get out of their zombie states, identify the causes of their illness (usually mercury "silver" amalgams were chief amongst them), and get back to life.

Soon I found myself listening to the stories of people with many other illnesses, all of which were supposedly of unknown causes, and I also began to hear stories about the suppression of treatments that work, such as chelation for cardiovascular disease and diabetic neuropathy, or cancer treatments without chemotherapy, radiation and surgery. I often wondered if I was caught in a nightmare and hoped to awake as soon as possible. All of this is a nightmare all right, but we are living in it wide awake.

Within less than a year I had entered a world I had not known existed: the dark side of medicine where ego and greed and power rule, and where ignorance is supported by ideology. I began to attend medical conferences, interview doctors and politicians and government regulators. My articles began to appear in health magazines, and rarely in mainstream publications, but I forged friendships with many excellent journalists in the mainstream whose help has always been invaluable—sometimes for information, but usually to get a story out that I could not get out by myself. I found to my surprise that I had left fossils and stone tools for a global war to achieve public health.

The life of a free-lance medical science writer is blessed by a lot of freedom to roam, search, and dig up the dirt. My editor at Toronto's *Vitality Magazine*, Julia Woodford, gives me maximum freedom to explore, because she shares my infinite curiosity for what's happening in this medical crime scene, and for the tremendous progress that is happening as well. Often my articles get published elsewhere later, in the US and Australia mainly, and even in the in-flight magazines of airlines (which is just great—the inside of an air plane is just about the worst chemically-saturated environment imaginable, and those people need this information most!).

I am asked so many times for copies of my articles by health activists, patient groups and (very gratifyingly) doctors who want to hand them out to their members or patients, that I decided to gather together topical articles likely to remain topical for a long time and make them into a book with updating information appended, as needed. They all deal with the theme of our environment and health.

But besides informing readers on environmental issues, this book is also a tool. Here is a mass of information and ammunition for patients and activists—who often are both. *You may photostat and distribute anything that is useful to you in this book without my express permission, as long as you give appropriate credits. In fact, I hope many readers will take to the warpath with this book.*

Reporting on Crime and Progress

The job of the journalist is to ask: "Is this really true?"

Unlike the Official Opposition in a government which questions, in line with its own party's principles, whatever the party in power is doing, a journalist is supposed to question the *whole* scene, including the opposition parties and their motives, and whoever is involved with the whole lot of them. The job of journalism is to question power, the status quo, and to doubt the reality of all appearances, in politics and all other human endeavors as well. Journalists work to minimize the powers of deception. There are great examples of what that looks like in the work of people like Linda McQuaig, CBC Radio's Michael Enright, Canadian Centre for Policy Alternatives' Ed Finn and colleagues, Michelle Landsberg, some fabulous people at CBC and the *Toronto Daily Star*, and blockbuster truth-sayers like Michael Moore of "Fahrenheit 9/11" fame, and Joel Bakan and the team that helped him make the documentary "The Corporation" (to name just a few of my heroes that come to mind; this is not intended to be a representative list which would be far too long).

But just as there are a few great doctors and a great many on automatic pilot, journalism has a lot of sheep and not so many lions. The jury isn't out, and perhaps never will be, on what's worse in any walk of life: active evil or tepid mediocrity.

For example, the research of Professor Joel Lexchin at York University in Toronto has shown that when it comes to reporting on pharmaceuticals, the media (even frequently the classiest among them) tend to take the press release from a drug company with all its propaganda, outright lies, and blatant sale's pitch, and publish it as fact. No nasty questions asked! (See section 5.)

Admittedly, the members of the media face the same problem as the individual: one often simply cannot believe that things could possibly be as corrupt as they really are. The learning curve involved in the recognition of evil is the steepest of all learning curves one encounters in life. Section 6 deals with this issue.

I remember an incident in 1999 when representatives of *Citizens for Choice in Health Care* and I were asked for a meeting with the health editors of the *Toronto Daily Star*. We had been providing them with information on serious problems in the medical licensing authority of Ontario that was, if true and if not exposed but allowed to continue unchecked, going to adversely affect the public interest in a big way. So, the editors asked to meet with us and discuss the possibility of publishing a series of articles designed to report on the failure of the College of Physicians and Surgeons of Ontario (CPSO) to act in accordance with its mandate. Ontario, having more doctors than the rest of Canada combined, basically sets the tone for the medical status quo in the country, so if there is something rotten at the CPSO, it is rather important.

The information we had available included many aspects of the CPSO's work and the contents of our files pretty much sizzled. Suddenly, one of the editors freaked right out. He burst out, "Are you telling me that I am supposed to believe the CPSO is not protecting my health and acting in the public interest? I can't accept that!" We were unable to answer this outburst, because he stormed out of the room. As a professional journalist he was supposed to become alert and interested at the mere possibility of wrongdoing. He was supposed to doubt that the CPSO, and all other institutions for that matter, are actually functioning the way they say they do. When he was gone, one of the fortunately more hard-boiled editors in the room said, "Don't worry about what just happened, let's get on with the info."

The *Star* decided to run with it. What we provided them with was just *one* major strand of the story (when something is rotten, there is always more than one witness available), including access to whistleblowers from within the CPSO, that resulted in the series "Medical Secrets". Over a period of two years, a whole lot of doctors from hell were exposed, who had caused tremendous damage, but were protected by the CPSO, often for many years and following many formal and well-documented complaints. *The Star's* articles resulted in these doctors losing their licenses and many legal actions being initiated by patients. At one point, the then Minister of Health for Ontario, Tony Clement, even phoned one of the principal reporters, Robert Cribb, to thank him for this effort and encouraged him to continue the expose, as such reporting was essential support for government reform. Clement then went on to do some much-needed clean-ups at the CPSO. Not nearly enough, but it was a great start.

Another off-shoot of this effort was the production of the *Glasnost Report* in 2001 by a group of medical organizations and patient groups. In Section 5 you can read all about that, and if you want to follow the leads provided there, you can read the *Star* series in the Internet. The Ontario story has its counterpart in the corruption in Health Canada's drug regulatory activity characterized by a near-total disregard for the existing legislation. The details of the public's demand to have these laws obeyed are described as well in Section 5 and 8.

The deception journalism is charged with exposing has many forms (Sections 5 and 6). Thus I may find myself interviewing a medical scientist who has become fully aware of *one* aspect of a deception and is appropriately outraged by it—such as a drug company hiding critical, potentially harmful research evidence under the subterfuge of "proprietary information", but that doctor may be unaware of the fact that the research into that specific medical problem was itself a deceptive exercise and totally unnecessary, because a cheaper, safer, possibly non-drug and far more effective treatment for that condition already exists. The current scandal involving the antidepressants, the SSRIs comes to mind. (SSRIs are so-called Selective Serotonin Re-uptake Inhibitors like Prozac.) See Section 6. It all depends on the doctor's training, how aware he or she is of a generally unconscious allegiance to a specific medical ideology, and what journals he or she regularly reads. Deception feeds on and counts on the presence of ignorance, and ignorance by definition simply means not knowing. Of course, the journalist is equally likely to be ignorant, as we all are.

A whole book on examples of this type of situation could be written—showing how the deception may include the drug sales representative who pushes a drug she might sincerely believe in, while being deceived herself by the manufacturer's marketing departments; the scientist who write the supporting literature is likely duped as well by raw data supplied in a deceptive, incomplete, or doctored manner by the manufacturer; and the patients in the trial from which the raw data came are also duped or have had their information distorted. The combinations and interconnections of these patterns are so varied and intricate, that the journalist can only hope to expose just one lie at a time.

So—this isn't easy. North on the journalist's moral and professional compass is where the question "Is this really true?" is found. That's all we have to go by and it works very well if we aren't afraid to follow where this compass leads us.

This web of deception sticks to everything that has to do with environment and health, the topic of this book. Drugs and their power to harm in the long run, while controlling symptoms in the short term, have now become an environmental problem as well, because they pollute the water, and not being bio-degradable, enter the bodies of people and animals for whom they were not prescribed, thereby doing a great deal of irreversible harm. I have explored this in more detail in my book *Hippocrates in the Land of Oz* (Kos 2004).

Cancer is the quintessential environmental disease. Only a cancer-promoting environment can cause its appearance. Even the genetically anchored forms of cancer and all chronic diseases, from asthma to multiple sclerosis, need a toxic chemical, heavy metals or a nutrient-deficient diet to trigger them. Just as all life can only exist within a very narrow range of temperature, humidity, and delicately tuned combination of gases, so health can only be maintained within a narrow range of essentials. Section 3 is devoted to cancer.

Even Down's Syndrome and many other genetically anchored diseases, require as prerequisites mothers deprived of important cellular nutrients (from what passes as food these days) to disrupt fetal development. It's really very simple: something never comes from nothing. Or, in the words of Hippocrates, the father of scientific medicine who lived in ancient Greece two thousand five hundred years ago, "Each disease has a natural cause, and nothing happens without a natural cause." (*Science of Medicine*, Hippocratic Writings). Sections 1, 2 and 3 will introduce you to some of what science knows about food, environmental toxins and disease.

However, the most serious and continuous exposure to environmental toxins comes from that cocktail of pesticides, herbicides, fungicides, heavy metals, radioactive waste, and antibiotics in our food, water, air, soil and from the subsequent food-processing, transportation and serving methods that further poison us and kill the nutrients our health and survival depend upon. Almost all of these substances are put into our bodies without our knowledge or consent and virtually none have been tested for safety; if they had—they wouldn't be in our environment. The same now also applies to childhood vaccines, which is why my article on autism (Section 4) is included in this collection.

Section 7 is devoted to Multiple Chemical Sensitivity whose victims throughout the industrialized world are fighting to have MCS recognized so that both treatment and legal compensation are possible. I am involved in this effort in Canada.

The good fortune is that medical science largely understands the nature of the damage from these chemicals, solvents and heavy metals, and the pathways have been determined by which they kill, or cause disease, or initiate birth defects. There is even a branch of medicine that started in the 1940s—when the chemical era itself began—which has systematically developed treatments and often cures, namely Environmental Medicine. Harvard Medical School has an entire department devoted to it, as do all major European universities. In the US, the UK, Germany and Japan hospitals exist that exclusively deal with environmental illness. Among the various medical journals reporting on the research of environmental medicine, the leading English-language ones are the *Archives of Environmental Health* and *Environmental Health Perspectives* in the US, and the *Journal of Nutritional & Environmental Medicine* in the UK.

The reason the articles in this book are like dispatches from a war-zone is because doctors who treat people damaged by this human-made toxic environment are taking on more than just a patient. The diagnosis, successful treatment and demonstrable recovery of each patient—repeated in thousands of cases—amount to a condemnation of the very basis of the world's economy.

All good medicine is, in principle, a *practical* moral force counteracting the abuse of humanity. Good medicine is at war with this chemical abuse.

However, when medicine becomes a business, as it now basically has become, it is in grave danger of becoming also an abuser. Medicine has become part of the sickness industry and often unconsciously, but also knowingly, has become part of that sinister aspect of the world's wealth-creating systems which create and maintain dependence. Nobody is more vulnerable to the almost always false advertising in medicine and the many useless and often harmful therapies than a seriously ill person. As the former editor of the *New England Journal of Medicine*, Marcia Angell, puts it in her new book, *The Truth About The Drug Companies*, "If prescription drugs are so good, why do they need to be pushed so hard? The answer is that good drugs don't have to be promoted very much. A genuinely important drug...sells itself."

While the marketing machine dupes patients into making billion dollar profits for the drug companies, the really curative therapies are consistently hidden from them by that same marketing machine that seeks to protect its largely useless products by ensuring the indoctrination of doctors and patients with pompous (self-serving) definitions of "scientific" medicine, as opposed to "unproven" or "alternative" therapies (whose medicines are unpatentable and hence unprofitable). The trouble for them is that truth does not support obscene profits, only lies do. A patient cured is a patient lost to business; as one overhead graphically showed in the March 2004 Canadian Forum on Pharmaceutical Marketing: "As a marketer, which is better for business? *Steady* continuous use of your drug, OR *occasional* use of your drug?" (Emphasis in the original.)

But there is hope. The fact is that nothing in Nature is uniform and totally predictable. The pessimist thinks he knows it's all rotten and always will be, but the pessimist is no more omniscient than the optimist. Corrupt organizations have whistleblowers, the promotion of obscene profits always backfires eventually, public outrage and political pressure exerted by organized activists is hugely successful, and everybody eventually trips over the most carefully constructed lies. Sadly, the human cost is horrendous, but helpful information is accumulating at such a fast pace, that more and more people may avail themselves of it before it is too late for them.

The Old Boys' Club of Standard Medicine is also wising up rapidly. I don't predict a perfect world of medicine for the near future, but Spring is in the air: I am impressed by the awakening of professional pride that won't put up with the sleaze anymore. In March 2004, the Canadian Medical Association hammered Health Canada and rebuked it for outright corruption. The CMA says Health Canada is complicit in "too often keeping quiet about buried evidence that questions drug safety and effectiveness."

The international committee of medical journal editors first laid down the law in September 2001 on conflicts of interest issues for the authors of research articles. Since close to 90% of all researchers are funded in some way by industry, this didn't work out too well and the sleaze continued. So they decided to go to the source of the mess and address the pharmaceutical industry itself, which has corrupted all research to a greater or lesser degree, so that basically there isn't a therapy or a drug on the market that isn't at least in part based on or tainted by fraud. The medical editors issued a statement published in all those major journals in their September 2004 issues. This informs the industry that they must register *all* their clinical trials from day one. What this means is, that they can no longer report only the data with industry-favoring results (or just their favorable-looking segments) and conveniently hide data revealing bad outcomes. This way, it is hoped with some justification, both the researcher and the sponsor will have to clean up their act. Obviously, this will benefit patients and the true toxicity of drugs and their lack of effectiveness may be revealed in time. It is hoped that this will then also give a chance for really useful research to be done and published.

Following the Canadian Supreme Court's 2001 *Hudson Decision,* which asserted the right of municipalities to determine whether or not to use pesticides within their boundaries, Canada also got new federal pesticide legislation. Both events provide reasons for optimism, especially since so many municipalities are fighting now to get by-laws passed that will stop the cosmetic use of pesticides and herbicides, and the whole of Quebec has already done so. All this activity to make our environment life-supporting again was assisted in a most timely manner in May 2004 by the report from the Ontario College of Family Physicians on the cosmetic use of pesticides and their causal role in childhood leukemia, asthma, cancer and neurological diseases.

As for the fight against disease-promoting foods, Italy has just passed a law that requires all educational institutions, from kindergarten to universities, to serve only 100% organic foods. Italy obviously has understood that investing in the future of the human brain begins with food capable of nourishing developing brains. This is just one of many examples of positive action. The stories in Section 7 deal with events that show that people are taking charge of their health and understand the political nature of medicine today.

I believe there is such a thing as progress and that we may experience it daily, if we wish, that we may cause it as well as participate in it, and that we can access its sources if we want to. Yes, that requires knowledge and the willingness to pursue information and go where it leads—to find out for your-self. I hope these articles provide a nice chunk of useful information to get you started.

We can choose *not* to be the fodder for other people's political ambitions, financial profit, or scientific ideology. We need not believe what we are told, even when we are told it in good faith, because we may be confident that even well-meaning people could be duped. We can choose to doubt. One of my favorite sayings is found in the 5th century BC Taoist text, *The Chuang Tzu*: "The sage steers by Chaos and Doubt."

I write in the hope of causing liberating disillusionment in at least some of my readers, and in order to offer them some tools to explore further and strike out on their own. Trust in authority, or herd mentality, in medicine always ends in injury and death. Hippocrates said, "A wise man ought to realize that health is his most valuable possession and learn how to treat his illnesses by his own judgment." The rest is up to you.

Sources

Sources of some of the ideas touched upon above which are worthy of your exploration:

M. Angell, *The Truth About the Drug Companies: How They Deceive Us and What To Do About It*, Random House, 2004

J. Bakan, *The Corporation: The Pathological Pursuit of Profit and Power*, Viking, 2004

M.N. Cohen, *Health and the Rise of Civilization*, Yale University, 1989

R. Firshein, *The Nutraceutical Revolution*, Penguin Bantam, 1998

J. Krop, *Healing the Planet One Patient At A Time: A Primer in Environmental Medicine.* 2nd ed., Kos Publishing Inc., 2003

M. Lappe, *The Tao of Immunology*, Plenum, 1997

M. Lappe, *Evolutionary Medicine: Rethinking the Origins of Disease*, Sierra Club Books, 1994

R. Porter, *The Greatest Benefit to Mankind: A Medical History of Humanity*, W.W. Norton, 1997

P. Radetsky, *Allergic to the Twentieth Century: The Explosion in Environmental Allergies—From Sick Buildings to Multiple Chemical Sensitivity*, Little Brown * Co, 1997

S. Steingraber, *Living Downstream: An Ecologist Looks At Cancer*, 2nd ed. Vintage Books, 1998

S. Rampton & J. Stauber, *Trust Us We're Experts: How Industry Manipulates Science and Gambles With Your Future*, Tarcher Putnam, 2001

M. Walker, *Elements of Danger: Protect Yourself Against the Hazards of Modern Dentistry*, Hampton Roads, 2001

1

Food

Five Reports on Biotechnology
and Organic Agriculture

The Montreal Event January 2000—Report No 1

Pigs won't eat it, deer avoid it, raccoons turn up their noses at it, mice can't be tempted to nibble at it—none will eat genetically engineered corn or tofu beans but seek out the real stuff in fields and barns. "What is it that they know instinctively that we ignore?" wondered a farmer speaking to agricultural journalist Steven Yankoton during his four-months investigative assignment across the Corn Belt researching genetically engineered (GE) food products for *Acres USA* (Sept. 18, 1999).

My first article on GE foods reported on the now famous "Montreal Event" that appears today, in retrospect, to have been the moment at which the GE tide began to turn against the corporate take-over of the food supply. The unilateral hijacking of the food supply was stopped, at least in its original ruthless form, in Montreal on that cold January day.

The popular demand for real food that nourishes and the rejection of the messing with poorly understood genes began in earnest in Montreal on the coldest day I experienced in more than 30 Canadian winters, namely on January 22, 2000. The temperature was minus 52 Celsius at noon in the downtown university area at which time exactly a demonstration was scheduled to commence to protest against the US-dictated decision not to label foods containing GE materials. This demonstration was to take place in front of the hotel in which delegates from 135 nations were meeting to discuss the labeling issue, and they were expected to do what the United States wished them to do.

The event and the protest were organized by Greenpeace, Council of Canadians, the Quebec Public Interest Research Group, and Biotech Action Montreal. The morning of this event had featured ten workshops at which scientists, international law experts, and activist from all over the world gave the whole truth and nothing but the truth concerning genetic engineering and the food supply to a crowd filling the lecture rooms to overflowing. Some 500 people had been expected. Almost 2,000 showed up.

The central problem, as explained by the delegates from all over the world, was "globalization without representation". The decisions being made by the World Trade Organization's member states are made basically without input from the elected representatives of those countries and in many instances are able to bypass those countries' courts. The WTO meetings are secret and their decisions are immune to local parliamentary debates. WTO courts have no transcripts or any mechanism of public oversight. GE foods are a major issue as they have been forced onto nations in this manner, food being of vital importance to international trade. The only action left at this point is grassroots protest and civil disobedience, and, of course, the refusal to eat this stuff—provided you can identify its presence.

Following the noon-time demonstration, the afternoon and evening programs' speakers included Maude Barlow, the British geneticist Mae Wan-Ho, a representative from Greenpeace in China, and American biotech critic Jeremy Rifkin. Interestingly, Maude Barlow was of the opinion that "we *can* turn this around", and indeed we did. Their presentations were followed by the advance screening of the National Film Board documentary entitled "The Genetic Takeover" which was introduced by its co-producer, Louise Vandelac, a professor at the University of Montreal.

The Montreal GE forum was entitled "Importing Trouble: Genetic Engineering and Trade". The theme of the presentations was summarized in a brochure for attendees as: "The makers of toxic waste, leaded gas, and silicon breast implants would like to fix you dinner…" referring to Monsanto, Dow Chemical, Novartis, DuPont and others who, in spite of their track record of injuring millions were now expecting the world to believe that their sole desire was to feed the starving billions of the planet by making agricultural methods more efficient through genetic engineering.

The brochure also informed the reader that about 60% of all processed foods in our supermarkets already contain GE foods—without our knowledge and consent—and that none have ever been tested for environmental safety or their effects on human health, as the internationally recognized Precautionary Principle requires. Furthermore, those studies that *were* done on safety issues had been suppressed in one of the most elaborate corporate mis-information campaigns to date. Thus, most of us unknowingly consume scorpion genes in tomatoes, soya and corn with various bacterial genes, potatoes with human and frog genes. Our digestive tracts, whose enzymes have been constructed by evolution over millions of years to deal with protein combinations within a specific range, have no way of recognizing and metabolizing these brave new human-made proteins. The opening frames of the NFB documentary screened that night showed the eerie image of a strawberry in the shape of a fish—not a sci-fi notion but a reality: genes from the cold-tolerant Arctic Char have been placed into the genome of the strawberry in the hope of permitting their growth in colder climates (it hasn't worked out).

On January 22, 2000, nobody knew that three years later independent scientists (meaning: not paid by biotech corporations) would prove that our gut cannot process GE corn, and as the intolerance is likely to apply to other GE foods, too. On April 4, 2004 the venerable science journal *Nature* suggested that organic farming would be the way of the future. Neither could anybody have known (though it was a hope then) that the food industry in Europe and Canada would rapidly respond and produce affordable processed organic foods and offer fresh organic produce in their supermarkets as well, thereby giving new meaning to the issue of labeling. One of the tasks suggested to the audience in Montreal was to write to Loblaws and ask its president W. Galen Weston to guarantee that his famous "President's Choice" line of foods would be labeled 100% organic. Although Mr. Weston did not do exactly that, i.e. label all produce as GE free, what he did do was to ensure that today, Loblaws offers a whole line of guaranteed GE-free foods to those customers who want it, and the line of products steadily increases. Most importantly, Loblaws' baby food comes in glass jars again to prevent harmful xeno-estrogenic substances in plastic containers from harming our babies, and harmful dyes, chemicals as well as refined sugars have also been removed. Gerber's guarantees GE-free baby food as well, and McDonalds went GE free in Europe to survive there economically. Indeed, the Montreal Event initiated the process of focusing on *all* food quality issues, starting with the GE issue.

When I reported on this event in the March 2000 issue of *Vitality* Magazine these developments lay still in the future and the main issue was how to avoid GE foods. My recommendation to my readers was then to "adopt a raccoon and take him shopping to sniff out the right stuff."

While the battle for earth-friendly food, and the need for all food to be in harmony with the imperatives of our biology and the earth's biochemistry, is certainly not nearly over, *choice* is a reality and the *right* to chemically and genetically uncontaminated food is firmly on the agenda of any discourse on agricultural issues in the world today. Indeed, as of May 2004 even the World Trade Organization has been forced into appointing a so-called dispute panel which has been charged with looking into the hundreds of thousands of protests against GE foods. Their task will be to evaluate the science upon which the original hijacking of the food supply was based—which was, of course, corporate "tobacco science", with the real science being firmly suppressed. Friends of the Earth, which organized this protest campaign is watching this process and you can find out all about this action, the WTO investigation, and future developments on **www.foe.co.uk** and **www.bite back.org.uk.**

As a result of the Montreal Event 2000 also, patent laws, once an arcane subject for specialists, became the subject of intense scrutiny. The public now questions the ethics and long-term effects of corporate patents being taken out on anything with DNA in it. Perhaps, in a hundred years from now, we will see the GE Food Wars as a dangerous adventure which, however, also resulted in educating the public that science, public health and corporate law cannot ever be left to those who solely wish to benefit from them financially.

Jeremy Rifkin, who more than two decades ago began to question the commercially exploitative direction biological research was taking, when the first patent for a bacterial life form was granted by a US court in 1980 to Ananda Chakrabarty and General Electric (see J. Rifkin's book below for the full story) is now often referred to as "the Ralph Nader of biotechnology". That is a supreme, though grudging compliment. Indeed, his message is parallel to Nader's, namely that these food stuffs are unsafe and a rip-off in any and all of their weird genetic combinations.

Following the morning's workshops at which people learned about genetic engineering from the invited delegates from all over the world, those willing to participate in the demonstration were taken in hand, as it were, most expertly by Greenpeace volunteers who had the preparations for this action organized to perfection: tables with sandwiches made on excellent European whole wheat and rye breads were ready and everyone was instructed—actually ordered—to eat. "You will burn calories so fast out there in that cold, you may not be able to stand it for more than half an hour if you do not eat," we were told. "You must eat!" Everybody ate. Extra hats, mittens and scarves were on hand and Greenpeace volunteers bundled people deftly if they believed them inadequately protected. Signs reading "Stop Genetic Pollution", "Biosafety Now", "Not in my Dinner!" were available in large numbers, and several hundred people grabbed these and moved on out into the bitter cold.

Just crossing the street was a supreme effort. The cold was so extreme, one could not breathe except through the protective layer of a thick scarf. The eyes began to water instantly, and any tiny part of exposed skin seemed to burn as if touched by fire. I felt terrible that I could not take part, but merely managed to make it across the road to the safety of a coffee shop. I was then still recovering from mercury and pesticide poisoning, and any extremes of heat and cold brought on double vision, impaired balance and serious breathing problems. I knew I was a potential liability to that effort.

The demonstration took place in front of the hotel in which delegates from 135 nations were meeting to commence a week of talks on the so-called International Biosafety Protocol—which had little, if anything to do, with safety. Simultaneously, the results of an opinion poll had been released which showed that 94% of Canadians do not want GE foods, if there are any doubts about their safety. The same results, showing consistently numbers above 70%, were obtained from opinion polls in many European countries, Japan and several Asian nations. The international delegates were made sufficiently nervous by this clear opposition that by 5 p.m, the following Saturday, January 29th, they arrived at a peculiar compromise: instead of acting in accord with the public demand of their own countries to label GE foods as such (which doubtlessly would have killed the GE food industry practically instantly), they decided to try and satisfy the big boys of the chemical industry *as well* as appease the clearly angry public of the world, from China to Canada, and allow labels reading "*May* contain GE products." This was a neat example of not getting off the pot...*and* not doing their business.

Virtually at once, European ports increased their use of GE testing technology and turned away GE food shipments on many, now well publicized occasions. This year, in 2004, most of the biotech firms closed their offices even in the UK where the government tried everything to force GE down its population's throats (*Nature* July 8, 2004). Since 1999, Canada lost its canola export to Australia which captured the market for GE-uncontaminated products in Europe, and the prediction made in 2000 by independent scientists, that GE plants would trigger rapid evolution of herbicide resistance and produce uncontrollable "super weeds", has indeed come to pass with disastrous consequences for Western Canada.

The GE battle was fought from the start with the same deceptive propaganda as all wars have always been fought. Indeed, in this case, too, "the truth was the first causality", as has often been said about war reporting. Similar to the sound bite of the 1970s, "freeing the world for democracy", in the GE food war it is "feeding the world", and just as the world was not keen on an American-style democracy back then, the world is not too keen on GE products from US chemical and seed corporations. Both American-style democracy and GE technology have in common the creation of dependencies instead of the promised liberation from oppression or want.

On the one side of this battle we find our governments supporting their GE-corporate clients and defending trade monopolies on *patented* life processes, thereby, ruling against the people's expressed will and the united opinion of independent scientists. Many of President Clinton's key staff and advisors had come to the White House from the board rooms of Monsanto and other chemical companies. Monsanto scientists developed most of the GE plants as well as the infamous bovine growth hormone.

Senator Eugene Whelan, who served for more than a decade under Trudeau as Canada's immensely popular Minister of Agriculture, told me that when he was in Ottawa, Monsanto was spending millions on lobbying in the hope of getting bovine growth hormone passed. This was unsuccessful, because the Health Canada scientists, led by Dr. Shiv Chopra, refused for more than a decade to waive the legally mandated requirement of proof of biological safety—something Monsanto did not wish to comply with, as this hormone is a carcinogen and hormone disruptor (i.e. gender bender), as was well known to scientists on both sides of this fight. Finally, the truth about this hormone became public though Senator Whelan's initiation of Senate Hearings into that whole smelly mess.

On the other side of this battle line are ordinary people who have suddenly noticed that breakfast, lunch and dinner may be politically charged events, and that what *looks* like food may not actually *be* food. Supporting ordinary people are scientists such as British scientist Ardai Puzstai and many others who were once forcibly silenced, the British Medical Association, the Sierra Club, the World Wildlife Fund, the Consumers Union and the Union of Concerned Scientists who include many Nobel laureates. This last group studied GE production and sales and concluded that 93% of all these efforts are designed explicitly to maximize profit for a few companies who were in no way planning to feed the world, as the propaganda asserted. On the eve of the World Trade Organization meeting in Seattle the year before, British geneticist Mae-Wan Ho and several hundred scientists submitted a letter to the WTO and President Clinton calling for an immediate moratorium on GE food production and research. Even the editor of one of the world's most prestigious but rather straight-laced science journals, *Nature*, opined candidly in the context of GE products and trade, that "free trade is not more important than the future of life on our planet."

The Canadian government began in the 1980s to subsidize GE companies, especially Monsanto, to the tune of $ 700 million annually with our tax money, but not with our permission. Canada and the US insist that labeling a product as containing GE is unnecessary because the government unilaterally and without a shred of independent evidence to support this stand, deems the stuff safe. Labeling it "would unnecessarily call attention to it, reduce consumer confidence, and adversely affect sales" (*New York Times* June 1, 1999). At the same time, the FDA obligingly changed its rules so that corporate-sponsored safety studies of their products are now "confidential" and not open to public scrutiny.

However, the Achilles' heel of all dirty tricks of this type always appears in the form of liability considerations (see last article in this section on the Schmeiser case): the mighty insurance industry will not insure GE crops because, as they point out correctly, no method of risk assessment exists for these strange materials. They are human constructs that replicate themselves, but their future potential liability is unknowable. Governments, in their frantic rush to make their corporate supporters happy and rich, have waived once mandatory regulatory requirements, which were designed to assess safety prior to approval and prior to letting something loose into the environment. The world's largest bank, the Deutsche Bank in Germany, understood the financial implications and announced in July 1999, that GE seeds should be perceived exactly like the nuclear power industry which is also uninsurable, namely as "an earnings nightmare" in the making. The bank correctly predicted that GE wouldn't work out financially, and that organic farming products would be sold at a premium instead.

The Food Wars were fuelled in large part by the fact that Monsanto's blockbuster herbicide Roundup (glyphosate) was due to come off patent protection by the end of the year 2000. While the main ingredient in Roundup is in fact biodegradable, its "inert" ingredients are listed with the FDA as toxic to the liver and the reproductive system. Indeed, in 1999 Swedish researchers reported that this herbicide triggers non-Hodgkins type cancers (the most numerous which have no known genetic anchor), and mainstream medical journals, such as *Cancer* have reported on various other cancers triggered by Roundup; type **glyphosate + cancer** into your Internet search engine for a full list.

In order to avoid a financial slump when Roundup becomes open to generic competition, Monsanto spent much of the 1990s to develop what's known as the "traitor" and "terminator" genes which have a genetically built-in dependence on Monsanto herbicide products to make saving seeds impossible. Their development caused an uproar throughout the world. In India, when the government approved experimental trials with these types of GE plants, protesting farmers committed mass suicide publicly in front of South Indian government buildings by drinking the allegedly safe herbicide Roundup. They were protesting the government's move to make the millennia-old tradition of the small family farm obsolete by supporting Monsanto's plans for mega farms. India passed legislation against GE seeds—which recently came under attack again, and it is not yet clear which way India will go on this issue.

Israelis fought the introduction of GE foods by referring to the days of Moses and rejected GE seeds calling the companies that make them "the new pharaohs". The European Union banned GE foods and later softened this stance by insisting on the labeling of those they were considering to permit. All this unexpected organized rejection caused Monsanto to lay off thousands of its scientists and reduce its research program drastically. Indeed, it was somebody whom they might have considered an ally, who asked them to stop all terminator research, namely the president of the Rockefeller Foundation. A WTO lawyer was outraged at all this grassroots interference and exclaimed, "How can we allow ethical and other irrelevant [!] considerations to interfere?"

The Food Wars represent a general awakening to a huge deception of which the messing around with genes is only one important component. Consider that in 1947 only 6 pesticide resistant agricultural pests existed. By 1999 more than 600 of these are known, even though 12 times as much pesticide is now being used than was the case 50 years ago. All of the efforts "to arm that little seed and send it out in the war against the environment", as Jeremy Rifkin put it, have failed and backfired. Scientific information now reveals that the so-called Green Revolution with its promise of higher yields through chemistry has caused a massive increase in quantity at the expense of quality: the soils degraded to the point where the nutrient value in the plants is decreased by 40% and more in key ingredients, such as magnesium and calcium.

The GE revolution made this situation worse and also brought with it the deceptive promise of less water consumption and reduced needs for herbicides and pesticides. In fact, water consumption has increased and so has the need for the chemicals because of the rapid resistance the pests evolved. Both the Green and the GE Revolutions have proven to be ecologically unsustainable and nutritionally undesirable. Worst of all, non-target creatures such as butterflies, ladybugs and bees, who are all important pollinators, are endangered in many areas because these agricultural chemicals kill their eggs. All this and the fact that important detoxifying bacteria in the soil are also being killed, and pesticide residues are constantly accumulating in soil and water, all point to an ecological disaster in the making.

The deception suffered by farmers appeared in the form of produce yields. Research published by the United States Agriculture Department showed in 1999 already, only 4 years after the introduction of the first GE seeds, that these plants consistently have a lower yield than conventional varieties (on average the yield is 14% less). Using freedom-of-information legislation, independent research showed that Monsanto knew this would be the case already back in 1996. Furthermore, certain plants, such as soya and potatoes lost their adaptability to sudden temperature changes due to the genetic engineering components introduced into them, thus causing serious crop failures. A certain GE cotton strain caused a failure of the pods to open, and Mississippi cotton farmers were compensated for their crop failure in a huge settlement with Monsanto in exchange for silence.

A striking fact is that the corporations dedicated to GE research and the deployment of these foodstuffs all specialize also in pesticides and herbicides *as well* as pharmaceuticals. Whoever controls genes, seeds *and* the sickness industry controls the world. Thus, as Rifkin pointed out that night in Montreal, these companies approach life as an "engineering challenge" and "force living organisms to meet standards of measurement, quality control, and predictable outcomes and utility". Logically, should such GE foods cause health problems, as pesticides already do, the pharmaceutical arm of this corporate enterprise can profit accordingly. This corporate agenda stands in stark contrast to Rifkin's view of the appropriate role of biotechnology: "the aim should not be to change the genome [of plants, animals and ourselves] to fit a dysfunctional environment, but to heal our environment, so it is healthy for all our genomes."

The National Film Board documentary shown that same night, following the demonstrations and supper, featured interviews with the scientists like Scotland's Ardai Pusztai who had been asked by the UK government to undertake safety studies on GE foods. Having helped with the development of the GE technology, Pusztai did not expect anything unusual when he began to feed rats GE potatoes. To his shock and total surprise, all organs and bodily systems were adversely affected suggesting that the GE potatoes were interfering with DNA replication. With the permission of the prestigious Rowett Institute in Edinburgh where Pusztai had worked for many years, he held a press conference announcing his findings. Upon returning to his office he found it gutted: computers, equipment, records—everything gone. The director of the institute informed him that Monsanto had asked him to fire Puzstai. The GE potatoes were a Monsanto invention and the Rowett is largely financed by Monsanto research money. Fortunately, history took a dramatic turn for the better when Prince Charles intervened and asked Puzstai to testify before the House of Lords. The GE debate moved center stage in Europe and activists everywhere became involved. One of the best websites for GE information and sustainable agriculture issues is the Prince of Wales site—which Prime Minister Tony Blair wanted Prince Charles to shut down! The Prince stood firm and told the PM to buzz off.

Like the Ancient Mariner in Milton's great poem, Ardai Pusztai and his scientist wife are traveling the world speaking about their discoveries, advising governments on GE policy issues, and encouraging those who dare to undertake independent research into GE safety.

The documentary also featured the stories of farmers duped by the false promises of the GE industry, and a detailed presentation of just exactly how genetic engineering is done and what its assumptions are. The most striking feature of this science appears to be its total lack of interest in evolutionary contexts. It views the properties of a creature (e.g. Arctic Char's ability to withstand very cold temperatures, or the rapid growth property of certain human genes, or the use of human colon cancer genes in food plants) as if they were interchangeable modules, as if they had not evolved within an environmental context that would obviously also have affected all other systems in that organism, not just the one property the scientist wishes to exploit commercially.

The machine metaphor, in which the parts are not dependent upon the whole, has been projected onto living matter resulting in neither an efficient machine nor in a viable organism. I sat through the screening of this Sorcerer's Apprentice tale thinking, "Those guys need to take a basic first level university course in evolutionary biology." Indeed, the lack of appreciation for context on all levels of human enterprises—cultural, economic, biological—is what characterizes this astounding obsession with the exploitation of everything that lives for the sake of a quick buck. The documentary got a standing ovation that seemed to last forever. The last time I experienced that in a theater was when Star Wars was first released. Let us hope the GE's Darth Vader has met his match.

On March 4, 2000, a few weeks after the Montreal Event, Senator Eugene Whelan spoke at an event entitled "The Future of Food" organized by farmers and environmental groups of the Stratford, Ontario, area. He appeared wearing his trademark 6 gallon green hat and spoke about his fears for Canadian agriculture and the government's commitment to an unproven, dangerous and uncertain biological technology—how "we are being sold down the river by jerks who know nothing about plants, soil and agriculture." He lamented the fact that Canada's famous canola oil, the development of which he had as Canada's agriculture minister shepherded through its many phases using age-old methods, had now been ruined through GE contamination and was no longer a valuable export commodity. "Who wants that junk now?" he asked. At one point he described buying some supermarket tomatoes, presumably the ill-fated FlavrSaver Monsanto scientists had created and which were taken off the market because people noticed quickly that they didn't taste like tomatoes. These tomatoes seemed to Senator Whelan, upon closer examination, somewhat "odd". He placed them on top of his fridge for observation. "Two weeks later," he said, "they were still sitting there on my fridge looking exactly the same as the day I bought them." He asked, "What the heck is this? Is this really a tomato? What's it going to do in my stomach?" He chucked them in the garbage, hoping, he said, the bacteria would know what to do with them.

Summary
The most significant known or suspected adverse health effects of GE foods are:
1. The research of Ardai Puzstai suggests that GE foods (e.g. potatoes) adversely affect the immune system, pancreas, reproductive system, brain, thymus and ovaries and may trigger diseases of various kinds.
2. GE foods and their residual pesticides and herbicides can trigger cancer and endocrine diseases.
3. In the general environment, GE plants promote antibiotic resistance in bacteria, thereby making our own medical use of them even more ineffective than they have already become.
4. The escalating use of these chemicals connected with GE crops will undoubtedly further degrade the soil and its beneficial bacteria, thereby also reducing key nutrient value. The key mineral magnesium, needed for more than 300 chemical reactions in our bodies is only available to us via plants that contain sufficient magnesium. Even prior to GE foods, magnesium became seriously depleted by ecologically unsound agricultural practices; a further depletion would be disastrous for all higher life forms.
5. The unexpected toxins produced by plants as a reaction to chemicals and in response to inserted foreign genes are subsequently ingested by us directly or via animals we eat, such as toxic GE cotton fed to cattle. This may lead to increased allergic disease in people.
6. Because GE plants promote the extinction of entire eco systems of insects, bacteria and plants they also promote the already serious biodiversity crisis. This reduces the genetic stability of all living things, including our own in the long run.

7. The use of GE organisms in pharmaceutical products, as currently considered possible, promotes the spontaneous appearance of new dangerous viruses which are extremely successful at exploiting the potential of new micro-environments.
8. Since it is now known that humans cannot digest GE corn, for example, all GE foods are likely to be phantom or "virtual" foods of no nutritional utility the health consequences of which can only be guessed at. The inability to process GE foods by our enzymes also allows for the very real possibility that foreign DNA will enter the blood stream with unforeseeable consequences for our own evolution, since we too are the products of a huge *co*-evolutionary event.
9. GE pharmaceutical products have potential uses for biological warfare, such as the virus-bacteria already found in many Gulf War Syndrome soldiers and their families.

Canada's geneticist and environmental activist David Suzuki said nothing but the truth when he bluntly observed with regard to the safety of GE foods on October 17, 1999, "When [corporate] scientists say these products are safe, they are either stupid or lying."

Sources and Resources

(See also bibliographies in following articles in this section)

The National Film Board documentary, *The Genetic Takeover* can be ordered from them directly: 1-800-267-7710 or through their website **www.nfb.ca**. Highly recommended is the following NFB documentary on the same topic which has been made since 2000: Clone Inc.. Also excellent are the following documentaries: *Beyond McWorld: Challenging Corporate Rule* by Just.In.Time Distributions 416-516-2472 and *Deconstructing Supper* by Moving images Distributions 1-800-684-3014 or www.movingimages.ca

L. Anderson, *Genetic Engineering, Food, and Our Environment*, Chelsea Green Publishing, 1999

J. Bakan, *The Corporation: The Pathological Pursuit of Profit and Power*, Viking, 2004

C. Barstow, *The Eco-Foods Guide: What's Good for the Earth is Good for You*, New Society Publishers, 2002

R. Burdon, *The Suffering Gene: Environmental Threats to Our Health*, McGill University Press, 2003

R. Cummins & B. Lilliston, *Genetically Engineered Food: A Self-Defense Guide for Consumers*, Marlow & Co, 2000

R. Heinberg, *Cloning the Buddha: The Moral Impact of Biotechnology*, Quest Books, 1999

M.-W. Ho, *Genetic Engineering: Dream or Nightmare?* Contiuum, 2000

J. Humphrys, *The Great Food Gamble*, Hodder & Stoughton, 2001

A. Jack, *Imagine A World Without Butterflies*, One peaceful World Press, 2000

C. Kneen, *Farmageddon: Food and the Culture of Biotechnology*, New Society Publishers, 1999

M. Lappe & B. Bailey, *Against the Grain: Biotechnology and the Corporate Takeover of Your Food*, Common Courage Press, 1998

M. Nestle, *Safe Food: Bacteria, Biotechnology, and Bioterrorism*, University of California Press, 2004

Garth Nicholson, Gulf War Illnesses: Role of Chemical, Radiological and Biological Exposures, *War and Health*, Helsinki, 1998

Testimony of Dr. G. Nicholson to the Committee on Government Reform and Oversight, United States House of Representatives June 26, 1997

G. Nicholson, Report on Kuwait, *Health Freedom News* 1998. Best source for all the research: The Institute for Molecular Medicine, 15162 triton Lane, Huntington, CA, 92649-1041, USA, Tel: 714-903-2900

S. Nottingham, *Eat Your Genes: How Genetically Modified Food is Entering our Diet*, Zed Books, 1998

A. Rowell, *Don't Worry It's Safe to Eat: The True Story of GM Food, BSE and Foot and Mouth*, Earthscan, 2004

Ardai Pusztai, *Report of the Project Co-Ordinator on Data Produced at the Rowett Research Institute* (Scottish Office, Agriculture, Environment & Fisheries Department (SOAEFD), Flexible Fund project RO 818, October 22, 1998. Online: **www.rri.sari.ac.uk**

J. Rifkin, *The Biotech Century*, Tarcher Putnam, 1999

W. Roberts et al, *Real Food for a Change*, Random, 1999

V. Shiva, *Biopiracy: The Plunder of Nature and Knowledge*, Between the Lines, 1997

V. Shiva, *Stolen Harvest: The Hijacking of the Global Food Supply*, South End Press, 2000

D. Suzuki & H. Dressel, *From Naked Ape to Superspecies*, Stoddard, 1999

B. Tokar, ed. *Redesigning Life? The Worldwide Challenge to Genetic Engineering*, McGill University Press, 2001

For the view point of the biotechnology industry no one-stop source is better than the gushing fantasy dressed up as science by M. Fumento, *Bio Evolution: How Biotechnology is Changing Our World*, Encounter Books 2003. It features an introduction by President Bush!

Websites with information on all aspects of GE:
www.canadians.org
www.gn.apc.org
www.gallon.elogic.com
www.healingourworld.com
www.policyalternatives.org
www.greanpeacecanada.org
www.safe-food.org

GMO and Organic Farming—Report No 2

Vitality Magazine June 2001

The timing is astonishing of the following three events: The *Royal Society of Canada* published its witheringly critical independent review of Canada's biotechnology policies in late January. Simultaneously, the international organic farmers' conference was held at Guelph University documenting the worldwide organic food boom. Also in January and February, the world renowned scientists who unknowingly initiated the now ongoing demise of the biotech industry, Arpad Pusztai and his wife Susan Bardocz, conducted a speaking tour through Canada telling of their research and how they unexpectedly discovered the potentially disastrous health effects of genetically engineered food plants. Finally, on February 16th in Ottawa, the *Council of Canadians* brought together activists, whistleblowers, and scientists from all over the world who brought forth huge amounts of political and health truths to a fact-thirsty crowd from all over Canada. On that occasion, the annual Whistleblower Award was given to Drs. Shiv Chopra and Margaret Haydon of Canada's Health Protection Branch for standing up to our government and saving us from genetically engineered and carcinogenic bovine growth hormone in the milk supply.

At Guelph the CEO of the *International Federation of Organic Agriculture Movements* (IFOAM *www.ifoam.org*), Bernward Geier provided the data from 105 countries showing how organic farming has grown in a mere 3 seasons from US $ 10 billion to 20 billion in revenues and, according to various government analyses, is expected to reach US $ 100 billion by the end of this decade. The organic movement started in 1924 in Germany with the philosopher Rudolf Steiner, and fittingly the headquarters of the IFOAM are in that country. The crowds cheered when learning that every university in Germany and Switzerland, and almost all major universities in Europe, have professorships and full departments with labs and independent, public research money devoted entirely to organic farming research.

Geier stated that *MacDonalds* in Sweden has gone organic, *Swiss Air* and *Lufthansa* are the first airlines to be totally organic, and the German government announced in late January that its official agricultural policy is now organic and pulled the funding plug on biotech agricultural research. The European Union has introduced legislation requiring labeling, making law what is worldwide reality already: most of Europe, Japan, Australia, New Zealand, Arabia, even China, many African countries and some South American countries all require labeling already. It was also learnt that Canada is quietly

(!) pouring millions into developing technologies to segregate GM crops from the real thing after having asserted for years that this could not be done. Now we have to—or we are not part of the global market any more: our major export product, canola, is at zero already in just 3 years.

The courageous agricultural professor, Ann Clark, who nearly lost her job at Monsanto-money-padded Guelph University for revealing that our government has done literally no safety tests whatsoever of GMO foods, described how organic farming is the ultimate challenge to globalization. She discussed the ecological disaster in Western Canada caused by the cross-breeding of regular rapeseed and genetically modified varieties; the hybrid is a "super-weed" and resists all known chemicals—something that wasn't supposed to happen according to the "tobacco science" of the biotech companies.

Bruster Kneen, editor of the excellent newsletter *The Ram's Horn* and author of the famous book *Farmageddon* (New Society Publishers 1999), provided wide ranging and detailed information on the efforts of biotechnology companies to gain total control in a few hands of the world's food supply—and how that control is coming unraveled through the worldwide grassroots movements demanding that "the world is our home, not the playground for corporate agendas".

In Ottawa, the *Council of Canadians* conference entitled, "Science and the Public Good" featured Ralph Nader who provided a magisterial overview of what activism in this area has done. (The entire conference can be enjoyed on CD ROM; call 1-800-387-7177 ext 250 for instructions). His wry humor alone is worth the Internet excursion!

Arpad Puzstai and Susan Bardocs, the Hungarian scientist couple told the story of their completely unexpected discovery of the potentially horrendous health effects of genetically engineered potatoes. Their experiments were funded by the Scottish agricultural ministry at 1.6 million pounds because the UK government had noticed that they could not find a single safety study on GMO foods anywhere. Not expecting anything serious, Pusztai and Bardocs who were trained genetic engineering scientists themselves, were stunned when they discovered brain damage, immune system dysregulation, precancerous changes in various cells and hormone imbalances in the test animals after only short feeding trials. With the prior written permission of their research institution, they went public with their findings, but were fired afterwards anyway by the Monsanto-funded Rowett Institute. They had worked there, in Edinburgh, for 3 decades and were internationally renowned for their work.

Prince Charles took note and asked the British parliament to have the

Pusztais testify before the House of Lords on their findings, an event that was open to the public. Thus began in the UK the revolution against GMOs that has taken hold all over the world. Theirs is still the *only* known safety evaluation in the entire scientific literature. The corporate research results are "proprietary information" and not open to scientific or government scrutiny!

The speakers from Brazil, Argentina, the US, and Asia told of their devastating experiences with corporate power which work to undermine their governments as well as the actions of courts and persecute individuals helping to turn the tide everywhere.

The event was crowned by the awards given to Dr. Shiv Chopra and Margret Haydon for having blown the whistle on our government's cavalier attitude to food safety. In their acceptance speeches they made it clear with grace and humor that they intended to keep blowing that whistle on behalf of Canadian and human health. Ralph Nader then observed, that he had met a great many whistle blowers in his career as an activist, but never any who promised to *continue* being a thorn in the side of the authorities.

Indeed, these are the best of times for a worldwide resurgence of common sense, and the worst of times for the corporate agenda of denial and deception that characterizes the push to deregulation of safety legislation and privatization of the common heritage of nature.

Genetic Warfare—Report No 3

Vitality Magazine July/August 2002

An emperor who went crazy started World War I. World War II was the project of a democratically elected chancellor who also went crazy and proclaimed himself Führer. Both took the world on a ride to hell. Now we are in the midst of World War III, and this time the Führers of biotechnology, with their mad scientists and greedy CEOs, are in the grip of so grand a megalomania, it makes Hitler look merely frightening and Emperor Wilhelm II look like a bully in a carnival suit.

Again the basic human right to chose one's fate is at stake, but unlike those previous conventional wars, this war centers on Life itself and who shall own and control it, who shall unilaterally decide the quality of the future. The genetic code of plants, animals and ourselves is what's at stake—and how much poisonous pesticides, herbicides and artificial fertilizer the world's population can be forced to accept. The poison gas of World War I was confined to the battlefield. Its solid form is on your dinner plate today, and you are no war hero when you succumb to cancer, but a mere statistic. What must be defended today, are the peaceful-looking supermarkets and pastoral scenes of the world's food-growing fields which have become the theatre of war and life.

Here is a report from the front which I visited at the international Organic Agriculture conference at Guelph in January and, in June, at the Council of Canadians' BioJustice conference in Toronto. There is cause for cautious optimism. The rapaciousness of the biotech industry is worse than ever, but the intelligence of the ordinary person, who won't be fooled or bought, and the determination of some of the world's greatest scientists are becoming any Devil's match.

Instead of guns and bombs, this war is waged with false advertising on a scale beyond imagining. Canada's Health Protection Branch (an oxymoron if ever there was one) in conjunction with the Food Biotechnology Communications Network puts out these little pamphlets informing us that the common soil bacterium, *Bacillus thuringiensis* (Bt), has been "used for years as an insecticidal spray in organic farming". Addressing those 92% of Canadians who, in poll after poll, consider the protection of the environment of top importance, they write that Bt is "an environmentally friendly pesticide because it is toxic only to specific types of insects, and breaks down to non-toxic substances." Without further ado, the next paragraph extols the virtues of Bt corn which produces this wonderful, natural toxin itself and cites marvelous scientific studies which supposedly showed how great this Frankenfood is for you, and me, and the world.

What Health Canada and their biotech buddies don't tell you, of course, is that pigs fed Bt corn go into false pregnancies, and even though their estrogen and progesterone levels are appropriate, there are no piglets. The Iowa Farm Bureau is horrified because more and more pig farmers reported this problem since October 2000. A doctor at the Center for Veterinary Medicine in Washington DC said, "We are working with a problem nobody has ever seen before. It's not in the books." You bet it isn't, and this is just the beginning of what's not going to be found in any medical book because nobody knows what this messing around with genes can do. Not even the mad scientists. And the biotech CEO's don't want to know and, most importantly: they don't want us to know what they don't know.

But never mind the pigs, how about the fact that Epicyte Corporation has developed a spermicidal corn that prevents human conception? Will it send women into pseudo-pregnancies, or maybe do wondrous things to men? Nothing is too absurd to imagine.

In addition to the hazards to agriculture, biodiversity and health posed by biotech products, their need for increased use (not *decreased*—as falsely asserted by the industry) of pesticides causes the quality of water to be threatened even more. As the biotech companies are also the world's largest producers of pharmaceuticals, those, too, contaminate the water with synthetic drugs finding their way into the food of people for whom these drugs were never prescribed—and what many of these chemicals do to animals and the soil is barely known. What *is* known, is that the world's waters are contaminated with enough antibiotics to render that load carcinogenic to many river and salt-water species.

The collateral damage of this current World War is everywhere, including in foods never targeted for genetic manipulation. One in four eggs in 1999 did not measure up to our food safety standards, and 50% of US honey contained the carcinogen phenol. In 2001 one quarter of our maple syrup was contaminated with the (banned) carcinogen paraformaldehyde, and more than half contained neurotoxic lead. "Drug residues in eggs, lead in maple syrup, and phenol in honey—Canadians can be excused for skipping breakfast" observed Burkhard Mausberg, the executive director of Environmental Defence Canada.

The big biotech companies spent US $ 50 billion within the last few years on just advertising genetically engineered food products—this figure does not include what they shelled out for lobbying politicians. The strategy is simple: make the process irreversible. "The hope of the [biotech] industry is that over time the market is so flooded that there is nothing you can do about it, you just sort of surrender," said the vice president of the strategic agriculture and marketing consulting firm Promor International. Having wrecked the original biological identity of canola already, Canada's chief export food, and created superweeds through the Roundup-resistant biotech crops which no known poison can control, the industry's next project is genetically engineered wheat. If that is released into the environment, the immense wealth it will generate at first for its creators will be matched only by starvation on an unthinkable scale—right here in North America. For us wheat is what rice is for Asia.

But not all business is created equal. Some of the largest producers of packaged food listen to the consumer, as good businessmen should. However, as the biotech bosses see it, if the consumer objects and is not lulled into compliance by the propaganda of advertising, brute force is next. Consider the following, reported in the *Ontario Farmer* April 2, 2002:

The CEOs of Weetabix and Canada Bread spoke out against GE wheat at a recent convention because of lack of consumer acceptance. They told biotech industry representative Paul Stevenson of the American Baking Institute they would not buy it. "Who is pushing for this stuff?" asked the CEOs, and Stevenson replied, "The company who has it spent a lot of money developing it, so they want to get it out." Weetabix's CEO Paul Millard countered, "So they are not listening to the consumer?" Stevenson smiled and replied, "I would say that's possible, yes." To their credit, Weetabix and Canada Bread stayed firm: they won't buy the stuff.

With Europe and much of Asia having refused biotech products, the industry's great hope for furthering the genetic pollution to the point of no return has been China. Its immense size, the gratifyingly large numbers of people trained not to object seemed a dream market. But deep down even the Chinese government's cult of obedience cannot short-circuit the powers of intelligent observation. Chinese scientists have reported that genetically engineered cotton, after the first five years of its use, has become an unmitigated disaster. Cotton is to Chinese agriculture what canola was to ours. The number of pesticide-resistant pests has increased and is out of control. Worse, the amount of pesticides and the variety needed to get any yield at all has escalated beyond their ability to pay for. They are recommending returning to their Confucian dictum: "The old tried and true ways are ever the best."

United Nations officers and scientists have the benefit of an unrivaled worldwide overview of what biotech does to local and global economies. The president of the UN's World Conservation Union, Yolanda Kakabadse didn't mince her words when she announced that GM crops are threatening the world's biodiversity. "Thousands of people in local communities are loosing their markets" and "are unable to substitute" their traditional products with anything else. She advocated an all-out effort to "support local varieties to support communities and satisfy global demand." (*Ontario Farmer* March 2, 2002)

The real scientists of the world, who are not paid by the industry, issued a statement recently signed by 136 of them, many Nobel laureates among them, coming from 27 countries: "Government advisory committees lack sufficient representation from independent scientists not linked to the industry," it said. "The result is that an untried, inadequately researched technology has been rushed prematurely to market, while existing scientific evidence of hazards are being suppressed, and little independent research on risks are being carried out." Among these scientists, incidentally, are those who originally developed the technology with which genetic engineering is done today.

Here two issues converge, as Dr. N. Olivieri pointed out at the BioJustice conference. As the biotech giants are aiming to control both agriculture and healthcare, their success depends on scientists whom they literally own, body and soul. Thus the pharmaceutical company Apotex tried to silence Dr. Olivieri when she noted fatal adverse effects in a drug she had been contracted to research. Under Apotex's pressure, the University of Toronto fired her, as did Sick Children's Hospital where the study was centered. Apotex sued her for $ 20 million in potentially lost sales. Scientists from all over the world were in uproar and voiced their condemnation. The Canadian Association of University Teachers (CAUT) published their *Olivieri Report* this year and advised government to take immediate steps to disconnect the interests of industry from those of research. Dr. Olivieri was re-instated into her university positions—and she counter-sued Apotex. She received a roaring standing ovation at BioJustice; indeed, our hope lies with people who will not bend to corruption.

Since our government supports biotechnology of all varieties, medical as well a agricultural, in spite of consistently negative public opinion (more than 70% of Canadians don't want biotech foods), a letter from you and me to those who pretend to be acting in our interest in Ottawa is in order: call 1-866-599-4999, or fax 613-941-6900, or e-mail **pmo@pm.gc.ca** and tell our Prime Minister we don't want our tax dollars to support this diabolical experiment. While we are at it, we ought to tell him also that we support the May 2000 federal environment report that recommended subsidies and tax deductions for farmers who want to convert to organic farming and get off the chemically addicted treadmill for their animals and plants.

In a daring and timely move, the organic farmers of Saskatchewan are suing Monsanto and Aventis, the two biotech crop giants, demanding "compensation for the damage caused to certified organic farmers resulting from the introduction of genetically engineered canola into the rural environment." They are also asking for an injunction to prevent the introduction of GE wheat. That asserts, that what is at stake, is "the right to grow organic crops, to serve organic markets, to eat GMO free foods, and to farm organically." Their legal claim is that "when Aventis and Monsanto introduced their GE canola, they knew or ought to have known of this crop's ability to cross-pollinate, spread and contaminate the environment, including organic fields." Indeed, this may very well be one of the most important court cases in all of western legal history. The judicial system is asked to prevent a crime against Life. Your donation is imperative and can be sent to SOD-OAPF, Box 1, Lisieux, SK, S0H 2R0. (*Note: As of October 2004, this case is still in progress and needs your support, even though GM wheat was withdrawn voluntarily by Monsanto; the case now centers on the disastrous contamination on many crops by GM varieties.*)

The good news is that organic farming is growing at a rate of 25% a year worldwide, said Gunner Rundgren, the current president of the international organic farming federation, IFOAM. There are now 750 organic farming organizations in 103 countries of which 50% are in Europe, 20% in Asia, 20% in Africa and less than 10% in the US and Canada. In May 2001 there were 2,230 organic farmers in Canada with Saskatchewan having the lion's share of 773. Ontario has more than 400. The problem is that there aren't enough of them to meet the exponentially growing demand for organic produce from the consumer.

At the Guelph conference some important myths were also dispelled. For example, European conventional farmers use *more* chemical fertilizers and pesticides than US farmers do. France uses the most among European countries, but has started to put on the breaks. On the other had, the Netherlands have decreed that within 10 years no pesticides may be used in agriculture at all! In May 2001 the Danish government invited the agriculture ministers of all of Europe who signed a declaration affirming that all of European farming should move towards 100% organic crops. Germany went through the most dramatic conversion experience: when Mad Cow Disease hit Germany, the agriculture minister resigned, the new one was a member of the Green Party (Germany has a coalition government with the Greens) and, responding to public demand as democratic governments should, within a week of taking office, she committed the country to an organic farming policy which is now in full swing. Finally, Japan is the world's third largest producer of organic foods.

The Quebec minister of agriculture declared last year that "organic is the way of the future", moving the province into supporting the transition accordingly. Brazil was the first country to refuse biotechnology completely, and they have now taken over from our canola market worldwide because theirs is not genetically polluted. But "organic" purity is itself a troubled issue. The air and water carries residues of pesticides and other toxic chemicals. The editor of *Alive* Magazine, Rody Lake, told an audience in Ottawa two years ago that she had her own organic produce tested. She grows most of her own food by the rigorous standards of purity required. Yet, the tests showed that her crops had 10% residues of pesticides, compared to supermarket produce.

The qualitative analysis of organic foods, not surprisingly, shows that in fact these crops contain dramatically less toxic residues compared to conventionally grown crops. The analysis is published in the peer-reviewed journal *Food Additives and Contaminants* and can be downloaded for free from www.biosciencearena.com. A Swiss study comparing over 21 years the yields of organic and conventional farming shows that the production of organic farming requires about 50% less energy, while the total yields are about 20% less than achieved by conventional methods. And if the nutritional quality alone were to decide this war, it would be won already: the *European Journal of Nutrition* (vol. 40, 2002) and the *Journal of Alternative and Complementary Medicine* published their respective studies, based on 300 comparisons, and showed that organically crown foods, on average have a higher nutritional content 85% of the time. For example, organic crops have 29% more magnesium, 27% more vitamin C, 21% more iron, 26% more calcium.

An old saying has it that the best revenge on one's enemies is to live well. This war can be won by political action, by spreading information, and by refusing the stuff that makes the earth and us ill and malnourished—indeed by eating well.

Sources and Resources

D. Suzuki & H. Dressel, *Good News For A Change: Hope for a Troubled Planet*, Stoddart, 2002 (most encouraging and good for fighting the environmental blues)

This Magazine (which I recently started subscribing to) is excellent in giving you the information on politics the regular news hasn't got the guts to publish. Check out www.THISmag.org

For the two excellent booklets, *Regulating Genetic Engineering for Profit* and *Galloping Gene Giants* which provide a first-rate worldwide survey of the genetic engineering mess go to www.polarisinstitute.org or order them by e-mail from polarisinstitute@on.aibn.org

K. Sullivan, *Organic Living in 10 Simple Lessons*, Barron's 2001

Dr. T. Barnard's taped lecture, from the January Organic Agriculture conference, on *Organic Foods and Better Human Nutrition* is a goldmine of up-to-date information on the importance of organic food to health. Available through Audio Archives of Canada 905-889-6555. Tape numbers 020125-280 & 281

The organic food home distributor *Wow! Foods* (formerly *Wanigan's*) can be reached through 1-877-926-4426

For organically grown meats and frozen vegetables www.nutrafarms.com or 613-549-1391 or 1-888-515-3846

For food safety and information on additives see www.consumersunion.org and www.biosciencearena.com

www.foodwatch.ca the web site of Environmental Defense Canada

Excellent on worldwide organics/GMO issues: www.organicconsumers.org

The website of the Canadian Organic Growers is www.cog.ca

For questions of verification of certification standards and enforcement see www.qaiinc.com

Organic Goes Mainstream–Report No 4

Vitality Magazine June 2003

The theme of the 22nd Annual Organic Conference was "Organic Goes Mainstream". Attended by about 1,700 people, it took place at Guelph University, one of the important centers in the current Food War; its agriculture department is heavily supported by the biotech industries. Guelph is, however, also the academic home of feisty Professor Ann Clark, one of the world's leading experts on that industry's record of unnatural acts against nature and consumers. Her web site **www.eaclark@uoguelph.ca** provides access to all that disturbing, rigorous international science about biotechnology that Health Canada works so hard to conceal from Canadians. Fun can be had (if you have a dark sense of humor) by comparing the facts on her site with the myths on her biotechnology-supporting colleagues' site **www.foodsafetynetwork.ca**—a name as oxymoronic as Health Canada itself, because the really important information is lacking.

The organic movement is in excellent health and the interactions between Mother Nature and biotechnology's Sorcerer's Apprentice are becoming increasingly interesting. It began with a delicious all-organic dinner sponsored by retailers of organic foods. Listening at my table to farmers from all over Canada discussing their daily rebellion against industrialized uniformity and determination to serve Nature's intent, I felt as if Dan Needles' "Letter from Wingfield Farm" had come to life. In those plays, Walt Wingfield, a Bay Street broker turned farmer, struggles to resolve the conflict between Money and Nature; but now life is outdoing fiction. Wingfield would be astounded to learn that on October 21 last year Debra Boyle, the president of the Organic Trade Association and CEO of Pro Organics, Canada's largest organic fresh foods distributor, was asked to open the trading of the NASDAQ stock market in New York's Time Square to celebrate the new laws governing organic food production and to salute organic food as today's commercial wunderkind, growing at 25% annually. (Industrial food revenues, by comparison, grow only 1 to 2% annually.) By the end of this year, the organic food industry will be worth US $ 25 billion, while annual genetically engineered crops are pegged at US $ 4.5 billion world-wide. Data published in BioDemocracy News (**www.organicconsumersw.org**) show that by 2020 most food sold in Europe and North America will be organic.

The keynote address was given by Dr. Thomas Cowan of the *Weston Price Foundation* from New Hampshire in the US. Weston Price is the father of modern nutritional medicine. His research was the first effort in the history medicine to show how food determines health in teeth, bones, organs, growth and reproduction. This research has grown enormously and become highly politicized because the principles of nutritional health are fundamentally incompatible with industrial intensive agriculture, the fast-food industry and refined foods—all of which are the source of chronic disease.

Dr. Cowan's work as a physician, he explained, is dedicated to the principle of non-violence which he extends in a startling and insightful manner to humans and viruses alike. He stated that a physician's oath, "first do no harm", is incompatible with the war metaphors governing medicine and food economics. Instead, if soil quality is protected from intensive, aggressive industrial farming, and if the natural requirements of plants and animals are met, then the entire food chain functions in such a way as to promote health. Disease in soil translates into disease everywhere, Dr. Cowan pointed out, as does a diseased cow whose milk and meat people consume. As for bacteria, viruses and parasites, they also are part of the great scheme of things and not inherently dangerous or useful. It has been said that there is no such thing as dirt, but that dirt is definable as matter in the wrong place. Similarly, the agents of illness are the result of imbalances primarily due to an exploitative approach to Nature.

Examples of imbalance as the consequence of violence are *Candida albicans*, a fungus normally present in our gut, which in the presence of a refined diet invades all bodily systems causing illness, even setting the stage for cancer; similarly, assaults on our immune systems through pesticides and toxic drugs can turn harmless viruses into deadly ones, and overuse of antibiotics promotes the evolution of unbeatable bacteria. These situations then result in a veritable arms' race with increasingly more toxic drugs being administered. Dr. Cowan provided several astounding case histories of thyroid disease, insulin-dependent diabetes and cancer, which he successfully treated with individualized diets to re-establish systemic balance, by using required nutrients and avoiding anti-nutrients. His motto is: "Don't treat illness, but cure everything."

Dr. Cowan described astounding supportive research results. Animals fed a diet equivalent in nutritional value to the one most North Americans obtain from standard industrial agriculture and processed food (SAD = Standard American Diet), caused bad teeth in the first generation, general reduction in bone density by the second, cancer and endocrine disorders by the third, and behavioral and brain problems by the fourth generation. When those damaged fourth-generation animals were fed a nutritionally optimal diet, the DNA was miraculously able to respond and slowly (very slowly) repair this entire cascade of degeneration. But it took seven (!) generations before a fully healthy litter of animals was once again born. The horror of these experiments is, as Dr. Cowan pointed out, that they provide a perfect snap-shot of the current state of human health brought about by the disregard for Nature's demands. The wonder of these findings is that Nature appears to have a clear idea of what a healthy and functional cat, cow, or human is and will return patiently, over several generations, to the original "model" whose integrity was violated by human greed and stupidity.

Dr. Cowan's identification of the violence inherent in industrial agriculture and biotechnology's illusions of power is right on point when considering new scary developments. Biotech company Morphotek of Pennsylvania has developed a technique called "morphogenics" which uses human colon cancer cells in order to speed up the evolutionary process in food crop plants, as reported by *Friends of the Earth* in November last year. Those mad scientists seem not to lose any sleep over how those cancer genes and their protein off-shoots are going to effect our metabolism and the food chain. Even if no disease is caused directly, indirectly such a violent speeding-up of plant evolution is likely to result in impairing its nutrient up-take, providing us with more dead food—as if we didn't have enough of that already. We already know from research into salmon forced to grow larger than Nature intended, through the introduction of certain human genes, that such animals become unnatural predators, have less essential fatty acids in their meat, and become susceptible to new diseases. The UK's *Independent* reported on March 30th this year that the only natural pesticide, Bt (*Bacillus thuringiensis*) has been so aggressively overused, that the pests it used to control have evolved enzyme defenses enabling them to feed and thrive on Bt instead. Scientists specializing in this area were predicting exactly this irreversible disaster, but the biotech industry and the EPA ignored them (*Nature*, March 6, 2003). Einstein's quip comes to mind: "The universe and human stupidity are infinite, and I am not sure about the former."

This violent economic philosophy justifies pouring annually 4.1 billion pounds of pesticides over the earth (at a profit of US $ 45 billion). Its effects show up in health statistics such as the Ontario study published last October in the *International Journal of Occupational and Environmental Health*. It reported that farm women are nine times more likely to develop breast cancer due to their continual exposure to the whole toxic soup of fertilizers, pesticides, fungicides and antibiotic growth promoters—all known carcinogens. Similarly, fish in the Great Lakes suffer at epidemic rates from liver cancers. The *Journal of Epidemiology and Community Health* in its October 15, 2002, issue listed the ten foods most contaminated with pesticides, warning us not to eat them: peanuts, cucumbers, meat loaf, popcorn, spinach, radishes, cantaloupe, butter, bananas, and squash. Worst of all are strawberries. It is true that we live longer, but it is also true that the populations of our industrialized world have evolved chronic diseases which were rare a few centuries ago and are completely unknown in the 5 million year old archaeological record of human evolution.

The shift from exploitative violence to an attitude of cooperation with nature was explored in the many workshops. These dealt with topics ranging from the restoration of soil health, to animal husbandry that does not speed up and unnaturally force growth and weight in animals with carcinogenic and endocrine-disrupting antibiotics, that make them and us sick, to the revival of traditional plant and animal varieties to boost genetic variety and restore soil health. Heritage breeds in both plants and animals are hardier, adapted to non-intensive systems, do not require artificial fertilizers, still have natural resistance to disease, and are adapted over thousands of years to local climates.

Sweden has given industry five years to show which of their 2,500 chemicals in agricultural use are actually safe. It is no longer up to the public to prove that these chemicals are harmful. In Canada chemicals are still innocent until proven guilty, but our new federal Pest Control Products Act at least made a few baby steps in the same direction by making industry accountable for all sources of pesticide exposure and requiring assessments of cumulative effects. The European Union has now banned the use of growth promoting antibiotics and reduced their use for disease control—indeed by 50% between 1997 and 1999. In January *The Ontario Farmer* distributed a special magazine insert providing information on how to control weeds the old fashioned way: through crop rotation, as the Old Testament asserted was God's will.

President Bush put a gag order on the Environmental Protection Agency's alarming report, earlier this year, showing that US-grown lettuce has 30 times the allowable limit of toxins on them, including rocket fuel. But Germany and the Netherlands have started the first organic fast food chain called "Real Mealz". The sheer volume of useful information is encouraging and cannot be downplayed. For example, the US National Institutes of Health journal, *Environmental Health Perspectives*, published a huge study last October (download from **http://dx.doi.org/**) showing the staggering difference in health and intelligence between children fed organic food to those who eat the organophosphate-laced supermarket stuff.

During a panel discussion the question arose as to who is going to feed the world. Professor Clark answered that the question assumes that there is somebody "who can make a hell of a lot of money by controlling the world's food supply". The real question should be, she suggested, "Why isn't the world feeding itself now?" She stressed, that whatever the answer to that question may be, "it will have nothing to do with genetics". The inequality in access to food is not due to insufficient genetic engineering to force Nature to produce more. Nature can produce all we need even now. Hunger has to do with exploitative economic policies, transportation and communication problems, wars, centralization of power, and the like. The solution is not to give even more power to that small group of about 1,000 billionaires and a few hundred trans-national corporations "who are poisoning our planet and undermining democracy" (*BioDemocracy*, Feb. 2003; also read the transcript of the CBC *Ideas* program of Sept. 17/18, 2002 in which Stephen Lewis of the United Nations provides a world-wide overview which reads like an answer to Ann Clark's provocative counter-question).

Ann Clark observed that we "need to stop governments from collegially assuming that whatever business thinks is good for it, is also good for the environment and our health." Indeed, the most astounding fact is our government rules consistently against the known will of the people. Canada is determined to make us the world leaders in biotechnology and sinks $ 700 million tax dollars annually into supporting this type of agricultural research—without a single study ever having been done on its safety or even efficacy! Survey after survey has shown that Canadians want mandatory food labeling to identify genetically engineered foods and be free to avoid them, but the government ignores this. The recently released federal report entitled *Improving the Regulation of Genetically Modified Foods and Other Novel Foods in Canada*, demands that the precautionary principle be implemented at once (as in Sweden and the EU), but then ruins everything by stating that "mandatory labeling would be problematic because of the cost to industry and potential conflicts would arise in international trade agreements." Well how about that? Has anybody ever thought that those trade agreements should be scrapped and that our freedom to chose what we eat takes precedence over those poor billionaires' interests?

In Europe the will of the people is not being ignored and GMO foods are not allowed. The US's saber rattling and threats to sue for profit losses caused a fabulous row and the EU's Development Commissioner P. Neilson observed: "If the Americans stop lying about us, we will stop telling the truth about them." The US has reason to fear great economic losses. The world won't buy their transgenic stuff. Monsanto laid off 700 scientists last year.

Since January 2001 GMO related stock has fallen by 50%, as more and more countries refuse it. China, long an enthusiastic supporter of GMOs last June published in its English language *China Daily*, the mouthpiece of the ruling Communist party, an article by Greanpeace on the ecological risks of transgenic crops. *Nature* observed (March 13, 2003) that that this was almost like asking Amnesty International to write on China's human rights record. China fears losing the European market and has had nasty experiences with the ecological effects of transgenic crops.

For us, the Food War is moving into high gear as the majority of Canadian farmers (**www.saskorganic.com**) are in the process of launching a class action to stop biotech companies from introducing transgenic wheat and ruining wheat ecology and the export market. Also, the case of Saskatchewan's organic farmer, Percy Schmeiser has been accepted by the Supreme Court. Monsanto claimed that Schmeiser used their transgenic seeds illegally. He never bought their stuff. It blew over from some other fields. Our Supreme Court has a good track record and setting the government's corporate sell-out policies straight. This decision could open up Canada for a non-violent economic food policy whose benefits would be felt very quickly in reduced health care costs as water, soil, and nutritional value in our daily food return to Nature.

Sources and Resources

M. N. Cohen, *Health and the Rise of Civilization*, Yale University Press, 1989
S. Fallon, *Nourishing Traditions*, 2nd ed., New Trends, 1999 (one of the best cookbooks ever)
M. Lappe, M.D., *Evolutionary Medicine*, Sierra Club Books, 1994
M. Nestle, *Food Politics*, University of California Press, 2002
W. Price, *Nutrition and Physical Degeneration*, 50th anniversary ed., Keats, 1989
Greenpeace, *How to Avoid Genetically Engineered Foods*, download at
  www.greenpeace.ca/shoppersguide/browse.php
On food safety see **www.ewg.org**
For organic food delivery services: **www.liferesearchuniversal.com/caorganics.html**
For tapes of the January 2003 Guelph conference call Audio Archives at 905-889-6555
CBC Ideas transcripts, call 416-205-6010

Make Mine Organic—Report No 5

Vitality Magazine May 2004

*"Necessity is the excuse of every tyranny," observed the 18th century
British Prime Minister William Pitt the Younger, when he failed to persuade
Mad King George to ease up on the economic repression of the American
Colonies; so they successfully revolted.*

Today, the biotechnology industry tries to persuade us that genetically engineered foods are absolutely necessary to eradicate world hunger, save the
environment, and bring us magical therapies through pharma-foods. The
situation is indeed dire, but mostly for the biotech companies whose allergy
to facts and truth is ruining their financial health; the world's hungry agree
with the world's over-fed that we need biotechnology about as much as a
belly-ache or cancer.

It looks like the decision by Monsanto, Aventis, Dow and Dupont to
pump US$50 million into advertising the benefits of biotech hasn't worked.
(*Washington Post*, April 4, 2000) Even advertising eventually does need the
support of experience, *and* evidence, to convince. January 2004 was a very
bad month for the biotech industry. The European Union rejected GE rice
known as LL Rice 62 because of serious environmental and health concerns;
the US Justice Department is investigating Monsanto and Pioneer for anti-
trust violations, or price fixing (*New York Times* Jan. 6, 2004); and in an
ironic twist of events, Monsanto was bullied for a change, forcing it to halt
sales of all Roundup-ready soya beans because the company is losing money
to the black market in countries where governments won't enforce patent
laws (*New York Times* Jan. 21, 2004).

Adding insult to injury, Swiss Re (which insures insurance companies)
published a report on GMOs stating they "pose the likelihood of new types
of loss patterns" and that the technology itself "represents a particularly
exposed long-term risk." Meantime, in Canada, not one but two earthquakes
began to rumble throughout the biotech industry. Firstly, on January 10th
the Canadian government abandoned one of its favourite private sector
buddies Monsanto on the GE wheat trials issue because Japan, the EU and
others had made it clear they wouldn't buy the stuff, or any other Canadian
wheat for that matter, if trials were permitted, as all wheat might then

become GE contaminated. And secondly, a week later, Canada's Supreme Court heard the case of Saskatchewan farmer Percy Schmeiser whom Monsanto accused of stealing their patented GE seeds when some blew over from a neighbour's field. A favourable decision for Schmeiser would establish that people have the right to farm as they have for the past 10,000 years by saving seed, that GE seeds do travel with the wind after all, and that the world's food supply may not be solely controlled by corporations. During cross-examination, the incisive questions posed to Monsanto's lawyers by the "Supremes" (as lawyers refer to these judges) illuminated the lies and deception of biotech such as to make the audience occasionally gasp. The decision has not yet been handed down.

On the weekend of January 23rd, farmers, scientists and journalists gathered for their 23rd annual conference at Guelph University to assess the progress of the organic movement. Here are some highlights from among the speakers.

The keynote speaker was George Siemon of Wisconsin whose co-op "Organic Valley" has become North America's largest organic food source grossing close to US$200 million this year. Siemon, who looks like the archetypal American farmer—tall, bony, wind-burned, huge rough hands—described with the humour and relaxed self-assurance of a Taoist sage his journey from a small organic milk co-op "with a mere wisp of a hope in 1990" to a nationwide organization involving hundreds of farms in 19 states providing 40% of the natural foods supply. Asked why more and more farmers join, he replied, "Rewarding work is rare. Everybody seeks meaningful work."

Success was not easy, being up against huge multinational bullies. Yet, as he pointed out repeatedly, the consumer runs the show; people want real food. In June 2001, ABC News conducted a poll showing that 93% of Americans want GMO foods labeled, so they can avoid them. This was confirmed by a Rutgers University poll a year later when 98% wanted labeling. Today, 30 million Americans buy organic food.

Real food means: no synthetic fertilizers (which reduce essential minerals for plants, animals and humans such as magnesium); no pesticides (which are toxic to all life); no genetic engineering (source of allergies, cancer and immune dysregulation); no prophylactic antibiotics in animal feed (prolonged use causes cancer in animals and humans and makes bugs antibiotic resistant—a currently unfolding medical disaster, especially for tuberculosis); no sewage sludge (full of synthetic medicines and frequent source of mutant disease agents); no irradiation (kills vitamins E and B). Furthermore, the farming methods used to grow real foods serve to stop soil erosion, prevent toxic run-off into the water supply, and protect biodiversity and human health.

Stewart Wells of the National Farmers' Union quoted Gloria Steinem's observation that "the truth shall set you free, but first it will make you miserable" when explaining how the Union had made the government miserable by digging up the (publicly-funded!) research truth (buried or ignored by Agriculture Canada) showing that the $50 to 100 million annual damage caused by certain weeds was in fact caused by Monsanto's pesticide Roundup.

The Union also repeatedly faced down the biotech guilt trip about the need to feed the world by pointing out that distribution monopolies are the problem, not the quantity of food produced. In Saskatchewan, for example, the number of food banks increases annually, even though 80% of all food produced is surplus and exported. (This province also has the largest number of organic farmers: 1,200 of them in a population of merely one million.) For the rest of North America, the number of organic farmers doubled since 1995. Since 2000, mainstream food producers such as Heinz, Gerber's, Loblaws and others all started hugely successful organic food lines—watched and tested diligently by Greenpeace and other NGOs.

Jennifer Sumner, who has taught at Guelph University since the 1970s, described the "corporatization of science". Biotech dollars pay for most research and so they claim ownership of the results. Unfavourable information is routinely suppressed. But the tide is turning: public and academic pressure has resulted in Canada's largest agricultural college opening a department for organic research.

Ken Roseboro from Iowa and editor of the excellent Non-GMO Source Newsletter, talked of the new challenge to organics: as demand is increasing at a steady 20% annually and organic foods have become a major economic force, the problem of unintentional GMO contamination has arisen in every product line. Interestingly, he referred to studies showing that genetically engineered food plants become weaker with every generation and die; Nature's quality control system can't be fooled, just like our healthy immune systems routinely destroy tens of thousands of improperly replicated (potential cancer) cells in our bodies daily.

This time I was one of the speakers at the Guelph conference, and being billeted as an "outspoken writer", I did my best not to disappoint. I reported on the health implications of genetically modified foods, the main areas being increased allergy, cancer risk, immune dysregulation, acute toxicity, delayed toxicity through increased pesticide residues, reduction in essential nutrients causing malnutrition, health hazards due to environmental degradation, and the creation of new viruses and other pathogens. (For a full discussion and all the scientific sources see the books listed at the end.)

Tyrannical corporations, in persuading people that their measures are necessary, to "feed the world", project enormous enthusiasm and flood us with images of a wonderful world to come; of course, dazzling visionaries and determined utopians don't want to it rain on their parade, and so it becomes essential to suppress contradictory information and dismiss it as just an irrelevant fly in the ointment one can pick out and discard.

Biotech companies have been exceedingly good at this, especially the suppression of contradictory evidence—a fairly easy task, since most research, medical, agricultural, and even much of the basic science supporting environmental research is dependent upon corporate funding. But what started as a few voices of caution has now become a flood. What began as a mere suggestion to be cautious in the 1999 statement by the world's scientific community, is now loud protest presented to the governments of the world, the World Trade Organization, the United Nations and the US Congress, all urging a total ban on biotechnology for food and in medicines.

Nobody worried about GMOs after their initial introduction in 1995 until Arpad Pusztai of the prestigious Rowett Institute of Edinburgh University, a key researcher and originally a promoter of genetic engineering, reported in 1998 that mice fed GM potatoes showed evidence of serious damage to all major bodily systems. Monsanto (the institute's major funding source) saw to it that he was fired. Fortunately, Prince Charles, who also happens to be the president of the British Medical Association, stepped in and had him testify before a special committee of the House of Lords. History may well one day see the heir to the British throne as the one who began saving the world's food supply.

Only about a dozen independent studies exist to date on health implications of GM foods (see review in *Nutrition and Health* vol. 17. 2003). Those show that due to the increased need for pesticides and herbicides, that such altered plants require, primary as well as secondary health effects result. While the biotech propaganda traveled on the environmental ticket by assuring the world that less pesticides would be needed for these pesticide-resistant plants, in actual fact 70 million additional pounds of these chemicals were used within just one year.

Due to the increase in chemical use, scientists wondered what pesticides in general did to nutrients: apples, it turned out lost most and sometimes all their vitamin C, as reported in the prestigious *Nature* (April 19, 2001). And, the much touted "golden rice", which allegedly had a high vitamin A content to eradicate blindness in Third World children, turned out to be an inhibitor of Co-enzyme Q_{10} synthesis (so the children could die of heart failure instead). Worse, as British geneticist Mae-Wan Ho pointed out, a person would have to eat 15 pounds of rice a day to get the amount of vitamin A required to prevent blindness, while the indigenous legumes, judged to be weeds by biotech companies and targeted for eradication with Roundup and other chemicals, contained a hundred times more vitamin A in just one regular serving in traditional meals (*Nature*, March 29, 2001).

British scientist Dr. Christopher Williams started calculating the worldwide health effect of GM crops, after demonstrating that the genetic alteration process, combined with the increased use of chemicals they required, resulted in serious essential mineral deficiencies (zinc, magnesium, iron). About 1.5 billion people were thought to already be in "sub-clinical decline" by 2000, which would show up later in impaired brain development, he reported to the British Economic and Social Research Council. And it became well nigh impossible to suppress some 8,200 university-based studies showing that GM crops have a significantly lower yield than conventional varieties. Research in the UK and in Venezuela showed that crops genetically engineered to be immune to certain pests caused these pests to adapt and then destroy the now totally defenseless crops; this raised the specter of agricultural catastrophe (*The Independent*, March 30, 2003). So much for feeding the world.

As early as 1995, the Chinese reported that stir-frying food in Canada's GM canola oil released carcinogenic chemicals (*Wall Street Journal*, June 7, 1995). Since then, animal experiments involving canola oil showed damage to the heart, kidneys, adrenals and thyroid gland; it is also implicated in the destruction of the myelin sheath protecting nerves (as in Multiple sclerosis). Remember that the next time you walk down the supermarket aisles carrying oils, maybe you best consider virgin olive oil instead.

When the biotech wizards came up with the bright idea in November 2002 of using human colon cancer genes to speed up crop growth, medical scientists everywhere woke up and the European parliament said, no thanks. In late 2003 *Nature Biotechnology* (vol. 22/2) reported that controlled experiments with humans had shown that GM corn passes through the human gut undigested, thereby providing no nutrition at all. Human digestive enzymes don't know what to do with those figments of human imagination coming down the pike. Even more refined research (*Environmental Health Perspectives* January 29th 2004) shows just exactly how the hormone-disrupting pesticides, so liberally used on GMOs, disrupt the chemical signaling in the body such as to interfere with normal gene activity. This week's *Nature* (April 22) seems to deal the deathblow to genetic messing-around in agriculture. In polite but clear language the cons (pun intended) are summarized, and no pros are left. The biotech party appears to be over.

Not quite ... big bullies with world-domination on their minds don't go away easily. The Council of Canadians is conducting nation-wide information workshops concerning the government's current move towards "deep integration" with the US. In a document entitled "The Canada We Want" they analyze the international treaties and tools (e.g. WTO, GATT, TRIPPS, NAFTA etc.) and show how these made possible the wholesale hijacking of entire sectors—from water privatization to food production. The organic movement is nothing less than enormously successful passive resistance against a dominant economic model of control and coercion. The COC also outlines how we can extricate ourselves from this system to avoid an escalation of this social and biological nightmare. We need to support the COC. Call 1-800-387-7177 and visit www.councilcanadians.org. Our personal health and running the world are too important to be left to mad scientists and somnambulant politicians. Send COC an e-mail to get a copy of "The Canada We Want" and find out how you can participate.

Sources and Resources
Rampton, S. & Stauber, J. *Trust Us, We're Experts! How Industry Manipulates Science,* Tarcher-Putnam, 2001
www.socialecology.com is Brian Tokar's site and contains the in-depth history of Monsanto
www.organicconsumers.org
www.cspi.net is the site of *The Center for Science in the Public Interest* (one of its directors is Marcia Angell, editor for 19 years of the *New England Journal of Medicine*), first-rate information provided by world-class scientists on GMOs, pesticides, environmental issues, the politics of medicine etc explains genetic engineering step by step
www.pbs.org/wgbh/harvest/engineer explains genetic engineering
The Greenpeace site for "true food shopping" **www.truefoodnow.org**

The Supreme Court's 2004 Decision the Schmeiser Case

Vitality Magazine July/August 2004

God and the Supreme Court work in mysterious ways. They don't follow a straight line, but somehow justice is slowly achieved, and they always offer great new opportunities for the doggedly determined. And so it is—and will be—with Saskatchewan farmer Percy Schmeiser whose canola fields were contaminated with genetically engineered seeds made by Monsanto. Schmeiser lost—sort of—against Monsanto, who would like to think they won, in the May 21 Supreme Court decision. It was mighty close: five judges ruled for Monsanto and four ruled for Schmeiser. Far from slamming the door shut on human rights and food safety, they opened up barrels of worms with which to renew our earth.

The Respondent: Monsanto

Since 1901 Monsanto has given the world almost all of the worst carcinogenic, neurotoxic, and teratogenic chemicals with which we have (usually unknowingly) poisoned our environment and made Monsanto rich. Its history as foremost "corporate criminal", according to the European research source CorporateWatch, began a hundred years ago with artificial sweeteners, ammonium nitrate fertilizers, styrene and polystyrene plastics (all carcinogens) and went on to worse with dioxin, Agent Orange, glyphosate (in the world's bestselling herbicide Roundup), the 2,4 D family of pesticides, PCBs, aspartame, bovine growth hormone, and—since the 1990s—a devil's kitchen of genetically engineered food plants; many more are still inside their laboratories in St. Louis, Missouri, such as their current "genetic improvements" to pigs (*Ontario Farmer* June 15) and plants that are supposed to deliver medicine and vaccines. According to R. Fraley, Monsanto's agricultural sector's co-president, "What you are seeing is not just a consolidation of seed companies, it's really a consolidation of the entire food chain." Not surprisingly, Europeans call Monsanto "Mon-Satan".

Monsanto's chemicals were used for war *and* agriculture, with war being at least an honest pursuit because its *stated* intent is mass-murder, while agricultural use of the same chemicals requires complex corporate strategies to disguise the *slow* poisoning of life through side-effects appearing much later. Not surprisingly, Monsanto also makes drugs which are generally also let loose on the market before *real* safety is established, a legally sanctioned business practice, as applicable legislation is not precautionary but damage control oriented. So, by the time the dead can be counted, companies have been laughing all the way to the bank.

In the early 1990s Monsanto spent US $10 billion to buy up seed companies and introduced genetically engineered products starting with bovine growth hormone Worldwide, 80% of all GM crops grown were developed by Monsanto. Whenever such a crop dramatically fails or causes environmental problems, Monsanto's deep pockets and their powerful connections with governments buy or enforce silence (see Tokar below). GE soya beans were the first to expose what Dr. Charles Benbrook calls "Monsanto's Big Lie": contrary to Monsanto's claims, they require 2 to 5 times *more* Roundup herbicide than conventional seeds, and instead of reducing the water needed, consumption increases (see his report on **http://nelsonfarm.net**). Ethical Investing lists Monsanto under "Health and Planet Destroying Products" and provides full information from the medical science literature and the documented ecological destruction to support their stance.

The Applicant: Percy Schmeiser

Schmeiser spent the past 50 years perfecting his canola crop through seed-saving and by following plant-breeding principles as old as agriculture itself. In 1998 Schmeiser's canola fields produced a mixture of his own and Monsanto's genetically engineered canola. The highest concentration was outside his property line in the ditch and some extended in decreasing concentration into his adjacent field. Many farmers had bought into the Monsanto promise that using its seeds would reduce the use of pesticides, protect their wells, cut costs and labor. It took just a few seasons for most farmers everywhere to realize that this was a false promise.

Open trucks carrying GM canola were passing Schmeiser's farm, and so began the problem of "volunteer" canola growing everywhere unbidden, and contaminating natural canola by crossbreeding. The US Department of Agriculture estimated that reliable methods of segregation would cost billions and be unworkable (*Boston Globe*, April 20, 2001). In Saskatoon, agricultural research centre Agri-Food Canada tested random samples of supposedly *natural* canola for contamination with GM varieties and found *none* conformed with the "mandatory genetic purity of 99.95%". Pioneer Hi-Breed confirmed that "100% purity, in genetic make-up…is currently not achievable for *any* agricultural product." (Remember the StarLink corn mess?) For Schmeiser this meant that a lifetime's plant breeding work was ruined quite literally forever.

Monsanto sued Schmeiser for patent infringement and the case made its way to the Supreme Court in January, a standing-room only affair. Especially interesting for me was overhearing so many attending civil servants freely expressing anger and outrage against the Canadian government's support of GMO technology. The press came out by the hundreds exceeding anything a movie star or sports hero could expect. Monsanto had as supportive intervenors various biotech organizations all claiming that research and the future of the human race was at stake if this patent was not protected for the sake of a "seed industry worth $ 100 billion". What *they* want to protect is *potential* profit. Seeds themselves have been most effectively protected for millions of years by God herself.

Schmeiser's supportive intervenors included the Council of Canadians, the Sierra Legal Defence Fund, the National Farmers Union and many more organizations from Canada as well as around the world. They supported the farmer's right to save seeds and they really knew something about farming—unlike the corporate camp. Interestingly, the Government of Ontario was an intervenor as well: OHIP was threatened by a law suit from Myriad Genetics Inc. for not paying royalties on a test for the genetic predisposition to breast cancer, and so Ontario sought legal clarification and wound up in Schmeiser's camp. The EU cancelled Myriad's patent in May, so OHIP is now off the hook, but other such patents are now also threatened.

The central issue was whether Monsanto's patent included the *whole* plant or just the *process* of insertion of an artificially altered gene causing resistance to the toxicity of Roundup. Schmeiser lawyer Terry Zakreski asserted that the patent granted to Monsanto in 1995 for GM canola clearly only covers the genetic *engineering process*, not the plant itself or even the plant seed, and that patented objects never self-replicate, only life-forms do, and that self-replication cannot be patented because then it is not a human invention anymore. If Monsanto wanted to sue somebody, they should sue another company, if it uses this insertion technique, but not a farmer who utilized the unpatentable natural growth and replication processes. Guelph University 's GMO expert Ann Clark asked, "How can the farmer be held accountable for something the seed trade itself cannot do?"**http://www. plant.uoguelph.ca/research/homepages/eclark/**

This is how: our government in 1995 not only granted Monsanto the patent for the canola gene insertion process, but **also** the "*unrestricted* release into the environment" without so much as a question about what might happen. The result: the rapid evolution of "super weeds" which neither Roundup nor any other chemical can kill, a world market that said, "We'll pass, thank you", and hopelessly contaminated natural seeds. Canada lost, and continues to lose a lot of money, farmers are faced with an insoluble mess, and Monsanto continues to make money until this wholesale exploitation strategy will at last no longer pay, a process that has already begun.

The judges needed to consider 1. a *Patent Act* not designed for biotechnology, 2. their own previous famous decision (the *Harvard Mouse* case), in which they had ruled higher life forms cannot be patented, 3. and the Canadian Biotechnology Advisory Committee 2002 report, which urges that the *Patent Act* should be changed so that contamination processes and self-replication are taken into account. That report points out that patent law never before had to deal with inventions that can do their own thing on their own time and don't stay put. Now, the Supreme Court's job is to interpret the laws made by parliament, and must therefore navigate between upholding existing laws and suggesting change to those existing laws. Supreme Court judges aren't nannies to whose skirts we can cling when big bad corporate wolves come salivating. We have to punch them out ourselves by demanding changes to the law.

The May 21 decision shows that five judges argued "...we are not concerned here with the innocent discovery by farmers of blow-by patent plants...in their cultivated fields. Nor are we concerned with the scope of the patent, or the wisdom and social utility of the genetic modification of genes and cells—a practice authorized by Parliament under the *Patent Act* and its regulations. Our sole concern is with the application of established principles of patent law to...this case." They go on: "The *Patent Act* confers on the patent owner 'the exclusive right, privilege and liberty of making, constructing and using the invention and selling it to others to be used.' Schmeiser was found to "cultivate" Monsanto's canola, that is to say: the stuff was on his land. These five judges found that he was using somebody else's property, because "our task is to interpret the *Patent Act as it stands*." Right—George Bernard Shaw famously said that most of the time "the law is an ass."

The four dissenting judges were led by Justice Louise Arbour who has just been appointed Human Rights Commissioner to the United Nations after her predecessor was recently killed in the bombing of the UN office in Iraq. She led a 1995 landmark inquiry into the abuse of women prisoners at Kingston penitentiary, served as chief prosecutor from 1996 to 1999 for the UN war crimes tribunals for Rwanda and the former Yugoslavia, indicted Slobodan Milosevic, overruled NATO generals who did not want to arrest war criminals, and forced the investigation of mass graves containing Serb victims. The UN is gaining a great person at the Canadian Supreme Court's expense.

Arbour et al argued that patent law is irrelevant because it is designed to protect an inventor's "*monopoly* over his invention". The question, they wrote, is whether growing a Monsanto invention *accidentally* in any way *deprived* Monsanto of that legally granted monopoly over their invention. These four judges found, that in no way was Monsanto's monopoly infringed, as it could go on making piles of money from people who buy their engineered seeds voluntarily. The judges cited the international treaty TRIP which states in article 27 (3) (b) that plants and animals can be excluded by member states from patentability—thereby delivering not only a blow to the Canadian *Patent Act*, but making it mandatory that it be harmonized with the treaty.

All 9 judges agreed that Monsanto had to bear the costs because Schmeiser had not profited in any way from this contamination. This ruling shows that all 9 judges had a very tough time. Both sets of arguments are sound and lay the groundwork for a whole new set of actions. In a weird sort of way Monsanto lost by winning. Schmeiser correctly pointed out that this will make it very difficult for Monsanto to keep suing farmers whose fields are contaminated, because this ruling also requires that Monsanto must prove that "a farmer has profited from" unwanted seed. "This decision has removed the teeth from their patent", he observed (indeed from all biotech patents) and pointed out that "now parliament will have to act, because we have a conflict between plant breeders' right and patent law."

That is true, too, because Supreme Court rulings, such as this one, which clearly identify a problem in existing law, cannot be ignored by Parliament. Something will happen now sooner or later to change the *Patent Act*. This is a great opportunity for those of us who want to get involved to do so.

It so happened that shortly after the *Schmeiser Decision* came down, the Supreme Court handed down another decision, and this one is a true zinger: on June 11, the Supreme Court ruled that corporations are fully accountable for the damage they cause to the environment through negligence or (greedy) intent. The Judges ruled that our environment, and everything that is in it, "should be valued on more than just a (potential) market value basis", said Sierra Legal lawyer Robert Wright, summarizing the decision.

Now consider the 18th century economist Adam Smith's famous "invisible hand" in the market which forced Monsanto to abandon its genetically engineered wheat (while still crowing over the *Schmeiser Decision*) because of world-wide opposition and flat-out refusal by several countries to buy *anything* edible from North America if *this* plan went ahead (because of the obvious contamination problem). The prospect of GM wheat was for the EU and Japan literally the final straw. In Australia, Monsanto had to abandon plans for GM canola for the same reasons. With Europe, Australia and most of Asia refusing most GMOs, Monsanto is hoping Africa will yield to their propaganda (BBC June 21). Given the long history of imperial exploitation of that continent, I am sure their wits will prove to be even sharper than ours, and they will have learned about Japan's Nagoya University research which reported on and detailed "Monsanto's fraudulent testing data for GE soybeans".

Patent law was designed at a time when 18th century polymaths invented gadgets and explored an uncontaminated world totally unlike ours today. Patents offered personal control of an individual's idea, not world control. Since corporations in the 20th century obtained the legal status of "persons", they became hungry giants who never can be satisfied in a world where the stock market demands infinite hunger and eternal growth.

Liability Law, however, carries the archetypal intent of establishing and enforcing *personal* responsibility, and nothing can ever be really new in that domain, not even biotechnology. Corporations are persons under the law and liability can be the fire that may destroy them. The concept of liability is ancient: here the god of the Old Testament growls from way back in the Garden of Eden demanding accountability. It is already doing so most notably in the pharmaceutical arena: New York State 's attorney-general Eliot Spitzer, famous for successfully indicting Wall Street fraudsters, is suing Glaxo Smith Kline for "deceiving doctors" with fraudulent drug research and for withholding negative information on drugs under development; he is doing exactly what finally brought down Big Tobacco (*Nature* vol. 429, June 10). It doesn't matter whether he succeeds or not—the process of raising liability on a grand scale has at least begun.

Simultaneously, the European Union stunned North America by tabling a law that would require *all* corporations to prove their products are safe *before* bringing them to the market. If it passes, this will be the most momentous change in the way the world does business.

Schmeiser asserts, "No one should have the right to release into the environment that which destroys the property of others." Zakreski is continuing legal action on behalf of Canadian farmers (see **www.saskorganic.com**) utilizing liability law, just as New York's attorney-general has done. Unlike the battle against corrupt pharmaceutical practices, agricultural issues have a great deal of precedent to draw upon. The two decisions the Supremes made in May and June will eventually, probably sooner than later, help to change patent law in Canada, and liability law will take center stage again as the correct weapon to use against all polluters, be they genes or giants.

Sources and Resources

How Monsanto became the "World's Most Unethical and Harmful Company": **www.corpo-ratewatch.org** and **www.ethicalinvesting.com**). See B. Tokar's history of Monsanto in *The Ecologist* vol. 28/5, Sept. 5, 1998, also available via his website **www.social-ecology.com.**

The Supreme Court decision is on **www.percyschmeiser.com**

For a fairly comprehensive bibliography on this issue see the one listed at the end of the first article in this section.

Update October 2004: *The Schmeiser case not only shows what problems have arisen due to the agendas of international trade agreements which are not interested in the complex problems brought forth by science, but this case also shows that grassroots action and determination are essential to humanizing the corporate agenda. Proposals have been put forward suggesting that patent law and laws governing corporate activities should include the proviso that profits may only be made as long as they do not harm the environment and human health. This contrasts, of course, wildly with what the entire corporate ambition is all about. However, there was a time when it was considered totally crazy to have an economy NOT based on slavery. The US of the mid-19th century could not imagine it and wound up having a civil war over this notion. We need to imagine an economy not based on exploitation. Currently, the world is using 20% more resources every year than the planet is capable of producing. We need to adjust our imagination accordingly.*

2
Poisons

Ottawa's ECO Summit 2000 and the New Pesticide Act

Vitality Magazine July/August 2000

Two thousand years ago, humankind was told, "Blessed are the meek, for they shall inherit the earth." Jesus meant non-violent people with gentle hearts. Today, within less than a century, "the meek" may turn out to be the roaches, mosquitoes, fleas, bacteria, and viruses and they may be the inheritors of the earth because they appear to be able to develop defenses against the pesticides meant to eradicate them. Humanity, on the other hand, may well succumb to the concoctions of three generations of chemists, if those who profit from these toxic substances filling our air, water and soil are not stopped fast. We, unlike the roaches and mosquitoes have no such defenses against chemicals.

On May 15th and 16th, 2000, the first formal Eco-Summit took place in Ottawa—a pesticide-free city. In fact, one can safely relax on the lawns of Rideau Hall's lovely grounds because Governor General Adrienne Clarkson won't tolerate pesticides, nor do any of the other official residences and Parliament's grounds have any pesticides either. Organized by Liberal MP Karen Kraft-Sloan, this was an environmental conference for parliamentarians and brought together MPs, doctors, lawyers and activists to join environmental experts in forging a plan to help avoid collective suicide by chemistry.

There was irony in the fact that the keynote speaker, Robert F. Kennedy Jr., one of the world's leading environmentalists with a breathtaking record of stopping polluters around the world, revealed that here, in pesticide-free Ottawa, "the Canadian government is engaged, at its own initiative, in secret talks with the US and Mexican governments to erode" the only provision in NAFTA "which allows citizens to force their own governments to enforce environmental laws." He added that "you should demand that these secret talks stop immediately." This revelation drew shocked gasps. Imagine, all those MPs sitting there didn't know this, and this American activist had to tell them! One of the MPs present and sitting in the front row was the Canadian Environment Minister. What did he know about this? Whatever he knew, he certainly kept silent.

Kennedy told of his childhood when his father, the US Attorney General during his brother President John F. Kennedy's administration, used to take him to visit his uncle in the White House. The most exciting part of such a trip to Washington was for the boy to see the enormous bald eagles that used to nest at that time on top of the capital's main post office. They are extinct today, he told the audience. This boy, who witnessed his father's assassination on television in real time, grew up to become the self-appointed restorer of the world's rivers. The great Hudson was so polluted in the late 1970s that it would burst into flames and be a river of fire for weeks on end. Today, because of Kennedy's efforts the river is full of fish again. His law firm trains lawyers who become political activists. They may chose to complete their legal training in the usual way, by articling, or by taking on the prosecution of a corporate polluter. This may take years, they need not win the case, but doing the job earns them their legal degree.

Kennedy observed that we are treating "the planet as if it were a business liquidation…to have a few years of pollution-based prosperity," yet true prosperity requires "investing in our environment as an investment infrastructure." In a true free-market economy, instead of the corporate-controlled economy we actually have, Kennedy said, polluters would "not be allowed to internalize their profits and externalize their costs", as the pesticide industry does worldwide. He pointed out that "the big shots", those faceless trans-national corporations, need to be faced down and told: "We are emissaries of the future. We want to know what you are doing with the things that don't belong to you, that belong to our children." Kennedy received a standing ovation that seemed unending—yet, not even one of the mainstream media even so much as mentioned his visit to Ottawa.

The following day, during the day-long environmental workshop for parliamentarians, the University of Ottawa's David Lean informed the audience that in the early 1970s the entire biosphere came close to very nearly being completely poisoned by PCBs. It was banned just in time. Yet, because PCBs travel by air and water, the highest concentrations are now found in the Arctic. There, sea mammals are so polluted that the Inuit are advised that on a daily basis it is not safe to eat a piece of meat larger than the size of a sugar cube. Sheila Watt-Cloutier, president of the Inuit Circumpolar Conference, commented that "we feel like an endangered species."

US scientist Joseph Jacobsen did groundbreaking research for the EPA over two decades that proved the disastrous effect on child development of PCBs and other toxic chemicals. His research has been duplicated internationally, including in Canada. The developing brain is defenseless against these toxins and becomes further contaminated by the fat-soluble chemicals found in mother's milk everywhere.

Renowned Canadian ecologist, David Schindler from Alberta, announced that within 50 years Canada's fresh water supply could be in crisis, and that by the year 2100 our fresh-water fish may completely disappear, if the relatively simply solutions that already are available are not implemented now. Schindler's research in the 1970s showed how acid rain renders lakes unable to support life and was the basis for world-wide legislative changes.

The impact of pesticides and industrial chemicals on the planet's ecological balance is profound, rapid and often irreversible. The poisoning and exploitation of the Aral Sea in the former Soviet Union caused starvation, rampant infectious disease and was an economic disaster. That event prompted the then Soviet president, Mikahil Gorbachev to found the International Green Cross which works for environmental disaster everywhere; he is its president now.

The world's ground water is polluted everywhere, mainly due to pesticides which travel through the ground in ways barely understood by science. Professor Ann Clark of Guelph University has shown how high intensity agriculture and its chemical addiction means that agriculture will be increasingly experienced as an environmental hazard. Soil dynamically interacts with light and heat, thereby sometimes greatly increasing the toxicity of these chemicals which then leach into the water supply around farms.

In 1947 six pests became resistant to DDT. By 1999 over 600 such pests, exposed to some ten thousand additional varieties of deadly toxins, began to thrive on them, even though application increased 12 fold. Their evolutionary clocks tick a lot faster and their generational turn-over is often a few days; that is not the case with larger animals, such as fish, birds and mammals; this evolutionary advantage enables the bugs to recombine their internal chemistry very rapidly to form defenses against synthetic poisons, and they can frequently even find ways by which those very toxins become nutrients for them. As a result, what we have connived to do unto others is backfiring onto ourselves such as to potentially wipe us out. Furthermore, because the genomes of pests can learn globally, today pesticide resistance is observed to occur within a *single* generation of these creatures, as they rapidly adapt to the deadliest poisons. It is the pests that are fruitful and multiply, while the daughters and sons of Adam and Eve are dying in an epidemic of diseases which destroy *our* nervous systems instead of the pests', our endocrine systems, our reproductive potential, our DNA's ability to replicate, and our brains—not theirs.

Stanford's Kay H. Kilburn, brain scientists, toxicologist and editor of the prestigious *Archives of Environmental Health*, became famous for proving how asbestos causes cancer. Today, his work shows that the brain is actually the target of all this toxic chemistry. "our civilization reeks with chemicals," he wrote recently. "Human health has been sacrificed to economic growth and profits, the twin idols of our time. We have perpetuated the myth that for human beings to be content and secure, chemical warfare is justified." He states categorically: "People must make peace with their insect coinhabitants of the earth."

In 1996 the US passed the Food Quality Protection Act which initiated reevaluation of all pesticides commonly found in homes and garden sheds. Led by Mt. Sinai Hospital's (New York) Dr. Philip Landrigan, the medical community informed the government that instead of the pests, our children are the victims. As a result, an entire class of organophosphates is now on the block, many have been restricted, banned or are being voluntarily withdrawn by the manufacturers. Dowe Chemical withdrew Dursban in the US, but in Canada it still is available and the company insists that some 3,600 studies supposedly exist proving it is safe. I was unable to find even one.

Duke University's neurotoxicologist M. Abu-Dania recently proved that even the notion of a "safe level" is a fantasy. There is no such thing as a safe level for any pesticide. He exposed lab animals to the lowest supposedly non-toxic levels of three commonly used pesticides consecutively without time intervals between the exposures, and he noted no observable damage. However, when the animals were exposed to all three of these chemicals simultaneously, all at those same low level concentrations, they all died. In the real world we live in, these very toxins are commonly found together in household insecticides, flea collars and lawn care products—and usually at much higher than "safe" concentrations.

One June 29th, 1998, delegates from more than 100 countries gathered in Montreal to initiate banning the so-called Dirty Dozen, namely the worst environmental toxins known as POPs (Persistent Organic Pollutants—because in practical terms they are eternal; they don't bio-degrade.) (**Note:** *the POPs Treaty became international law in March 2004.*)

In the UK proof of nervous-system damage sustained by thousands of farmers from organophosphates used in sheep farming forced government action. The Countess of Mar (currently the living representative of the oldest peerage in the UK going back in an unbroken line to the 10th century) is a sheep farmer herself as well as a member of the House of Lords. She nearly died from using this stuff. Under the care of a physician trained in environmental medicine, Dr. Jean Munro of the Breakspeare Hospital outside London, she recovered and went on to lead the Lords in achieving a moratorium on "sheep dip" (a total ban has since then been imposed).

The Countess wrote to me on March 9th: "You seem to be having very similar problems in Canada. Truly independent scientists' findings are always ignored in favour of those of the industry-funded scientists. I have made speeches in parliament citing intellectual corruption as a severe handicap. Those of us who know we are right must simply go on in the hope that, one day someone in authority will see the light." Indeed, some people in Canada are seeing the light and will succeed if we, the people, help them.

Liberal MP Marlene Jennings and her daughter learned their eczema was caused by chemicals in mosquito repellents. Wishing to use non-toxic natural products, she found to her dismay that Canadian licensing regulations assumer only the use of toxic chemicals, thereby preventing natural substitutes from being marketed. As a result she championed the Private Member's Bill C-388 to ban all cosmetic use of pesticides—especially to get them out of reach of children in any form. This started the ball rolling for legislative renewal so that the current pesticide legislation is brought up to date.

By the way, the highest infant mortality rate—almost 9 for every 1,000 live births—is in Saskatchewan, a province which also has the greatest number of breast cancer cases. That province has the most intensive use of pesticides in Canada.

Asked how to deal with the compulsive dandelion hater, Marlene Jennings said, "We stopped asbestos, we took lead out of gasoline, we stopped land mines, we led the world in the fight against tobacco—why can't our citizens learn about pesticides?" Right on, Marlene! The assumption that people can act intelligently in their own and communal interest be smart is the very spirit of democracy.

Speaking of the annual war on dandelions, the May/June issue of the *International Journal of Integrative Medicine* has an article by L. Alschuler who lists that very plant's verified medicinal uses, one of them being also involved in cancer therapy. "When asked which herbs are indispensable, most herbalists would certainly name the dandelion," she writes. "Observing that "the entire plant is therapeutic," she cites supportive clinical studies and discusses its biochemistry. Different parts, at various times of the year, produce chemicals used as a diuretic, a source for steroids, an anticarcinogenic in breast cancer therapy, to prevent recurring kidney and gallbladder stones, and in the treatment of colitis, asthma and eczema.

As for pesticides in agriculture, the following gives pause for thought: Charles Walters, editor of *Acres USA* wrote to *Alive* magazine in June, that "weeds are an index of what is wrong and sometimes of what is right." The presence of weeds such as lambsquarters and pigweed tell the farmer the crop will thrive because harmful insects will stay away; the presence of cocklebur informs that the soil's phosphate levels are good. The three-foot deep dandelion roots transport calcium and minerals to the surface and enrich our food. Grassy weeds like foxtail prove soil pH is imbalanced, but compost and aeration fix that without chemicals.

In June 1999 the Standing Committee on Environment and Sustainable Development, chaired by MP Charles Caccia (PC) began the formal re-evaluation of pesticides and published its report on May 16, 2000. It turned out that more than 7,000 approved pesticides in Canada have not been evaluated in more than thirty years, most of them never, in fact. The old *Pest Product Control Act* guarantees complete confidentiality to the manufacturer, with regard to sales, use patterns and even toxic reactions. This Act is nothing less than a gag order on the government and also prevents all independent health and ecological research, which necessarily would adversely affect sales. Canadian doctors testified before the standing committee that they can not get even the most basic information from the Health Protection Branch or the manufacturer, even in acute emergencies. In desperation, they routinely phone the EPA in the US, where the availability of complete toxicology data on pesticides is already mandatory.

"It is high time," the report states, "that paramount interests be placed above the business interests of pesticide manufacturers." Most radical of all, the report recommends that legislation be passed to allow the government to inform the public of health hazards without asking the manufacturer for permission. As these manufacturers are usually trans-national corporations, Article 1711.5 of NAFTA gives them the same protection from responsibility to the public as does Article 39.3 of TRIP (Trade Related Aspects of Intellectual Property Rights). Both treaties are subject to the World Trade Organization's rules which prevent disclosure of data on agricultural chemicals. Do we dare hope that Canada will protect its citizens from the World Trade Organization's global economic gang-rape?

Here is one example of what the WTO is all about in practical terms: after Kennedy had spoken and the crowd dispersed along the many corridors of the Parliament Building's centre block, I was delayed speaking to one of MPs and was therefore one of the last people to leave the ball room where this event took place. To my surprise, I found myself walking behind the Minister of the Environment, David Anderson, who was on crutches because of a skiing accident.

He was walking slowly and engaged in conversation with another MP. Because of they took up the width of the corridor and as the thick red carpeting made my presence behind them not noticeable, I overheard the following: the MP was taking the Minister to task in a friendly but clearly disapproving way over having recently caved in on taking out a chemical added to gasoline to make engines run more smoothly. In the past lead was used for this purpose, which was removed because of its carcinogenic properties and replaced by benzene, which is just as carcinogenic, as well as yet another chemical which is especially implicated in childhood cancers, namely MMT, this being the one discussed at this moment. "I can't understand why you didn't stand firm on that," the MP exclaimed. The Minister's reply was preceded by a groan: "Listen, I tried and tried and I fought this all the way," he said. "And then the WTO got in the act. Nobody had told me they could! Well, and then it was all over."

Under certain provisions of the WTO, *future* lost revenues take legal precedence over national health and environmental concerns, even if those concerns are enshrined in national law. Canada was successfully sued. So, when we elect an MP, in fact he or she can do very little.. (*Note: for technical reasons, not health concerns, MMT has now been removed from gasoline.*)

Caccia's report also recommends that organic farming should be encouraged through tax incentives and that Chemical Sensitivity Syndrome (another name for MCS or Multiple Chemical Sensitivity) should receive "legal recognition". Wow!!! Every Canadian should read this report and jam the government's fax machines and e-mail servers with ecstatic support.

The Official Opposition will, however, go down in history as having missed the boat most embarrassingly: their appended critique extols the virtues of pesticides, perfect lawns and business consideration. Did they read the report? What about *their* children's future?

In the Eco Summit round-table discussions with physicians and international law experts it was most interesting to learn how frustrated parliamentarians are in trying to get something done. Brian Emmet, Canada's first Commissioner for the Environment, lamented that even the most serious of environmental concerns simply do not get the attention of the press. He also chided Ontario for its lax handling of polluters and lack of environmental law enforcement. The cozy relationship between "the big shots", as Kennedy called the trans-national corporations, and the top most levels of our government is so secretive that even the rest of our government doesn't know what to do. MP Kraft-Sloan observed in an article she recently wrote for *The Hill Times* (April 10) that prodding for changes comes primarily from non-governmental organizations, not government, which should be in charge. Government, she wrote "keeps putting out little fires" instead of "making a dent in the changes facing us."

Ecologist David Schindler said that Canadians have to take back their government's agenda if we wish to survive.

We stand at a crossroads. US presidential advisor on cancer prevention, Sandra Steingraber, observed that the pesticide industry fosters a huge deception, namely that their products are necessary. The truth is out now, everywhere, and needs action to support it. Mikhail Gorbachev, the man who ended the Cold War, in writing about his efforts with the International Green Cross he founded in 1988, observed: "I reject the view that things will somehow work themselves out. I am convinced that mankind can meet the environmental challenge, if all of us join the cause, if all of us act." That means that in every kitchen, bathroom and garden the Chemical War must stop. Now.

Summary Information on Pesticides, Herbicides and Fungicides

In animals and humans they are: *endocrine disruptors* ("gender benders" and infertility); *mutagenic* (cause severe genetic mutations in fetus); *genotoxic* (kill DNA); teratogenic (cause birth defects and brain damage in fetus); *immunotoxic* (disrupt immune system); *carcinogenic* (cause cancer, especially leukemia and brain cancer in children); cause of *retardation* in children; *behavior altering* by affecting specific brain areas (violence, ADHD, depression).

Specific diseases known to be caused or triggered by pesticides: all cancers, even genetically predisposed ones; *Parkinson's, endometriosis, leukemia, brain tumors*, certain *kidney diseases*, most *liver diseases, autoimmune diseases, ADHD*.

The environmental cost of lawns (from F.H. Borman et al, *Redesigning the American Lawn*, Yale, 1993): a lawnmower pollutes in 1 hour as much as driving a car 425 km; 30-60% of fresh urban water goes on lawns in North American annually; about US $ 5 billion is spent on lawn fertilizers annually; about 600 million gallons of gasoline are used for lawnmowers annually; about US $ 700 million are spent annually on pesticides. All this for about 25 million acres of residential lawns. Lawns are major contributors to greenhouse gases and climate change and the increasing world-wide deficit.

Sources and Resources

K. Bock & N. Sabin, *The Road to Immunity: How to Survive and Thrive in A Toxic World*, Pocket Books, 1997

T. Colborn, *Our Stolen Future*, Penguin, 1997

R.F. Kennedy Jr. & J. Cronin, *Riverkeepers*, Simon & Schuster, 1997

S. Steingraber, *Living Downstream*, Addison Wesley, 1998

J. Wargo, *Our Children's Toxic Legacy*, Yale, 1998

The government report, *Pesticides—Making the Right Choice*, May 2000, contains the source list from the medical literature on the diseases and condition s listed above.

The US EPA can be reached at 703-305-5017 or **www.epa.gov/pesticides/biopesticides**

Update October 2004: *The new pesticide act did become law. It is surprisingly good and useful. For an example of how you can use it yourself, to stop the cosmetic use of pesticides in your area, as the whole of Quebec has already achieved, read the next item following this article. In May 2004, the Ontario College of Family Physicians published their report, providing proof that pesticides cause childhood leukemia and asthma among many other illnesses. The doctors urge people to eat organic and stop the cosmetic use of pesticides. Simultaneously, the US government completed its first series of investigations into which toxic substances are found in people throughout the USA. It turns out, every person carries a minimum of 13 such toxic substances in their bodies, all neurotoxic, carcinogenic, or hormone disrupting or all three. The details and how to get this information are provided below.*

Working to Stop the Use of Pesticides

The following is a presentation made by my husband in June 2004 before the town council of the Town of Orangeville near which we live. This is a work in progress; the mayor is supportive. This provides helpful information on pesticides, the new federal pesticide law, international efforts and scientific sources. It may serve as a guide for those who want to initiate such ban in their own area. For videos and other educational material explaining the scientific basis for banning pesticides contact CAPE (Canadian Association of Physicians for the Environment): **www.cape.ca/toxics/pesticideskelly.html** *and WHEN (Women's Healthy Environments Network), a registered charity (No. 11926 2533 RR0001)* **when@web.ca** *or visit* **www.whenvironments.ca**. *Call 416-928-0880 or 416-960-4944.*

In Support of a By-Law Banning the Cosmetic Use of Pesticides in the Town of Orangeville, June 2004

by Robert K. Ferrie, M.D. (519-927-3206) member of CAPE

On Scientific Consensus

The *Ontario College of Family Physician's* 2004 report asserts that pesticides and herbicides must be stopped because of the documented adverse health effects. Their documentation is solid and they are supported by medical organizations all over the world.

They are also supported by the *World Health Organization* which has convened **this month** in Europe a meeting of health ministers from governments all over the world to establish new guidelines for environmental toxins relative to the health of children and women in particular.

The OCFP findings are also supported by *Health Canada* and *Environment Canada* as well as the Canadian courts; the *Supreme Court* decision of 2001 known as the *Hudson Decision* being the most important one. It gives every municipality the right to prohibit the use of synthetic pesticides and fertilizers. The court action undertaken by CropLife against the City of Toronto has been thrown out by one court already and because of the Supreme Court's decision does not stand a chance in appeal either.

The *Health Canada* website has a great deal of information on pesticide reduction and the scientific support for such needed change. Of special importance is their information on the **new standards for toxicology**. In the past the idea was "the dose makes the poison", now we know that synthetic chemicals are harmful to certain groups at certain specially vulnerable times and that—across the board—repeated exposure to small amounts (each exposure being below the old toxic threshold) causes the serious damage, i.e. cancer and neurological and developmental diseases. The leader of *Health Canada*'s agricultural research team, John McLachlan, is quoted on their website as follows; *"Instead of one plus one equaling two, we found that one plus one equals a thousand-fold."* Furthermore, *Health Canada* provides a 122-page document entitled *Basic Knowledge Requirements for Pesticide Education in Canada*, 2004 edition. Alternatives to chemicals are strongly recommended.

The OCFP is also supported by *Canada Mortgage and Housing Corporation* whose fact sheets on pesticide harm and reduction strategies can be downloaded from their site also: **www.cmch-schl.gc.ca**. It provides a complete list of all the non-toxic products currently available in Canada.

The OCFP is further supported by the US Centre for Disease Control whose data are published in *Chemical Trespass* (a copy was provided to you earlier). An average of 13 toxic chemicals are now found in all individuals, the highest concentrations being in women and children because these lawn care products are almost all estrogen mimics (that explains the women) and are taken up in larger quantities by growing children.

The OCFP is supported also by the leading universities in the US. Cornell, Harvard, Michigan State, Oregon State, University of California at Davis and the US National Agricultural Pesticide Impact Assessment Program run a website called EXTOXNET through which they provide the same kind of health hazard information as is contained in the OCFP report.

On the law and government responsibility

First: The fact that every person in North America has 13 or more toxic chemicals in the body means that **government regulatory agencies have completely failed to protect us.** None of those toxic chemicals are in our bodies with our consent and none should be in our bodies. All of them are known to cause harm. The clean-up process through education, changes in legislation, court decisions and new medical therapies is now beginning.

Second: In a democracy action does not happen from the "top down". Governments that act from the top down are called totalitarian. In a democracy the people initiate change, which finally results in the formulation of laws and court decisions. The *Canadian Pesticide Act* was reformed because scientists, doctors, and grass-roots citizens' groups demanded change. The political process worked rather well in this case, but the price paid by millions of people who were adversely affected by these chemicals was high. In fact, Canada's cancer burden alone is such that our national health care system cannot meet the demand and the cost is escalating such that we are in danger of bankrupting Medicare with just cancer alone. We now know that at least 2/3 of all cancers are due to environmental toxins, especially pesticides, herbicides, fertilizers and industrial solvents—not because of smoking or other life-style factors.

Because of the enormous financial implications, this process of education and reform is understandably slow and often corrupted. Currently, *Health Canada* faces law suits for negligence in the range of $ 13 billion dollars. In their annual meeting this year in May, the *Canadian Association of Journalists* identified *Health Canada* as the most secretive and undemocratic institution in Canada. In March of this year, the *House of Commons Standing Committee on Health* and the *Canadian Medical Association* rebuked Health Canada for virtually ignoring the legislation under which they must ensure the safety of drugs and products of all kinds that have the potential to affect human health. They specifically praised the whistleblowers, such as *Health Canada's* Dr. Shiv Chopra, Dr. Margaret Haydon and Dr. Brill-Edwards who made Health Canada's corrupt collusion with the industry public.

Therefore, both is true: government agencies can be criminally negligent AND they can be made to do their jobs through the pressure of citizens and scientists. Often this has positive results, such as the new *Pesticide Act*. But we—you and I—must be the source of change, not the government.

The new *Pesticide Act* enshrines the 1998 international Precautionary Principle which in its treaty form was ratified by Canada; it states: **"When an activity raises threats of harm to human health or the environment, precautionary measures should be taken, even if some cause and effect relation ships are not fully established scientifically…the proponent of that activity, rather than the public, should bear the burden of proof."**

Our new *Pesticide Act* also enshrines all the scientific principles raised by the OCFP report, such as identifying specially vulnerable groups, that nontoxic substances are preferable at all times, that synthetic pesticides are indeed harmful to health, etc. There is nothing in that act that defends the use of synthetic pesticides, fertilizers and herbicides. It is designed to minimize damage everywhere.

The Canadian government also passed the so-called **Westray Bill C-45** in March of this year which amends the criminal code such that employers are now 100% responsible for the safety of workers. The legal opinions on this bill have already made the case that this includes chemical trespass and injury at the workplace. Since lawn-care employees have the highest rate of prostate cancer, we are likely to see some cases in court soon.

Last week the Supreme Court handed down a decision that allows corporations to be sued for damaging the environment. The *Sierra Legal Defense Fund* stated: *"This case will have repercussions well beyond forestry law to air pollution, water contamination, oil spills and the like—indeed any case where a natural asset is held in common for the benefit of everyone and is harmed by corporate negligence."* This applies directly to the water and air pollution pesticides are causing in communities and which have resulted in all these chemicals being found in our bodies.

On the alleged "other side"

There is no "other side". There is nothing that justifies the use of synthetic pesticides, herbicides and fertilizers. They do not protect us from anything at all. A dandelion does not cause cancer, does not damage the fetus, or even bring on an asthma attack. There is no weed in nature that does any of this. The cause of asthma lies in reduced immunity due also to cellular damage which then over-sensitizes the person. The *National Film Board* made a documentary in 2002 on how the pesticides used in potato farming in PEI is the cause for that province's high asthma rate, especially among children. Pesticides cause plenty of cellular damage as well as compromise DNA replication of healthy cells.

The fact is that, according to the House of Commons Committee report of May 2000, of all pesticides/herbicides produced, 9% goes on lawns; the remainder is used in agriculture. **However, 56% of the industry's total sales profits are derived from just lawn care products**. Lawn care products are sold at a higher margin of profit than agricultural pesticides. No wonder, the industry is fighting back.

The industry often makes the claim that "pesticides are safer than salt." A Canadian regulatory directive # DIR 96-02 forbids this comparison because salt is a nutrient and pesticides are not.

The industry also routinely claims that if there was cause to worry about pesticides, the government would have already done something about it. First, the government acts when the citizens want it to, as I have already said. Second, the government did act, and these new actions are not favoring the industry, especially not the new *Pesticide Act*.

Industry also often asserts that there are more carcinogens in our foods than in synthetic chemicals. They usually cite the work of a famous scientists Bruce Ames. What they don't tell you is that since Ames discovered natural carcinogens in food, the anti-carcinogens which neutralize them in the same foods have been discovered, and we now know that the cooking process completely neutralizes those natural carcinogens. Finally, none of those natural carcinogens actually cause cancer, as subsequent research showed, because the natural cancer-fighting systems in our bodies, evolved over millions of years, take care of improperly dividing cells. Only synthetic pesticides and herbicides (as well as other environmental toxins) actually attack our natural, genetically provided cancer fighting systems. Ames has acknowledged all this research.

The industry presents the health concerns of doctors, citizens and grassroots activist groups as ill-informed, alarmist etc. The Weed Man even had the nerve to attack the Supreme Court's 2001 Hudson Decision as being the result of having listened to "idealistic propaganda"! However, all of those who object to pesticides do not derive any financial benefit from their protest. We only have our health and the health of our patients and towns to gain by stopping the use of pesticides, not financial profits.

The manufacturers and franchised lawn-care companies have a great deal to lose, and the sooner they do, the better for our children, our future and our collective health. Natural lawn-care business will fill the vacuum.

On what you can do and what will happen as a result.

It is within your power to pass a by-law that prohibits the cosmetic use of pesticides and herbicides. The *Hudson Decision* specifically allows you to do so. It only take s a phone call or a quick search on the website for the City of Toronto or the Province of Quebec and you can down-load the texts of their anti-pesticide ordinances. Furthermore, you are supported, apparently by a great many people in Orangeville in such an action, if *Canadian Tire* is any indication! Their lawn care department informed us that they have been selling non-toxic alternative products for two years, they are all cheaper than the chemical toxic ones, and they sell better than the traditional ones! *President's Choice* no longer sells any synthetic lawn products as of December 2003.

Secondly, you are **mandated** by the new *Pesticide Act* to educate the public on safe home and garden practices, as for example the Town of Caledon is already doing. My wife Helke Ferrie, who is a medical science writer, and I as a doctor are most willing to help you with any public education project you may design. We have an excellent educational video produced by the *Canadian Alliance of Physicians for the Environment* which would be helpful to you.

Finally, if you take a pro-active stance in the elimination of pesticides from Orangeville you will, without a doubt, achieve what **Sweden** already has as a country: they started to phase out pesticide use twenty years ago and their cancer rate has dropped rapidly so that they now have the lowest rate in Europe. Similarly, in **New York State**, when certain pesticides were limited about a decade ago, the birth weight and brain size of newborn babies returned to their normal values such as doctors were used to seeing before pesticides came into use.

We would be pleased to assist you in any way we can, and be assured we will not go away until the use of pesticides and herbicides stops.

PACKAGE FOR EACH COUNCIL MEMBER

1. A copy of the 4th of a series of 7 articles published in 2002 by the **Canadian Medical Association** on the topic of the health effects from environmental pollution and how to treat such patients. This article summarizes the health effects of pesticides and establishes basic treatment protocols. These protocols are still evolving. This series of articles is based on the

research and treatments done over the past decade at the University of Toronto's Environmental Health Clinic and the government funded Environmental Health Clinic in Nova Scotia.

Significance: This publication sets a new standard of care and has resulted in the doctors of Canada incorporating into their practices the advice to their patients to stop using pesticides, herbicides and synthetic fertilizers and to turn to alternative lawn care methods which are not detrimental to health. This is equivalent to the declaration of war doctors declared on smoking. There is no medical compromise on either smoking or pesticides, and the facts established so far will not go away, be found flawed, or be diminished by further research.

2. The relevant passages from the May 2000 **Standing Committee on Environment and Sustainable Development** of the Government of Canada. This report resulted in the new national *Pesticide Act*, which became law in December 2002, and served as one of the basis for the Supreme Court's 2001 *Hudson Decision*.

Significance: This report established the benchmark of the internationally agreed-upon scientific facts about the nature and extent of harm pesticides, herbicides and fertilizers do. Significant is the table on page 41 of the hormone disruptors (the process by which cancer is caused), which includes the very ones the synthetic lawn care industry continues to deny as being harmful, such as 2-4 D. Since this report was published, the scientific consensus now also includes glysophate (active ingredient in Roundup).

3. The **cancer statistics** for Ontario up to 1995 as published by the Registrar General of Ontario in 1998 and the world statistics for breast cancer and all cancers from the *World Health Organization* up to 1997. The greatest increase in cancer rates is among children.

4. An article by Michelle Landsberg from *The Toronto Star*, October 25, 2003. The reference to the **Quebec teenager Jean-Dominic** is important; his efforts were crucial to stopping the use of cosmetic pesticides in the Province of Quebec.

5. A summary information on the question of **"inert" ingredients** in pesticides and herbicides. While this refers to US standards, these apply to Canada because the manufacturers are transnational corporations usually headquartered in the USA.

Significance: the new Canadian pesticide law requires the publication of these *inerts* and some manufacturers have begun to comply with this requirement. Because the new Canadian pesticide act also requires a review of all pesticides—old and new—the inerts will now be publicly known and, beyond a doubt, result in many products being taken off the market. That process will, however, take years, and children, pregnant women and sick people cannot be expected to wait.

6. The chemical data on **2-4 D**, its action, ecological effects, health effects on animals and humans, and the list of the **22 inert ingredients** which damage liver and kidney function, harm developing fetuses, cause infertility, skeletal abnormalities, anemia, cataracts, genetic defects in laboratory animals, fatal respiratory failure, and together, as a mix they are now the known to cause cancer.

   Note: this is the 2-4 D sold in stores; this is not the 2-4 D contaminated with dioxin which was used in Vietnam as a defoliant and was known as Agent Orange, and it is obviously not for sale for lawn-care purposes.

   Significance: until recently we did not know what harm 2-4 D can cause because the industry was not compelled to reveal the full slate of ingredients. Our new pesticide act is changing that now.

7. The chemical data on **Roundup (glyphosate)**. This is the updated information package and includes the recent proof that Roundup is carcinogenic, specifically being associated with breast cancer in both women and men (male breast cancer is rising exponentially every year). The **11 "inerts"** are listed as well.

8. The National Office of Pollution Prevention of **Environment Canada** has a terrific website devoted to pesticide reduction: **www.pestinfo.ca.** Basic information on this site is provided here. It shows how the NGO's of the supposedly most radical stripe (e.g. World Wildlife Fund, Sierra Club etc.) are endorsing this effort by our government and actively taking part in it. The information on the health dangers of pesticides and herbicides are so solid, that such a joint effort is possible. Of special importance is the *information package for municipalities* by which they can learn how to pass by-laws in accordance with the Hudson Decision and how they can educate the public to change their chemical addiction.

9. The second important website is that of **Pesticide Free Ontario www.pesticidefree.ca** which is linked to the government sites and is especially useful with regard to by-law projects and clarifying the junk science with which the industry keeps confusing people.

Green Spring Cleaning

Vitality Magazine May 2001

If cleanliness is godliness, we need a redefinition of the word "clean". For sparkle and shine may signal that brain death is steadily progressing in your home, and your sweet smelling fluffy laundry may be at war with your immune system—to say nothing of that weed-free garden which is helping to give everybody cancer within a radius of a several kilometers.

To tell a woman how to clean her house is rather like telling a man what car to drive; deeply ingrained habits are as difficult to give up as hard drugs. To suggest that your home is an immaculate toxic dump and your good intentions ignorance is pushing one's luck, I know. Before venturing into the minefield of spring-cleaning practices, let us invoke religion's aid.

Two thousand five hundred years ago, the Buddha taught the world that suffering stems from ignorance. Puzzling, until one learns that ignorance gives rise to suffering through being stuck in habitual thoughts and resistance to careful consideration of cause and effect. Similarly, Jesus, five hundred years later, pulled no punches: before healing a desperate, bedridden cripple, he asked him first the stunning question: "Do you want to be healthy?" That story haunted me when I myself started on the road to recovery which required revolutionary changes in habits, as I, too, had an immaculately toxic household.

Because of the overwhelming evidence that all illness is either caused or triggered by our chemical inventions, and the realization that ignorance is not bliss, the US National Centre for Disease Control and Prevention recently began a large-scale project of testing the population annually for exposure to toxic substances in the environment through blood and urine samples. They test for heavy metals (mercury, lead etc. which damage the nervous and immune systems), the carcinogenic indoor air pollutants (tobacco, solvents etc.), the equally carcinogenic pesticides (including those now outlawed, as some are generationally transmitted), and phthalates (endocrine disruptors found in plastics and detergents). Over the next few years, it will be possible to see disease patterns correlating with life styles and geographic areas (see CDC's web site **www.cdc.gov**).

While much of the toxic sludge our world is financially addicted to, comes from industry, possibly as much as two thirds of this witch's brew is found in our kitchens, bathrooms, garages, closets and gardens. They all share the nasty property of doing their deadly work awfully slowly and usually through low, frequent exposure.

Before we take a walk through the house and scare ourselves silly, it is important to be reminded of a concept fundamental to environmental medicine, namely "total load".

The body's capacity to rid itself of toxic substances is immense; it took evolution millions of years to build this amazing system. Living things have had to deal with organic and inorganic toxins for millions of years, but since the Industrial Revolution we have increased the toxic load astronomically.

Why, one wonders, is there always the jolly old grandfather who smokes his cigars and is healthy till he dies in his sleep at 90? People often ask, how come everybody eats the same stuff in the family, yet one has asthma, another migraines, a third varicose veins and a fourth absolutely no problems. Charlotte Gerson, daughter of the famous cancer expert Dr. Max Gersen, pointed out at a workshop in Toronto last year, that one reason cancer has increased so dramatically in children is that their livers can no longer detox the massive environmental load; indeed they are born with such toxins in their bodies. Most people born up to about 30 years ago were able to develop their immune systems and retain the functional health of their livers before the massive onslaught of pesticides, heavy metals, insulation materials, the fluoride craze and the overuse of antibiotics. All this, combined with a diet overloaded with immune-destructive refined sugar and processed foods, which is essentially dead, is the source of our modern Pandora's Box of illness.

It's all about that proverbial camel's back: if you don't have mercury amalgams in your teeth and don't get exposed to smoke, your liver and kidneys can handle a lot more. If you eat organic food and take vitamins C and E and minerals like selenium and magnesium regularly, you might survive a toxic office building without trouble, while the person in the next cubicle, who lives on processed foods, succumbs to environmental illness.

Similarly, the spring-cleaning discussed below must be seen in terms of individual applicability. However, there are a few toxins that are so bad, you are asking for trouble for yourself and all your differently constituted family members: smoking, solvents (especially habitual use of nail polishes and removers), fluoride, chlorine, kerosene heaters, open gas flames of any kind, and mercury amalgam fillings. It is a waste of breath to argue: the evidence is overwhelming. Get rid of them.

Bathroom/Laundry

Only a small sample of the known facts can be touched on. The law does not require listing "inert" ingredients in just about everything that's found here and they are almost never inert. The New York Poison Control Centre published a report showing that 85% of all warning labels are inadequate.

Most household cleaners, especially Windex, contain butyl cellosolve which is absorbed fastest through the skin; it is toxic to blood cells, kidneys and liver. Deodorizers usually contain dichlorobenzene, now found in 95% of all children tested; it causes birth defects and is toxic to lungs and mucous membranes. Make-up used frequently during pregnancy raises chances of childhood brain tumors by 60%; in 1987 Germany outlawed the offending substances in all cosmetics—not so here. But we are not the only ones ready to die for beauty: Queen Elizabeth I painted her face white, as was the custom in the 16th century. The paint was lead-based and she died from classic lead poisoning.

Many of the chemicals found in perfumes are also listed as hazardous-waste chemicals by the EPA. The petroleum-based chemicals in perfumes are cheap, while jasmine petals cost roughly a thousand dollars per pound. You can probably only afford the first type, until you get sick from the second—especially since most perfumes also contain the carcinogen benzene.

Hair dye, especially the dark shades, are responsible for at least 20% of all non-Hodgkin's lymphoma cancer cases in women, according to the US National Cancer Institute. Men's hair dyes are even worse: they usually contain acetate, which is not only a known carcinogen, but its presence in the body enhances the effects of other environmental carcinogens. Pregnant mothers using hair dye increase their kids' risk of cancer ten times.

Phosphates in laundry detergents are banned in Europe, but here it is still a matter of choice which you buy. Laundry softeners and anti-cling materials almost always contain carcinogenic benzene and, especially in children, often cause eczema. Fluoridated toothpaste is one of the craziest inventions ever: fluoride, a nuisance by-product of the chemical fertilizer manufacturing process, is more toxic than arsenic and lead and a really efficient way to induce immune disease. See Yiamouyiannis' fabulous medical-political expose.

Consider what Dr. Kaye Kilburn has to say. A professor of medicine and editor of the prestigious *Archives of Environmental Health*, he became world famous for discovering and proving the carcinogenicity of asbestos; he is considered one of the foremost authorities on chemical brain injury. He wrote in 1998: "Detergents and cleaning agents must be chosen with care to avoid chlorine, ammonia and other brain-violating chemicals ... perhaps the most harmful cosmetic chemicals are the solvents in polishes for fingernails. [They] are extremely hazardous with their methylethyl ketone, acetone and other brain solvents, so they must be forsworn and considered the worst of surface coatings."

If you really want to know what is in each and every item in your bath and laundry (by brand name, no less!) get yourself a copy of *The Safe Shoppers Bible*). It is exceedingly accurate: none of those cosmetic, detergent, and food producing industrial giants have so far been able to launch a law suit against its author, world renowned cancer researcher Samuel Epstein. To find what to buy instead, a list of great resources is listed below. The healthy (and almost always very much cheaper) alternatives for every vanity and practical need exist. What's more, you will be in the glamorous company of the likes of Nicole Kidman, Jane Fonda, Tom Cruise, Meryl Streep, John Travolta, Al Gore and many more who swear by many of those products (not as paid ads), because they are committed to environmental truth. The money saved on commercial cleaners could go into organic food.

Kitchen

It comes as no surprise, that here we find the neurotoxic polishing materials and aromatic detergents, the endocrine disrupting plastic cling wraps, and neurotoxic (and carcinogenic) formaldehyde producing dishwashing detergent. Formaldehyde is found in disinfectants, germicides, defoamers and even food preservatives and vaccines. It is a known asthma trigger. Only rats are not affected by it, as they can metabolize it. Not being a rat, three years ago I picked up the towel and threw out the dishwasher when I had had enough of the nightly low-grade headaches and the struggle to keep my balance. Our family of 7 (of three generations) washes everything by hand while having a grand old family-time with raucous conversation and laughs every night. Formaldehyde-free dishwashing detergents have finally arrived, but we like it this way much better. This Spring, throw out all cleaners whose ingredients you can't pronounce and give your liver, brain, and kidneys a chance to spring-clean themselves. The Canadian Mortgage and Housing Corporation provides excellent healthy house kits.

Living and Bed Rooms

It is possible to clean your rugs and curtains without shortening your lifespan: vinegar in the water work wonders and non-toxic detergents are available. It has been estimated that 10 % of foam rubber pillows in your bed after six years consists of dust mite dung and dead mites: sweet dreams! Replace with cotton ones. If you have pets and also suffer from allergies, but refuse to give up the pets, daily vacuuming will go a long way, I know: we have seven cats and 2 big dogs. Better still: replace wall-to-wall carpeting with cotton or wool scatter rugs. Resist dry cleaning those curtains, or anything else if at all possible because you need that common dry-cleaning fluid perchlorethylene quite literally like a hole in the head: prolonged exposure causes irreversible brain damage. "Green" dry cleaners already exist in Toronto, so check the Yellow Pages, or replace with washable curtains.

By now it is clear that human life is painfully challenged by solvents, detergents, aromatic chemicals of many kinds, and just about by everything from the petroleum industry. Not only is this relentless effort to make things perfectly clean, perfectly white, perfectly sweet smelling, and perfectly perfect, bad for health, it also often confers on bacteria the ability to evolve more effective defenses. PineSol, a popular floor cleaner, was shown to trigger antibiotic resistance in E-coli (the stuff of the Walkerton crisis) by then 13 year-old Canadian Merri Moken in a science project. She is at Princeton University now (*Globe & Mail*, Feb. 3, 1998).

If you really want to know all about those paints and varnishes in your garage or basement, read the labels very carefully. "Only to be used in well ventilated conditions" ought to give you the creeps right away. Check out the non-toxic equivalents in the information provided below which will also help you deal with mold in basements, closets and bedrooms; it produces carcinogenic benzene fumes. Farmers in Europe used to say that damp houses are cancer houses.

Garden and Office

Lawn mowers cause as much air pollution as cars: get one with a catalytic converter, if yours is aging. The use of chemical pesticides is quite simply criminal: we should all move to Halifax or Ottawa where they are forbidden. Non-toxic alternatives are available and cost a lot less.

There are some great and inexpensive air filters available which can sit on your desk or plug into your car's cigarette lighter. Many companies offer regular ozone filtration services for your photocopiers, printers etc. The EPA has repeatedly found that indoor air quality is at least ten times worse than even polluted city air. A friendly discussion with the boss about using non-toxic cleaners will get his attention when he/she learns they are cheaper.

What to do?

For the pro-active type who enjoys irritating people for their own good, I suggest talking to your Canadian Tire manager and requesting (not just once, but several times) environmentally friendly, non-toxic materials. The same might work with your supermarket manager—eventually. Politically, you can really make your mark: On December 10, 2000, initiated by Greenpeace, an international treaty was created that, when ratified, will ban the use and production of the world's most toxic chemicals, the so-called "Dirty Dozen" or POPs (persistent organic pollutants). That includes everything mentioned above. If ratified, phase-out will take 4 years. This May, ratification is being negotiated in Stockholm. To ensure that we begin to spring clean this planetary home of ours, write to Environment Minister, the Hon. David Anderson and Hon. Gilbert Parent, Canada's Ambassador for the Environment at House of Commons, Ottawa, K1A 0A6, and urge them to sign it. (*Note: Canada signed this treaty and it came into effect in 2004.*)

Sources and Resources

Kilburn, K., M.D., *Chemical Brain Injury*, Van Nostrand Reinhold, 1998

Rogers, S., M.D., *The E.I. Syndrome*, SK Publishing, Sarasota, 1995 (best single volume source on spring cleaning your body and restoring your health)

Rogers, S., M.D., "Total Wellness", Prestige Publishing, PO Box 3068, Syracuse, N.Y. 13220, 1©800©846©6687/315©455©7862. Simple the best medical newsletter in North America (monthly, annual fee $ 40).

Thornton, J., *Pandora's Poison*, MIT, 2000

Yiamouyiannis, J., M.D., *Fluoride*, Health Action Press, 1993

Allergy Shop, 2285 B St. Laurent Blvd. Unit 2, Ottawa, 613©737©5183

American Environmental Health Foundation, P.O. Box 29874, Dallas, Texas 75229

Store: 241 350-8942 for info on products also for sale in Canada

Berthold & Bond, A., *Clean and Green: The Complete Guide to Nontoxic and Environmentally Safe Housekeeping*, Ceres, New York, 1990 ($ 13.95)

Clarus 1-800-425-2787, for home and offices devices to neutralize electro magnetic field pollution

Bower, L., *The Healthy Household*, 1995, The Healthy House Institute, 430 North Sewell Road, Bloomington, IN 47408, 812-332-507 (also have excellent books on home building, ventilation etc.)

Lawson, L., *Staying Well in A Toxic World*, Lynnwood Press, Evanston, 1993

Randolph, T. M.D., *An Alternative Approach to Allergies*, Harper Collins, 1990

Steinman, D. & Wisner, R., *Living Healthy in A Toxic World*, Berkeley Publishing Group, 1996

Steinman, D. & Epstein, S. M.D., *The Safe Shopper's Bible: A Consumer's Guide*, Macmillan, 1995

Update October 2004: *One of the unexpected, amusing, and empowering developments with regard to the toxicity of cleaners and cosmetics is that "green" companies offering non-toxic alternatives no longer just label their products as environmentally friendly, biodegradable, not tested on animals, unscented, and so on, but they give us an education in chemistry. You may never have heard of,* **say sodium lauryl sulfate** *(SDS) and therefore not know it is harmful until you are informed about its absence in a dishwashing detergent made by* Nature Clean. *A large pink sticker informs the buyer that this detergent is free of SDS. Similarly, deodorants have suddenly become available that inform you they do not contain* **propylene glycol** *–so, there's your homework! Look it up by using your Internet search engine: type in the chemical's name and add +* Safety Data. *After that experience, you might want to take everything in your home's bathroom, kitchen cupboards and garages and look up all those words you can't pronounce and study their safety data information. It will undoubtedly result in the most thorough house-cleaning you have ever done. Be sure to get rid of everything you now know to be toxic in the hazardous waste disposal, not the regular garbage.*

Pressure Treated Wood
A Little War on God's Island

Vitality Magazine July 2002

In May of this year there was a War in Heaven. It was a short war and it was won with a flourish. One of God's own islands was in great danger of an attack by the neurotoxic poisons copper, cadmium, and arsenic. A few months earlier, on snowy, moonlit New Year's Eve 2001 three couples happened to meet by chance for a memorable gourmet meal a few hundred yards from the planned site of attack. They had no idea that the great Manitou, after which Manitoulin Island is named, had decided to inspire these three latter-day Musketeers to prevent this disaster. (Manitoulin means literally "island of god".)

For the past 24 years, my family has vacationed on Manitoulin Island, one of the world's great magical places. One of its grand sandy beaches at Providence Bay is several miles long. Part of that beach has an undulating boardwalk, almost a mile long, which dreamily dances over the dunes along the shores of Lake Huron. There the chatter and cries of Canada Geese, ducks, and seagulls fill the air, deer come to drink at night and raccoons fish for crayfish by the light of the moon. During the day, children build elaborate sandcastles and one time, one sculpted an enormous mermaid. People of all ages wander through the soft sand, and barefoot lovers wander along the boardwalk watching the sun set into the lake and taking in the scent of the wind-sculpted pines that line the boardwalk. These Manitoulin dunes are home to several hundred species of flowering plants usually found only at sea shores, attracting many botanists for scientific study every year.

This Spring the owner of the Providence Bay Home Hardware store suggested to the town council that the boardwalk needed to be protected. He offered to sell them several hundred gallons of "Copper II", a wood preservative made from petroleum distillates containing copper, cadmium and arsenic—neurotoxins and carcinogens all. It is used to make pressure-treated wood and to treat raw wood so that it becomes like pressure-treated wood.

In combination, these chemicals have the additional horrific property of changing over time to become increasingly toxic, as University of Florida researchers recently published. The timing was peculiar, too. All Canadian and American producers of such wood preservatives and pressure-treated wood, announced in January, in response to overwhelming scientific evidence and public demand, that these products would be phased out completely by 2004—something already the case in Europe since the late 1980s. Oddly, the Home Hardware owner is one of that company's directors and must have known about his company's voluntary phase-out decision and the reasons for it. Could it be that the prospect of taking thousand of gallons of unsold Copper II to the hazardous waste disposal in Sudbury, instead of selling it, had something to do with this? We'll never know.

Anyone interested in knowing what this set of chemicals can do need only watch "Erin Brokovich" played by Julia Roberts for which she won an Oscar. The research done by that feisty lawyer, which resulted in hundreds of millions of dollars' worth of compensation payments, paved the way for this universal voluntary phase-out before governments have even put legislation in place.

Copper is toxic to aquatic life. As it leaches out of the treated wood, it causes cycles of destruction followed by regeneration every few months, but it is unknown for how long this cycling goes on, and if some other chemical attacks the spawning eggs as well, recovery is not possible at all. To humans, copper is neurotoxic and enters our systems through contaminated drinking water. *Cadmium* is a carcinogen and one of the main causes of Parkinson's, now a well-established fact in mainstream medical research. Medical journals have published data since the early 1980s, showing how cancer is caused in men working with pressure-treated wood. *Arsenic* is deadly in every conceivable fashion and one of the causes of ADHD in children, if their mothers were exposed to it while pregnant. Its mode of action appears to be by damaging the pathways which allow the body to maintain the proper essential fatty acid status. Arsenic's preferred mode of entry is via the skin and breathing.

Thus, pregnant women walking through the sand at Providence Bay, children on the swings sets treated with Copper II, immune-deficient people on cortisone, old people with lowered immunity, and people with respiratory problems seeking the clean air of Manitoulin Island were going to be hit by an invisible toxic wave designed to kill termites and winding up killing them. Only more slowly. The dose ingested by a termite is proportionately mammoth for it. The amount breathed in by us allows us to recover, only to unleash its effects in a heart-attack weeks later or maybe in a kid from hell 9 months from now.

On May 8, I got a call from Greg Niven, the creator of that marvelous New Year's Eve dinner and owner of the quaint School House Restaurant in Providence Bay. Chef Greg and his wife Heather had recently become parents of a little girl who joined their preschool-aged son. Greg was clearly in a state of high alarm. "The local hardware store wants to sell hundreds of gallons of wood preservative to the town," he told me. "That stuff is deadly! Tomorrow the town council is meeting to vote on this, I must get some first class information to them at once! The last time the town sprayed the boardwalk some 5 years ago, every breath hurt for about a week after! We need help—fast!"

Greg and Heather happen to read my _Vitality_ articles regularly, and so they figured I might be able to suggest some tried and true activist tactics. That proved to be a correct hunch. Within an hour I had put them in touch with super-effective activist Debra Barrie in Smith Falls, an expert on the health effects of preservatives. Debra spearheaded the movement that has resulted in the Canadian building industry's voluntary phase-out of these products. Debra's health is severely compromised by years of exposure to the arsenic fumes of burning pressure-treated wood, but she uses every ounce of energy to stop this terrible health hazard. Go to her website and be amazed!

By the time another hour had passed, Greg had informed the island's newspaper, _The Manitoulin Expositor_, whose reporter Neil Zacharjewcz interviewed Debra and me and began calling the town councilors—the single most effective way to get any politician's attention. Greg also called the local doctor, Dr. Maurianne Reade. She and her husband had sat at the table next to ours and we had spent part of that New Year's Eve night chatting about the Reade's native Yukon and our shared love for Manitoulin Island. Greg and Heather had joined us to show off their lovely new baby girl. What we didn't know, until we all read the excellent May 15th article in the _Expositor_, was that my physician husband and Dr. Reade are both members of CAPE (Canadian Association of Physicians for the Environment). Thus Providence Bay most providentially was blessed with an on-the-spot physician knowledgeable about environmental toxins and motivated to do something about them.

Greg's political conscience proved to be as zesty as his marvelous dishes: off he went in person to as many councilors as he could reach before the sun turned the sands of Providence Bay turned pink and sank into Lake Huron. The next day, the chef and the doctor attended the council meeting to learn about the fate of Providence Bay's boardwalk. The message had got through: although public comment is not part of the protocol of such committee meetings, Dr. Reade was asked to comment, which she did most ably.

The councilors quite correctly replied that 15 years ago, when the boardwalk was built, nobody knew about these toxic horrors, and not much was known even 5 years ago. Now that they knew, they weren't about to persist in such harmful actions. When *The Expositor's* editor read reporter Neil Zacharjewicz's article and came to the description of wood preservative being absorbed through the skin, she said, she felt "her arms tingling". That prompted her to put the story on the front page with an inch high headline.

One week later, my husband and I walked along the boardwalk after a wonderful dinner at Greg's and—for now at least—once more the spirit of Manitou spreads its peace over the island. This summer, children will frolic on the swings, women will walk on the sand, lovers will wander along the boardwalk, and the magic will be complete.

Sources and Resources:
Debra Barrie: e-mail at **deborahbarrie@hotmail.com** and her website: **www.sympatico.ca/pbarrie**
www.thestar.com/conwatch for Consumer Watch information
The book on pesticide alternatives by S. Tvedten, *The Bug Stops Here* (2002) is available for
   downloading totally free of charge, in HTML or PDF formats, on
   www.thebestcontrol.com. You can e-mail its author at **steve@getipm** for further questions.
For house and garden environmental information e-mail
   HealthBuildingNetwork@yahoogroups.com
For the relevant data safety sheet information on any toxin of your choice and, specific to
   this article, on arsenic, cadmium and copper contact *The Journal of Pesticide Reform* at
   infor@pesticide.org. Their website is at **www.efn.org/~ncap/**
The original article on the toxicity of pressure-treated wood, which started the world-wide
   concern about its use, was published by neurologist H.A. Peters in the *Journal of the
   American Medical Association* May 11, 1984

The Folly of Fluoride

The information following below tells about the still ongoing battle to get the Region of Peel to stop fluoridating the water supply. My husband, Dr. Robert Ferrie, and I became involved in this issue when a town meeting was announced in May 2004 for the purpose of expanding the fluoridation of water into those areas of the Region of Peel where private wells are the main source of water supply and, consequently, the few households obtaining municipal water in those areas, could be hooked up to a fluoridation system. Now I realized that the rest of the Region was already fluoridated, and stopping this practice has become one of my ongoing projects.

Having a grand-son whose teeth are mottled from the excessively high levels of fluoride in his area's drinking water and knowing about the world-wide scam involved with fluoride, both my husband and I were appalled and we went to the meeting. To our surprise, there were very few people present. On second thought, that was not so surprising because, after all, we have been told for decades that fluoride is good for us and it is found in all super-market-sold toothpastes, to say nothing of the perpetuation of fluoride's alleged beneficial properties by most dentists who are on automatic pilot with regard to carcinogens just like most doctors are regarding the harmful health effects of environmental toxins in general.

We were shocked when the Region's health officer, Dr. Dr. D. McKeown, got up and made a power-point presentation which was from beginning to end at best an excellent advertisement for the fluoride industry, but totally untrue with regard to the claims made about fluoride's properties and benefits to health. The worst of it was, that he expected his audience to simply believe him—without a shred of supporting scientific evidence cited.

Below is the article my husband published in the local paper. These summarize what is currently known about fluoride. The truth will hit the fan in a big way in August 2005 when the *American Academy of Sciences* will publish its comprehensive review of the world literature on fluoride in its prestigious *Proceedings*. Meanwhile, the Mayor and the Council of the Town of Caledon decided to shelve the fluoridation plans for the time being.

By fortuitous chance an in-depth investigation of the fluoride issue was published by a famous British investigative journalist, Christopher Bryson. The book is highly recommended and comes with an introduction by Theo Colborn of the World Wildlife Fund: *The Fluoride Deception*, Seven Stories Press, 2004.

Doctor Comments on "Myths"

Caledon Citizen, June 2, 2004
By Robert K. Ferrie, MD

On May 6 the Town of Caledon held a meeting to obtain public input on the proposed by-law to fluoridate the water. About two thirds of the residents in Caledon Township are on wells and one third are supplied with municipal water which could, therefore, be treated with fluoride. Bolton is already fluoridated—much to the surprise of residents who called the Town office wondering when and how this had come about; apparently it was fluoridated just before the recent *Clean Water Act* came into force and even before the 2003 Region of Peel's study on the dental health of children in this area was published. This happened at a time when hundreds of municipalities across North America have stopped fluoridation (142 cities in Canada) and most of the members of the European Union have banned it. Hence, justification for fluoridation is, to say the least, mysterious.

I am a physician practicing in Alton and my wife is a medical science writer and publisher of books on health and environment. We attended the May 6th meeting and presented our objections to fluoridation. The currently available international scientific literature shows beyond any doubt that fluoridation is ineffective as a preventive measure against tooth decay and seriously harmful to the immune system and it is a known carcinogen at even minute levels. We urged an open discussion of **all** the available information, especially also to the residents of Bolton, so that legally mandatory informed consent is observed.

At this May 6 meeting Dr. D. McKeown, the Medical Officer of Health for the Region of Peel and primary author of the 2003 *Children's Dental Health Report,* stated that it would reduce the incidence of cavities amongst the children of this area if the water was fluoridated. The allegedly supporting evidence was very troubling indeed.

For example, he handed out a list of six so-called "myths" about fluoridation: fluoride, according to Dr. McKeown, is (1) not a by-product of synthetic fertilizers, (2) is not contaminated with dangerous impurities, (3) is not corrosive, (4) is not a poison in low concentrations, (5) is not used in rat poison, and (6) does not cause osteoporosis, cancer, immune diseases, cognitive and neurological problems in children. However, the safety data information published on the Internet by **all** the manufacturers of the very fluoride used in municipal water systems state exactly the opposite on the first 3 "myths". As for the 4th "myth", standard poison manuals list fluoride as toxic even in low concentration, and regarding the 5th "myth", chemical analyses readily available from the manufacturers of the home and garden various pest control products include fluoride as a main ingredient.

Most troubling is the assertion that fluoride does not cause all those diseases ("myth" no 6). Neither at this meeting nor in his report did Dr. McKeown provide even a shred of evidence to support his assertion that fluoride is safe or effective. Not even one scientific source to support those alleged 6 myths was provided. Apparently, we are simply supposed to accept his unsubstantiated opinion on the basis of pure trust. What completely astounded us was his bald assertion that the *American Medical Association* supports water fluoridation. Dr. Charles Gorden Heyd, the AMA's past president, recently said, *"I am appalled at the prospect of using water as a vehicle for drugs; fluoride is a corrosive poison that will produce serious effects on a long-term basis."* The current position of the AMA is that the safety of fluoride, at any dilution, cannot be proven.

Totally surprising is the fact that the Ontario Government's 1999 commissioned *Locker Report* was not mentioned at all either. That report came to the following cautious conclusions:

"The magnitude of the effect...is often not statistically significant, and may not be of clinical significance... Canadian studies do not provide systematic evidence that water fluoridation is effective in reducing decay in contemporary child populations. The few studies of communities where fluoridation was withdrawn do not suggest significant increases in dental caries as a result." (Page 4)
" The main limitations of current research on the effectiveness of water fluoridation are its exclusion of adults and elderly and failure to consider quality of life outcomes. Since water fluoridation is a total population strategy, its benefits to the population as a whole need to be documented."(Page 62)

In 1993 one of the most prestigious research institutions in the world, the *American Academy of Sciences*, recommended that research be done in those areas pertaining to fluoridation where gaps existed, i.e. from cancer to developmental problems. Now, the *Academy* is completing its comprehensive analysis and the report is due August 2005. Reports by this internationally recognized scientific body are fair, unbiased and reliable because no industry funding is ever involved in their research projects. All currently available international medical and toxicological research on fluoride in dentistry is available on **www.flouridealert.org** .

University of Toronto professor of preventive dentistry, Dr. Hardy Limeback, said about the Peel Region's report on dental health, that fluoridating the water here could only be kept to non-toxic levels if all residents were informed first that no child may use fluoridated toothpaste and if it could be made sure that all soft drinks are also free of fluoride—pre-conditions that are clearly not possible.

At the very least one could expect the Town of Caledon to obey the Precautionary Principle of international law, to which Canada subscribes, and which would demand that in this case no steps be taken to fluoridate the water until the 2005 *American Academy of Sciences'* report is published and residents are made aware of its conclusions.

The observation, that the teeth of children exposed to fluoride are mottled but have less cavities, was first made around 1900 by dentist Dr. Frederick S. McKay in Colorado. Examination of the water led him to conclude that naturally occurring fluoride was the reason. Medical science was at that time not as advanced and the science of epidemiology was in its infancy. It is disturbing to have the same simplistic association of fluoride and tooth decay presented as adequate a century later. Most importantly, even the type of fluoride Dr. McKay studied is no longer the one that is now advocated for the same purpose. Hence, fluoridation of water for prevention of tooth decay remains an unproven hypothesis—which is exactly why the worldwide data from the World Health Organization are consistently presented as being inconclusive—in contrast to Dr. McKeown's assertion.

The Peel report assumes that lack of fluoridation is "the most likely cause" of the observed dental problems. However, lack of fluoride has never been shown to be the cause of anything—dental health or any other health issue. While *fluorite* (spelled with a "t") is a naturally occurring substance in the earth's mineral deposits, and as such might be biologically necessary, the *fluoride* under discussion is the by-product of a man-made substance, and NO man-made substance has ever been shown to be biologically necessary. Fluoride is not a biologically necessary substance, such as selenium, iron etc. There are also no studies showing that areas where *naturally* occurring fluoride is lacking, produced any kind of health problems in the resident population.

During the discussion the question was raised by council members whether pesticides may have something to do with dental health. Indeed, medical literature shows that pesticides and artificial fertilizers cause serious depletion of biologically necessary minerals without which teeth and bones in animals and humans cannot develop properly and become vulnerable to bacterial assaults and osteoporosis. The most serious depletion being in magnesium and bio-available calcium which now, according to EPA and EU reports, is depleted to the point where people in North America only get 40%

Discreptancies between the REGION OF PEEL REPORT ON CHILDREN'S DENTAL HEALTH and our information

1. Source of fluoride (alleged fiction 1)	Region of Peel asserts that fluoride is not a by-product of fertilizer/ pesticide production	All available information contradicts this; see attached manufacturers' data sheets which clearly state its derivation being from phosphate fertilizer
2. Contamination of fluoride (alleged fiction 2)	Region of Peel asserts that **hydrofluorosilicic acid** is not contaminated with impurities	Industrial safety data show that this specific type of fluoride is contaminated with arsenic, a known carcinogen, which would increase the risk of cancer in the Caledon area by 1 in 10,000 people. (*Pharmaceutical grade* fluoride is prohibitively expensive.
3. Corrosive nature of fluoride (alleged fiction 3)	Region of Peel asserts that fluoride is not corrosive	The corrosive nature of fluoride is responsible for mottled teeth and the manufacturer's safety data state it is corrosive
4. Poisonous nature of fluoride (alleged fiction 4)	Region of Peel asserts it is not a poison and that it becomes poisonous, like many other substances, only at a dose-dependent level	Fluoride is generally classified as a poison and like many other environmental toxins, it is not only dose-dependently toxic, but cumulatively so through steady exposure to *small* amounts; poison manual list it as such regardless of concentration
5. Use of fluoride in poisons (alleged fiction 5)	Region of Peel asserts that the fluoride recommended for water fluoridation is not the same as that used in rat poison etc.	This type of fluoride is indeed used in many types of pest control products as well as in pharmaceutical drugs which have been taken off the market because the fluoride in them killed people
6. Fluoride as health hazard (alleged fiction 6)	Region of Peel asserts that fluoridated water does not pose health hazards and is not toxic at low dilutions.	The international medical, dental, and epidemiological literature provides overwhelming proof that it is a *major* health hazard and has been found to be so in many countries and for many diseases and developmental conditions.
* Scientific support for its use	Region of Peel has provided **no up-to-date scientific support** in its published report on which it bases the recommendation to fluoridate the water in Caledon. Most of the supportive sources cited are organizations which, in fact, either are no longer supportive, or are debating the issue in their published research, or provide inconclusive information.	The mainstream medical literature is so alarming that, *at the very least,* the precautionary principle must be invoked and any move to fluoridate the water should be put on hold. At this point in time only the UK, USA and Canada still advocate the use of fluoridation (142 cities having rejected it); the rest of the industrialized world appears to have doubts which can hardly be purely arbitrary.

of the international RDA for magnesium. As a consequence, the *American Medical Association* last June recommended that everybody—on conventionally or organically grown diets—needs to supplement with this and other minerals and vitamins in order to have at least the RDA's. This would be a measure the Region of Peel ought to look into and support, instead of adding a known poisonous substance to our water supply.

The acidity in the saliva, which is a contributing factor in cavities, is known to be caused by too much refined sugar in the diet. Last April, the *World Health Organization* published a report on refined sugar and showed its causative links to dental health, diabetes, and obesity; the WHO called for a reduction in refined sugar for everybody by at least 30%. Before deciding to use a known toxic substance such as fluoride, which is of uncertain relevance to tooth decay, a 100% harmless pilot project in Caledon would be easy to design and cheap: take 100 volunteer children who eat no refined sugars for two years with 100 junk-food diet kids and compare their teeth at the end of that time period. Acidity of saliva and number of caries could be measured at the beginning and end of the project.

No—You're Not Cooking With Gas!

Alive Magazine, December 1997

In 1986 the United Nations persuaded 24 countries to start controlling the emissions of carbon monoxide in transportation and industry. This has been quite successful. However, indoor air quality has been shown to be as much as 10 times worse than outdoor air.

According to research by the Environmental Protection Agency (EPA), one cause of indoor air toxicity is the propane and natural gas appliances which produce odorless carbon monoxide as well as nitrogen dioxide, a reddish-brown gas with an ac rid odor.

Back in the 1950s, after years of careful observation, a remarkable physician, Dr. Theron Randolph, noted that women using gas ranges developed a specific complex of symptoms and illnesses. Dr. Randolph noted the prevalence of depression, apathy, circulatory problems, confusion, fatigue, memory loss and intractable infections—all of which were often dramatically restored, once exposure to gas stopped. More than 800 of his patients removed their gas ranges and he published the astonishing results.

Since women statistically suffer the most from depression, I wonder how many would no longer use antidepressants if they stopped cooking with gas.

Dr. Randolph is also the pioneer who founded the American Academy of Environmental Medicine and moved the Kennedy administration to organize the first air quality conference in 1961. Eventually, this led to North America's clean air laws. But the much worse indoor air quality was not considered until very recently.

J. Spengler of the Harvard School of Public Health provide that nitrogen dioxide was far more prevalent in the home and work place than on the road. By the late 1980s, EPA studies made industry take note. Because of this, gas ranges no longer have pilot lights and carbon monoxide detectors are now readily available. These detectors, however, do not show you the levels of nitrogen dioxide.

Research shows conclusively that nitrogen dioxide inhibits respiration by attacking the mucous membranes of the lungs; it decreases brain activity by interfering with the transport of oxygen; it causes oxidation of unsaturated fatty acids in cell membranes to form highly active free radicals whereby protein structure is altered (hence antioxidants prove helpful); finally, it forms nitrosamines which are potently carcinogenic.

Nitrogen dioxide can accomplish all of the above with as little as 0.1 parts per million per cubic meter of air, and it does so by the same route as carbon monoxide: they both bind with your blood's hemoglobin to form methemoglobin, which causes hypoxia, an acute oxygen shortage in the blood.

People most at risk are those with reduced cardiovascular ability, such as fetuses and young children, elderly people, asthma and autoimmune disease patients, and even healthy individuals who are adjusting to a higher altitude. All others are at risk through chronic exposure, even at very low levels.

Nitrogen dioxide can cause not only short-term distress, but also long-term structural damage to the brain. The olfactory system reports to the brain faster than the digest system.

Our sense of smell is directly wired to a most important structure deep in the brain, namely the limbic *system.* There, the hypothalamus regulates body temperature, heart rate and hormone production; the amygdala monitors feelings of self-preservation; the cingulated gyrus mediates emotion, humour and affection; the hippocampus "installs" new learning and controls memory. The immune system is also activated in part via smell.

When I became sick and was told by my doctor that one of the main sources may very well be my gas cook stove, I telephoned the head offices of various gas companies in the Toronto area to find out what they knew about the toxicity of gas. At first I was told, "Oh no! Natural gas and propane are definitely not toxic." But after a pregnant pause, I was asked, "By the way, is there anyone in your family who suffers from asthma or an autoimmune disease?"

"Why?" I asked.

"Because if that's the case, we are not even supposed to install a gas range, and at the very least you must have a range hood vented to the outside."

I got rid of my gas range within 48 hours and am now cooking on a glass-top electric range—the safest way to cook. The improvement in my health was dramatic.

I admit, that I regretfully parted with my gas range, which was an enormous old-fashioned enameled beauty equipped with two ovens (and four pilot lights!) dating back to the 1930s. I had painstakingly restored it myself to full working condition. Now the Stratford Theatre in Ontario added it gratefully to their prop collection, where it will do perfectly for those depressing modern classics so often set in kitchens in those very years when Dr. Randolph was observing women getting depressed, suicidal and sick—and began to wonder if the gas range had something to with it.

Sources

T. Randolph, *Environmental Medicine—Beginnings and Bibliographies of Clinical Ecology,* Clinical Ecology Publications, Fort Collins, 1987

T. Randolph, *Human Ecology and Susceptibility to the Chemical Environment*, Charles C. Thomas, Springfield, 1967

For practical information contact the *Healthy Home Institute* at 430 North Sewell Road, Bloomington, Indiana 47408, USA or phone 812-332-5073 to request their excellent publications.

3

Cancer

New Perspectives In the War on Cancer

Vitality Magazine September 1999

In 1971, U.S. President Richard Nixon declared war on cancer. The army of recruited scientists assured him cancer would be beaten by 1990. It and the Vietnam War were fought in the spirit of "search and destroy" to free the world of communism and cancer. Both wars were lost. While communism transformed itself unexpectedly, cancer now claims the lives of one in four, and one in two people will develop it. Some cancers have increased several hundred percent in the last 30 years, especially in children for whom it now is the leading cause of death. The greatest, and most recent, increase is in hormone-dependent cancers of the breast, prostate, and testicles.

Cancer is the most expensive illness, cost for treatment having almost reached the U.S. $5 billion mark annually in North America. Yet over the past 40 years treatments have barely improved and survival rate is no better. Every 12 seconds a woman dies of breast cancer. Worldwide, nearly every family has been affected by cancer. Two recent ground-breaking events in Ontario brought interesting new information on the battlefront in the war on cancer. *Everyday Carcinogens: Stopping Cancer Before it Starts* was a conference held in Hamilton in March, and the five-day *Second World Conference on Breast Cancer* was held in July in Ottawa. Experts are in agreement that the causes of cancer are known and that the answer lies in prevention. It is a wholly preventable disease. But less than 3% of the annual U.S. National Cancer Institute's budget is spent on prevention, and even that amounts to only the blame-the-victim variety, even though cancers *un*-related to smoking, drinking, lack of exercise, etc. have increased the most. No funds are spent on prevention at all from the $100-million budget of the Canadian Cancer Society; not a single grant application last year dealt with prevention.

Internationally-acclaimed oncologist, Dr. Samuel Epstein of the University of Illinois, stated in his keynote address to the Health Canada sponsored conference at McMaster University in Hamilton: "Preventive oncology is an oxymoron. We have so much information on cancer prevention which we are not using. I wouldn't give a damn if we didn't do any more research for the next 50 years." Epstein went on to say that "The worldwide cancer epidemic is primarily the responsibility of the cancer establishment, comprised of the American and Canadian Cancer Societies and the National Institutes of Health of both countries. On their boards sit people who are directly connected to the very industries that are known to produce carcinogens (ie. pesticides, carcinogenic drugs, and industrial xenobiotics).

More than 200 experts from 55 countries presented at these two recent conferences. Presentations included evidence to show that cancer is big, big business and access to the "market" (our bodies) is fiercely fought over pre- and post-diagnosis of cancer. Some pharmaceutical companies profit both ways: Zeneca's annual revenues from the cancer drug Tamoxifen are at $470-million; the same company also makes over $300-million annually on the carcinogenic herbicide Acetochlor and other chlorine products.

Current treatments were mostly judged by the delegates as failures ("same old slash, burn, and poison," as UCLA oncologist and surgeon Dr. Susan Love refers to the standard cancer therapies of surgery, radiation and chemotherapy) while interest was great in new and totally different treatment approaches.

Several presenters focused on the danger of getting cancer from regular mammography and the failure of preventive drugs such as Tamoxifen which Dr. Epstein described as "a rip-roaring liver carcinogen" because over the long term it increases the chance of developing liver cancer dramatically. These scientists also exploded the prevalent myth that early detection is the answer. Rosalie Bertell, the internationally respected radiation expert, provided evidence to show that mammography causes more cancers than it detects, and that even those tumours which it does detect are at least seven years old by the time this crude method finds them. Regular mammographies cause cumulative radiation damage, especially in pre-menopausal women.

The second myth, that cancer is ultimately genetic, was rejected by all on the basis of world-wide epidemiological evidence which shows that the horrendous increase in cancer has happened in a mere two generations, faster than can be expected by evolutionary mutation. Dr. Susan Love puts it bluntly in the documentary film *Exposure*: "We are born with perfectly good genes, and then something comes along to screw them up." That "something" are the environmental toxins on which the wealth of the world seems to depend, from agricultural to military practices.

Cornell University ecologist Sandra Steingraber states: "A cancer cell is made, not born." Documentary film-maker, Nancy Evans, echoed this scientific fact poetically by observing: "We have become the bodies of evidence." Medical science is in agreement that radiation in any form (from bombs to microwave ovens) causes cancer and has worked out the biological basis for the carcinogicity of pesticides.

The path to cancer begins with a toxin entering the body where detoxifying liver enzymes begin their work. These can defuse water-soluble toxins readily, but not those which bind to fat cells (e.g. pesticides). In metabolizing these toxins, liver enzyme systems act like a double-edged sword by also making toxins out of some of the chemicals not previously toxic (e.g. benzene). It is these metabolic toxins, created by our enzymes, that are able to bind with cellular DNA where they cause mutations and cancers. Once this process has begun, all other bodily defenses, such as tumour suppressor genes, are also destroyed. Then oncogenes are prevented from supervising correct cell replication and repair, and finally the so-called "spell-checker" genes are altered, causing them to mess up the DNA/RNA base-pair process. Cancer cells proliferate, create their own blood supply, thrive on estrogen, and finally kill the host.

All delegates agreed with Devra Lee Davis, internationally renowned toxicologist and epidemiologist of the World Resources Institute in Washington, D.C., who spoke primarily on the need to adopt the precautionary principle. This would require that industry would have to prove that a new substance causes no harm; currently, North American law requires that citizens have to prove a substance is dangerous before it can be banned or restricted. In Canada, for example, between 1994-96 a staggering 1.4 billion pounds of toxic chemicals were released into the environment legally; of these, 280 million pounds were known carcinogens, each requiring to be banned through citizen action, one at a time.

The common theme of both conferences was that our current social and economic system is the ultimate cause of cancer. The requirements of human biology cannot be made to harmonize with the priorities of a world economy in which pesticides are of central importance. Our biology also stands no chance against the world's enormous military death machinery which depends on radiation and heavy metals. Already thirty years ago, the World Health Organization declared that at least 89 per cent of all cancers were caused by pesticides, radiation, and other toxic chemicals in our environment.

Dr. Samuel Epstein, whose research was key to banning DDT in 1973, and whose assistance to Canada's Health Protection Branch was recently vital in Dr. Shiv Chopra's efforts to ban (carcinogenic) bovine growth hormone here, pointed out that all of us now carry more than 500 different compounds in our cells, none of which existed before 1920, and that "there is no safe dose for any of them". Breast milk in western countries is so dangerously contaminated with dioxin, a carcinogenic byproduct of incinerating plastics, that it would not pass U.S. Federal Drug Administration safety standards, were it a bottled substance. In six months of breast feeding, a baby has absorbed the maximum life-time "safe" limit of dioxin in its cells.

Epstein is a world-class medical activist whom the powers-that-be dare not ignore because his credentials are so gilt-edged as to be dazzling. Epstein's membership in the medical establishment's "old boys club" is solid, yet he has spent the last two decades giving those old boys hell in every international forum imaginable. A professor of occupational and environmental medicine at the University of Illinois, he published some 300 primary research articles and, at Harvard Medical School established the first environmental toxicology registry. He is a consultant to governments around the world on environment and human health.

Last year Sweden, one of the world's most environmentally conscious countries, invited him to address their parliament on "anything that happens to be on his mind lately". Epstein outlined a plan for cancer prevention for the coming century: 1. all substances known to be carcinogenic in animals should be so identified on the packaging of foods, cosmetics and household products; 2. the monthly water bill should list all carcinogenic substances found; 3. the public must have full disclosure of all the ties to cancer causing-industries of board members of cancer societies and research institutions; 4. funds should be available to cancer research only if *preventive* public health implications can be shown to flow from such research as well. While unflinchingly confronting the current health disaster unfolding in our poisoned world, he seems to enjoy hammering home the truths that have the potential to heal us. "I was brought up as an orthodox Jew and was taught that social justice is our primary duty." With a twinkle in the eyes he added, "Ever heard of Don Quixote and his windmills?"

Asked which country responds the most to the need for prevention, he replied "Germany." Why? While in North America cancer research is almost exclusively funded by pharmaceutical companies, making cancer a stock-market commodity, in Germany a lot of research is publicly funded and science is not gagged totally. While American pharmaceutical companies control much of the "cancer industry" world-wide, they meet great resistance in Europe from health freedom groups as well as from doctors. In Germany, Epstein explained, there is a generational split with the post-WW II generation having started the *Green Party* as a conscious challenge to American corporate "biodevastation"; they politicized prevention as reflected in their antinuclear power and anti-pesticide stance. The *Greens* now hold the balance of power in Germany.

For Steingraber, U.S. presidential advisor on cancer prevention and author of the best selling *Living Downstream*, cancer has "become a human rights issue" which can only be tackled with "old-fashioned political organization". That is why "scientists are now going directly to the public." The earth has been made "chemically addicted" and all life is being poisoned, Steingraber states. The epidemic rise in cancer has basically taken place within one generation, those born after World War II, and it is especially childhood cancers that have risen by several 100% since the 1970s.

For those cancers which have increased the most, early detection methods do not yet exist, she pointed out. "We now have more two-year olds with brain cancer than ever in history," Steingraber explains, "and every year the number of childhood cancers increases of the year before." Wild animal data show the same trend. And children and wild "animals do not hold stressful jobs, smoke, drink, eat bad diets, or fail to exercise." Blaming the victim explanations for our current cancer epidemic cannot be maintained, especially since the cancers NOT related to smoking are so dramatically on the rise. Today, one in 2 people is expected to get cancer, and one in 4 will die from it.

"A cancer cell is made, not born," she states. Cancer is triggered by organochlorines, dioxins, solvents (and radiation). Since the end of World War II, each of us on this earth carries in our bodies detectable amounts of hundreds of varieties of chemicals. Breast, milk in western countries is so dangerously contaminated with dioxin that it would not pass FDA standards, were it a bottled substance. Mothers on the Eastern seaboard and the southwestern US (the most highly industrialized parts) are advised not to breastfeed past 6 months, as the baby by then has the maximum life-time amount of dioxin in its cells.

Dioxin is the byproduct of incinerated old vinyl siding, plastic window blinds and the like. It is in our soil, water, air and food. Dry cleaning fluid, a carcinogenic and neurotoxic solvent, is detectable in amounts above standards of safety in the breath of most North American city dwellers. Organochlorines, invented to gas prisoners in Auschwitz, are now used on lawns everywhere in even greater amounts than in agriculture. Certain cancers, not surprisingly, effect especially golf course workers and farmers.

"At heart of the chemical industry," Steingraber explains, "lies a great deception", namely that these herbicides and pesticides are necessary." In another landmark book, *The Spoils of Famine*, she showed how the so-called "green revolution" created the escalating world-wide poverty in the Third World. *The Practical Farmers of Iowa* proved her point: they use no pesticides and have consistently shown to have higher yields while saving a lot of money, for pesticides are expensive.

Steingraber, in discussing the genetic fallacy of the causes of cancer, points out that one generation cannot sprout cancer genes. Instead, she eloquently observes: "What runs in families does not necessarily run in blood. And our genes are less a set of inherited tea cups enclosed in a cellular china cabinet, than they are plates used in a busy diner. Cracks, chips and scrapes accumulate. Accidents happen." She drives home the point by adding that most members of her family have had cancer, including herself who survived bladder cancer (one primary cause: dry cleaning fluids). But she was adopted.

Asked about how genetic research and the epidemiological facts of cancer incidence known today can assist each other, she answers, that whatever we eat, drink, breathe and touch very soon becomes part of the dynamic genetic system of the body. Toxins contained in mothers' milk will soon become part of the total toxic burden of the child which the DNA and its repair mechanisms attempt to neutralize. Genetics gives us the mechanisms, not the cause, nor even the answer.

The answer is prevention. A young mother herself, Steingraber feels strongly about implementing the precautionary principle; we need not wait until we have perfect scientific proof before we stop contaminating our environment. After all, smoking was declared a hazard to health a quarter of a century ago, but the genetic proof did not come until 1997. We stopped allowing faeces to contaminate our water supply 150 years ago, long before bacteria were known. "A woman's body is the first environment," Steingraber states. "Whatever contaminants are in a woman's body find their way into the next generation. I think there is no better argument for the precautionary principle."

Yet she is optimistic. Dry-cleaning fluid, which can cause many cancers including bladder cancer, which she survived, is among those substances that may be completely phased out in the foreseeable future. She is also impressed by the intensity and intelligence of the "wave of social change" in agriculture, animal husbandry (organic farming has become a multibillion dollar business), people's increasing rejection of pesticides, as well as grassroots and international opposition to cancer as an inevitable price of progress.

Davis ended her presentation with a quote from the Talmud which catches the spirit of these conferences poignantly: "It is not for us to complete the task. But we must begin it."

Steps to Preventing and Curing Cancer

The following recommendations are drawn from the enormous amount of information these conferences provided; many are also part of the current publications of cancer researchers and the World Health Organization.

Avoid Known Cancer-Causing Sources:

1. Do not smoke, or tolerate smoking in your family's presence.
2. Avoid excessive exposure to sunlight and ultraviolet rays.
3. Do not consider breast implants.
4. Do not use dark hair dyes; check out safe alternatives.
5. Avoid perfumes, air-fresheners, and perfumed deodorizers. If they contain benzene, aluminum, lemon-scented chemicals, or lack a full list of all ingredients to permit a check-up in a toxicology manual—do not use them.
6. Treat all cosmetic products with extreme suspicion until you have proof positive that they contain no known carcinogens; safe alternatives exist.
7. Avoid dry-cleaned clothes; contact 1-800-667-9790 for safe cleaners.
8. Do not drink or even bathe in chlorinated water; fit your home with a de-chlorinating device.
9. Do not drink fluoridated water, or use fluoridated toothpaste.
10. Avoid electromagnetic fields (EMUs), especially for children. EMUs have been linked to childhood leukemia and brain cancers. Use appropriate protection on your computer screen; do not use microwave ovens; avoid living near hydro towers.
11. Do not use hormone disrupting or mimicking substances such as chemical pesticides, herbicides, fertilizers, fungicides and bug killers.
12. Do not use cleaning, polishing, renovation materials in your home that list unspecified "inert ingredients". If they have toxic warning symbols, require calling "a doctor if...", are "corrosive", give special disposal instructions, or require "well-ventilated areas" for use—look for substitutes. If you cannot avoid some of these substances (e.g. oil paint, furniture stripper, car maintenance materials, etc.), wear the best charcoal-filtered mask available and minimize exposure, especially to skin and lungs.
13. Reduce consumption of salt-cured, smoked, and nitrate-cured foods.
14. Do not use the meat or dairy products from animals routinely treated with antibiotics and raised with hormones. According to Dr. Epstein, such milk products are among the most reliable cancer causing agents currently known. Safe, certified organic milk and meat products are widely available in health food stores and some grocery stores.

15. Never heat shrink-wrapped foods or food in plastic containers. The plastic molecules migrate into the food when heated. They are xenobiotics.
16. Avoid food additives, especially Red Dye No. 3 found in most junk foods and many pop products. Avoid emulsifiers such as carrageenin; do not consume hydrogenated vegetable oils or margarine (to my knowledge there is no margarine on the market that is safe).
17. Limit sport fish consumption to the guidelines provided seasonally by the government.
18. Do not drink or eat foods that contain sugar substitutes such as Nutra-Sweet, aspartame, etc. and avoid refined sugar which usually contains silicon. Unpasteurized honey, maple syrup, brown rice syrup are healthy substitutes easily available.
19. Avoid antibiotics, unless your doctor has done the necessary test to identify the exact bacteria this antibiotic kills (except in extreme emergencies, e.g. meningitis); keep treatment period to a minimum.
20. Avoid prescription drugs unless your doctor also gives you a photostat copy of the full drug information from the annually updated CPS (Canada's drug dictionary which every doctor has in the office.
and explains this information to you; if the drug requires regular liver function tests, insist on discussing alternatives or keep treatment to the minimum.
21. Avoid birth control pills, anti-hypertensives, antidepressants, hormone replacement therapy in pill form (toxic to the liver), and do not take Tamoxifen preventively; get the full data on those drugs; check them out first on the Internet and at www.preventcancer.com.
22. Do not invest your savings and RSPs in known cancer source polluters such as Dofasco, Stelco, Algoma Steel, Domtar, Bayer Rubber, Shell, Nora Chemicals, Imperial Oil (these are just some of the worst offenders).Inform yourself about Ethical Mutual Funds, etc.

Doing Something Constructive about Cancer

1. Have your mercury amalgams removed by a dentist trained in the proper protocol (Visit the website of the International Academy for Oral and Medical Toxicology to find out about a dentist trained by them working near you: www.IAOMT.org)
2. If you are overweight, have your hormone levels checked and find out if you have food allergies. Over-exposure to estrogen, lack of progesterone, thyroid problems brought on by pesticide exposure, or an adaptation to allergenic foods (wheat products and refined sugar are frequent cause of

obesity, which promote cancer through excessive estrogen and pesticide storage).

3. Exercise regularly and moderately.

4. Eat cruciferous vegetables (cauliflower, brussels sprouts, broccoli, etc.. *always* from organically grown sources.

5. Buy your foods in glass containers, avoid cans and plastic.

6. Take supplements, especially vitamins C and E, beta carotene (natural source, not synthetic.and minerals such as selenium and magnesium; check out the literature and take charge of your health. If you need hormones, consider primarily natural ones and/or trans-dermally administered varieties in the smallest possible doses; they bypass the liver.

7. Join a health or cancer activist group; for a full list call Canadian Environmental Law Association at 416-960-2284 (e-mail: cela@web.net.   or contact Women's Network on Health and Environment, 736 Bathurst Street, Toronto, Ont. M5S 2R4. Join the Council on Canadians which has been extraordinarily successful in stopping corporate power from becoming total—613-233-2773. Join Pollution Probe, respected internationally, they get things done—416-926-1907.

8. Start a pesticide education group in your neighborhood, demand from your MP and MPP mandatory toxicology disclosure of all chemical ingredients being sold today; approach your local golf course manager and discuss alternative ways of maintenance; go to your city council and get them to explore alternatives to chlorine in public swimming pools and to put a stop to the use of chlorine and fluoride in the water supply.

9. Read the *Journal of Pesticide Reform* for basic, reliable information. Read Steingraber's *Living Downstream*, 2nd ed., 1999 (paperback). Read R.N. Proctor's *Cancer Wars*, 1995. Don't go shopping without Dr. Epstein's *Safe Shopper's Bible*, 2nd ed. 1999, or *Additive Alert*, Alive publications, 1999. If you have reason to be concerned about cancer, read Dr. Epstein's *The Breast Cancer Prevention Program*, 2nd ed., 1999, and give it to your daughters, women friends and others.

10. If you have been recently diagnosed with cancer, search the web and the literature for the latest alternative treatments; your doctor is no doubt sincere, but possibly functions on automatic pilot, especially if he or she relies on drug representatives instead of the medical journals.

11. Thoughtfully consider, but carefully doubt all information (including this article.) and start your own search. Only a determined consumer revolt and informed resistance will turn the cancer tide.

The Cancer Industry

Vitality Magazine November 2000

If we actually lived in a free-market economy (the illusion our politicians sell), and if science was really our guiding light, we would not have the current mess in cancer therapy. Instead, we would have access to the full information and would be able to choose what works. However, the truth is the cancer machine is churning out immense profits, while patients are treated as mushrooms—kept in the dark and fed bullshit. Simultaneously, cancer therapies that work are ignored and dismissed behind pompous mutterings which warn of "unscientific and unproven therapies".

For decades the world's finest minds worked to find the cause of cancer and, indeed, they found it where Rachel Carson told us long ago to look: in our tobacco-pesticide-chemical addicted and radiation-heavy-metal contaminated environment. Those

fine minds have since also proven the biology of cancer, and the merchants peddling its causes have moved into denial overdrive. To prevent cancer requires transforming the world's economic philosophy from exploitation to stewardship: children's healthy brains will have to be more important than pesticide sales; industry will have to agree that healthy breasts and prostates are more important than sales of plastic products. Furthermore, Canadian agriculture will have to consider the high rate of stomach and colon cancer among our farmers more seriously than high yields dependent on toxic nitrates and atrazine (see *International Journal of Epidemiology* no. 28, 1999), and the Canadian government will have to stop manufacturing and selling their bone cancer producing Candu reactors. As well, we need to rid our homes, foods, and workplaces of the entire infernal list of industrial and everyday carcinogens (for this list call the U.S. Environmental Health Information Service at 1-800-315-3010, and see *Scientific American*, Feb.1998, "Everyday Exposure to Toxic Pollutants").

This is not proposing utopia—but disposing of deadly garbage, all of which serves only two purposes: to inactivate our natural tumor suppressor genes, and drive the world's economy—a major part of which is the cancer industry. Our priorities will have to do more than shift: we need to welcome an earthquake.

To treat cancer effectively will require that doctors, currently mostly on professional automatic pilot, and governments in bed with industry, reject their puppet status and stop the puppeteers—cancer industry's pharmaceutical companies, cancer research centers, and the cancer societies—from treating cancer as a gold mine. There is such a thing as divine wrath—that anger that seeks to expose the Big Lie because the time has come for serious truth-telling. We need to look closely at those who confront the cancer machine, and offer cures and prevention. And those of us who have cancer need to think very carefully about what we are willing to believe and no longer willing to endure.

Since 1998 German medical science is in crisis because several internationally leading scientists committed major research fraud. Government appointed scientists are sorting out the damage. Reporting on this ongoing investigation, the science journal *Nature* described in its June 22, 2000, issue the clinical implications. German medical scientists manipulated experimental data so as to make a new technique for speedier recovery from chemotherapy in bone cancer patients appear authentic, thereby allowing higher doses. The new technique is fictitious as is the efficacy of high dose chemotherapy. The survival rates usually cited are equally massaged: now five years after diagnosis is considered "survival" (it used to be seven years).

Dr. Zoltan Rona in Toronto recently reported that the majority of chemotherapy specialists won't allow their families to take chemotherapy. A whopping 81% of them would not consent even to drug trials. While chemotherapy has limited effectiveness in some types of childhood leukemia and colon cancers (around 7% of those), it does nothing to enhance quality of life or prolong life in all other forms of cancers. The president of the American Chemical Society, Dr. Alan C. Nixon stated recently, "As a chemist trained to interpret data, it is incomprehensible to me that physicians can ignore the clear evidence that chemotherapy does much, much more harm than good."

In 1990, U.S. $3.53 billion were spent on chemotherapy; by 1994 business was booming with an increase to U.S. $7.51 billion—while the cancer rates increased exponentially. The side effects are so debilitating that 20% of patients become suicidal, and recent comparative data show that high dose chemo does nothing to help breast cancer (*Medical Post*, June 1, 2000). Yet another side effect is the high rate of miscarriages among the nurses and female doctors who handle and administer chemotherapy drugs (*Medical Post* Sept. 28, 1999).

The situation is no better with regard to radiation which is notorious for killing the cancer but destroying brains—especially in children (in prostate cancer it causes impotence). As for mammographies, it is now acknowledged that they do nothing for early detection, but can actually cause cancer.

In recent years, Tamoxifen was hailed as a great breakthrough in breast cancer treatment and prevention. Its huge international trial involved tens of thousands of women. Its developer, V. Craig Jordan won many prizes for it from the pharmaceutical establishment. With great fanfare it was announced in 1990 that the trials would be stopped because observed benefits could not ethically be withheld from the world any longer. What they didn't say, was that the trial was broken off because too many women

were getting liver cancer. In fact, Tamoxifen is a carcinogen. In 1992, the *New England Journal of Medicine* reported that Tamoxifen appeared not to be so great after all. In 1999 the equally famous mainstream journal, *Science*, reported the drug's carcinogenic properties. Of course, the pharmaceutical companies tell us that a new and improved version is in the pipeline based on beta carotene (!), the known cancer preventing nutrient, which slightly chemicalized could be patented.

Turning to the trendy illusion of the genetic basis for cancer and the sci-fi promise of manipulating the genetic code therapeutically, I was struck by an amazing synchronicity of events: on July 13 this year the *New England Journal of Medicine* published the results of an astonishing study; 90,000 identical twins were studied for 28 different types of cancer to determine whether genetics or environment play the greater part in the development of cancer. Not surprisingly, the conclusion is that "the environment has the principal role in causing cancer". So, we have to clean up our backyard after all. That same day's edition of *Nature* ran articles showing the immense efforts by scientists itching to find a genetic cure for cancer—even though our genes are exquisitely responsive to and dependent upon the environment. Sci-fi medicine is irresistible it seems, even to money-strapped governments: Ontario's health insurance plan covers genetic testing for hereditary cancers since April of this year. Yet, less than 2% of cancers have a hereditary component, and as oncologist Samuel Epstein has pointed out, that means that those people are more vulnerable to environmental toxins than the rest of us. We wouldn't even know about such genetic vulnerabilities if our world was clean and fit for all our genomes.

One of the worst cases of deception is found in the official journal of the Canadian Oncology Society called "Cancer Prevention and Control." It is, of course, financed by pharmaceutical giants Novartis, Smith Kline Beecham and by their colleagues at Health Canada. I read every issue. It literally has nothing—ever—on prevention, and as for "control," just whom are they kidding? This nonsense goes to every doctor's office, most of whom have not noticed that these emperors have been stark naked for a very long time.

There are many more lies, deceptions and misconceptions about cancer treatments worthy of the public's attention, but there also is a lot of exciting news on treatments that work. Consult the list of books at the end of this article. Dr. Carolyn Dean recently observed that she is a great believer in genetics and is looking forward to the discovery of "the gene for stupidity".

Burton Goldberg, who publishes information on the science, efficacy and availability of non-toxic medicine, recently testified before Congress on a highly effective treatment developed by Dr. Joseph Gold in 1969 from a chemical called hydrazine sulfate. It blocks a liver enzyme generally enslaved by the cancer growth process, thereby promoting tumor growth. It works, but cannot be patented. When the clinical trials at the University of California in Los Angeles confirmed its efficacy, the National Cancer Institute undertook an even larger investigation. By deliberately tampering with the protocol developed by Dr. Gold, they wound up with a lot of dead people and successfully discredited hydrazine sulfate. Journalists brought out the truth by 1995. An FDA investigation confirmed it. Then the NCI succeeded in altering key statements in the report and lobbied Congress to ban the treatment—by November of this year. Goldberg and many other health freedom fighters went before Congress and revealed the details of the fraudulent report.

Dr. Abram Hoffer, who cured hundreds of cancer patients with a Vitamin C regime, tells of a National Institute of Health study done by a Yale University medical scientist showing that Vitamin C causes all manner of harm. Hoffer requested the sources, since annually more than 2,000 scientific articles are published on the clinical applications of vitamin C, none of them showing harm. The reply he received was simply, "Oh, that was just a mistake." It was never corrected, however. (Curiously, it is common practice to provide laboratory animals, especially monkeys and apes, with 50 times the RDA of vitamin C to ensure they are healthy for the experiments.)

"Science and medicine advance funeral by funeral," Burton Goldberg observes. New discoveries are implemented only as the establishment with its vested interests of prestige, careers and money, dies off—along with their patients. Treatments that work are dependent entirely upon patients who question, doubt, and refuse to go along with the status quo. Your doctor does NOT necessarily know best—you may be given chemotherapy simply because your doctor doesn't want to be sued or have a fight with the authorities. In California, for example, it was forbidden by law to treat cancer by any other method except cut, burn and poison (surgery, radiation and chemotherapy.) until July of this year, when the law was repealed through overwhelming public pressure. In the early 1900s, W.S. Halstead (1852-1922) proposed the dogma that still informs cancer medicine: that the tumor is the problem and must be treated, not the patient in which the tumor has evolved. Consequently, all current treatments offered are easily divided into those that treat the patient, so the tumor or metastases can be effectively reversed, and those which attack the tumor and wind up killing the patient later, too, in most situations.

That said, it is very important to heed the wise statement by famed nutritional medicine physician, Dr. Atkins: "Patients with cancer who seek either orthodox or alternative approaches are entrusting their lives to doctors who are playing with half a deck." For example, surgery by itself can be a highly effective cure. But nothing will replace a thoughtfully informed and critical patient.

Great insights and therapeutic modes arise wherever compassion and the quest for truth take precedence over complacency and greed. And indeed, the greatest breakthroughs in cancer therapy come from scientists trained in the mainstream. The coffee enemas, for example, which some "alternative" cancer therapies employ, were developed in rigorous controlled studies in German universities before World War II, when it was discovered that coffee stimulates the liver to produce cancer fighting enzymes most efficiently when approached through the bowel. The science proving the effectiveness of nutrition in cancer therapy is published in all the top journals of the world; my filing cabinets are full of them.

Treatments developed by Dr. Max Gerson, Hulda Clark, Dr. Nicholas Gonzalez, as well as the Japanese macro diet, the oxygen therapies (see Dr. Majid Ali's books) which dissolve tumors because cancer is an anaerobic phenomenon (Otto Warburg won the Nobel prize for that proof in the 1920s), Gaston Naesens' 714-X treatment, Dr. Burzynski's peptide therapy, the orthomolecular mega-vitamin therapies, and the herbal therapies all have a rigorous scientific basis and excellent clinical results.

But why so many therapies? Because carcinogens attack in different ways and different places, in bodies which have huge variations in predispositions, nutritional status, pre-existing bodyloads of toxins, and varying healing potentials. Yet, when you study the therapies that work (see list below), they have three essential elements: they detoxify, they fortify the body, and they strengthen the immune system. In short, they renovate the damaged house, instead of searching for an intruder under the couch. They have understood the great 19th century doctor Sir William Osler's observation, "The physician without physiology and chemistry flounders along in an aimless fashion, never able to gain an accurate conception of disease, practicing a sort of popgun pharmacy."

I spent the summer immersed in books on the history of medicine—a very sobering experience that makes one grateful to be alive today—and came to the unexpected conclusion that we are living in the midst of the golden age of medicine. We have choices our ancestors never dreamed of. It takes an open mind and a fearless curiosity to benefit from what is available—and the determination to protect that freedom of choice.

Sources and Resources

W.J. Diamond et al., *Cancer Diagnosis: What to do Next*, Alternative Medicine.com publishers (Burton Goldberg Group), 2000

W.J. Diamond et al., *Cancer: An Alternative Medicine Definitive Guide to Cancer*, Future Medicine Publications (Burton Goldberg Group), 1992

R. Moss, *Cancer Therapy: The Independent Consumer's Guide to Non-Toxic Treatments and Prevention*, 9th edition, Equinox, 1999

Cancer Control Society, 2043 N. Berendo St., Los Angeles, CA 90027, phone 323-663-7801

M. Ali, M.D., an in-depth interview with him done by me are available on video from Consumers' Health Organization of Canada at 416-490-0986

Environmental Health Information Service of the U.S. government provides the full list of all officially recognized carcinogens. Call: 1-800-315-3010

H. Clark, *The Cure for All Advanced Cancers*, New Century Press, 1999. Available through Consumer's Health Organization of Canada where you can also obtain a video with her lectures and an interview done by me. Call 416-490-0986

M. Gerson, *A Cancer Therapy*, 6th ed., 1999, Gerson Institute. Call 619-585-7600, e-mail: info@gerson.org

A. Hoffer, *Vitamin C and Cancer*, Quarry, 2000

E. Nussbaum, *Recovery from Cancer*, Avery, 1992

P. Quillin, *Beating Cancer With Nutrition*, Nutrition Times Press, 1998

CAPE: Canadian Association of Physicians for the Environment, 613-233-1982

Pollution Probe, 416-926-1907

FACT: Friends of Alternative & Complementary Therapies (they help find alternative health practitioners), 416-299-9569

The Cancer Treatment Controversy

Vitality Magazine June 2002

A cancer diagnosis can really ruin your life—not necessarily because of the cancer, but because the treatment mill of the Cancer Establishment may grind you down. In that vast and impersonal cancer industry you will find yourself smoothly shunted through the cut (surgery), burn (radiation) and poison (chemotherapy) routines, to use the words of cancer activist, oncologist and surgeon Dr. Susan Love. Done with those routines, you become a statistic. Thirty-five years ago, when my husband left medical school, he had been taught that real "survival" in cancer meant ten years disease-free after cessation of treatment. By twenty years ago that definition was downgraded to seven years, and now it is five years—and cessation of treatment is not mentioned any more; you may be sick as hell during that entire time and taking drugs worth a king's ransom, but according to the statistics, you are a survivor. You will be listed as a survivor even if you die the day after the five years are over.

Meanwhile, cancer incidence is rising exponentially—everything we touch or ingest is laced with *known* carcinogenic chemicals found in different concentrations and combinations in pesticides, food preservatives and enhancers, cosmetics, furniture, cleaners, and prescription drugs. Despite standard medicine's high-tech-magic-bullet philosophy mortality rates have not changed since the 1950s and recovery rates are equally dismal, with a few exceptions. Back then, one in 20 people was expected to develop cancer. Now, it is one in two.

Early detection is more myth than fact. Indeed, by definition "detection" means you've already got cancer, so this is hardly preventive. By the time a mammogram finds a tumor, it is on average already 9 years old and likely to have spread. Medical researchers at the University of Toronto, C. Baines and A. Miller undertook a comprehensive worldwide analysis of the data for a 25 year period and found that the claims made for early detection are at best wishful thinking; at worst they are hazardous to your health because of the great number of false positive results leading to unnecessary aggressive cut, burn and poison protocols.

What has increased even more than the cancer incidence itself is the sophisticated art of bullshitting the public. For example, anastrozole (Arimidex) advertisements show a woman holding a star-shaped pill with the caption "Put survival in the palm of her hand". In fat print below it claims "56.1% survival". That percentage results from massaging of non-facts:

cancers for which this drug is used kill in a median time of 26.7 months. Taking this wonder-star pill prolongs life by 4.2 months which is statistically insignificant (Moss, 2000).

About half of all prescription drugs are carcinogenic (Moore 1998) and most cancer drugs themselves are carcinogenic, such as the infamous Tamoxifen (Epstein 1999); in fact, Zeneca, the company that makes it and other cancer drugs used world-wide, qualifies all by itself as a first rate carcinogen: Zeneca is one of the world's largest producers of pesticides. Totally shocking is the fact that cancer experts themselves avoid their own treatments at all costs. In the late 1980s, the chief of staff of the world's most prestigious cancer research center, the Sloan Kettering Institute, said when he was diagnosed with cancer, "Do anything you want—but no chemotherapy!" He had spent his life developing chemotherapy treatments. Another bigwig of the same institute sent his mother to an alternative cancer clinic in Germany. Recently, oncologist R.E. Witts of the National Cancer Institute observed about the *Manual of Oncologic Therapeutics* (the practitioners' source book for all mainstream cancer therapies), "One may hope that in another 10 or 15 years medical progress will make this read like an archaic document from the Middle Ages."

Lies are fed by grand illusions and tend to be very lucrative. The editors of one of the world's most prestigious medical journals, *The Lancet*, observed on April 6, 2002, in a most damning editorial, that drug companies "have much to celebrate" because spending on drugs soared by 17% in just 2001 alone, bringing the total to US$ 155 billion, doubled since 1997. The scandalous connections between doctors, researchers and drug manufacturing, the editors concluded "has put the whole of medicine in disrepute." And it is cancer that provides the biggest pot of gold on which research money, prestige and careers depend. Hence, it is hard to find an oncologist who really wants to cure you or even knows how: the focus is muddied by research priorities and information flowing exclusively from the drug industry. The former commissioner of the US Food and Drug Administration (FDA) observed bluntly: "Everything is tainted [in medicine as a whole and cancer care in particular]. Almost every doctor in academia has something going on the side... I don't know what they are getting as far as financial return, stock, money, whatever, is concerned. I have no authority to find out. I certainly don't know what they are getting under the table." (Moss 2000) For the most comprehensive overview of just how lucrative your cancer—not your cure—is, see Epstein's books and the hot new mainstream publication by a professor of medicine who seems not to mind living dangerously: J.S. Cohen, *Overdose*, Tarcher, 2001. It is vital to know who benefits from your illness and not its cure, so you know what and whom to avoid.

The truth shall make us free through knowledge of the facts. The truth shall some day also make us free of cancer. All the causes of cancer are known; we are capable right now of preventing all cancers, even the genetically mediated ones, and we have at our disposal truly effective treatments that work often even for the worst cancers. Amazingly, these treatments are comparatively cheap—very bad news for the cancer industry. And these treatments are not patentable—which, given the huge space cancer occupies in all of medicine, may cause a revolution. Medicine without patents means it returns to serving humanity and ceases to be the lucrative death industry it has become. Doctors who use non-patentable treatments and have no ties to any industry are the only doctors one can trust.

HOW TO SEARCH

The first step to recovery from any serious illness is a mental shift without which nothing positive can happen. That mental shift involves the rejection of the victim stance and the decision to take charge. After all, with every second person likely to develop cancer, we are all in this together. Indeed, a good doctor works with you every step of the way. The standardized conveyor-belt -type delivery of therapy leads directly to the funeral home—"to a conventional death", as one alternative medicine oncologist observed. Blind trust is equivalent to blind death.

Fortunately, the information, on treatments that work, exists and is readily available with little effort. A large bookstore is the best start. The websites given below are gold mines of information, providing everything from the hard science to the cost of all aspects of treatment which are surprisingly cheap. The truth in science and in life tends to be simple, elegant, uncomplicated, low-tech, and of universal application. Whether your diagnosis is terrible and confirmed, or uncertain and possibly false-positive—you do not need to be an oncologist to make an informed choice. Cancer is an intelligible process that requires eyes wide open and totally focused attention.

Beyond doubt, the best single source of information is that compact little softcover, *Cancer Diagnosis: What To Do Next* by Burton Goldberg's Alternative Medicine publishing company. Written by doctors specializing in cancer and untainted by industry connections, it provides an overview of cancer treatments, which work and why, what potholes of abysmal ignorance exist on the road of standard care, which tests are reliable and how to understand them. Most important for those already in the cancer mill, you learn in what limited circumstances the orthodox cut- burn-and-poison routines do work and how they can be made to work even better, with less horrible side effects. Indeed, there are a few childhood cancers, some forms of uterine and colon cancers, and a few special situations in which plain surgery and some chemotherapy, combined with high-powered nutritional regimes, do help.

DR. NICHOLAS GONZALES

Several cures for cancer were developed over the past 10 years. Just like the observations by ancient Greek astronomers, repeatedly confirmed, that the sun—not the earth—is the centre of our solar system, the discoverers of a new understanding of cancer were ignored or dismissed as lunatics. Then came Galileo. Sure, the Pope put him under house arrest, but he could not stop the big change in understanding that followed. Like Galileo, Dr. Gonzales is from the establishment. Armed with an Ivy League medical education and mainstream publications, he studied under world famous immunologists and cancer experts. He wears only pinstriped suits. Like Galileo he has spent a decade in virtual exile. The New York medical licensing authorities tried to take his license away. He kept on treating cancer patients, and they didn't go away to become statistics, but went back into life and told everybody. Now Dr. Gonzales is unstoppable. Curing cancer with nutritional and detoxification regimes, he is turning the world of cancer upside down. He has refused several six-figure book proposals. He is not interested in money or fame. Dr. Gonzales is a doctor down to the marrow of his bones—and that's a divine obsession.

In 2000 President Clinton mandated the National Institutes of Health to commence research into complementary medicine. Harvard researchers had reported that half the population was using alternative medical care, and 7 out of ever 10 cancer patients were secretly using them (see the excellent book by the NIH complementary medicine section's director Dr. James Gordon, below). Clearly, this was a popular movement demanding to be understood. Dr. Gonzales had spent two decades researching nutrition and cancer and experimented with the protocols of pioneers considered quacks.

Then Dr. Gonzales challenged the medical establishment to investigate his treatment of pancreatic cancer. "If my results work, they work. If not, I'll walk away," he said. The preliminary results of this carefully controlled research project, fully supported by the NIH, were published recently showing that Dr. Gonzales' therapy, focused on organic nutritional protocols, vitamins and supplements, enzymes, detox regimes and NO chemotherapy, surgery or radiation, wins hands down over the orthodoxy. "I am offering a primary treatment for major cancer. You don't do chemotherapy and Gonzales. You do one or the other. I have been referred as the doctor of last resort—and perhaps I am" he explained in an excellent *New Yorker* article (Feb. 5, 2001; available on his website). He rejects the polarization between "complementary" and "evidence-based" medicine. For him there is only one medicine and it's testable, verifiable, affordable, and it works. His wish is to be back at the Sloan Kettering Institute and see cancer care renovated totally. We may all get his wish. The shocking fact is, however, that even though there isn't a shortage of pancreatic cancer patients, Dr. Gonzales is having a hard time getting these to his NIH program, because US oncologists loose about $ 30,000 per patient in income, if they refer the patient to somebody else.

THE GERSON INSTITUTE

During World War I, a medical researcher at the University of Heidelberg, Dr. Max Gerson, one of Dr. Gonzales' sources, began to develop a nutrition and detoxification regime for cancer. Among his famous successes were Albert Schweitzer and his wife. Having fled Germany under the Nazis, he continued his practice and research in the USA. Following Hiroshima and Nagasaki, US legislators were burdened by deep guilt and doubt which led to their enthusiastic support of suggestions that radiation might also have some beneficial effects. Thus radiation and then chemotherapy, those attractively dramatic high-tech treatments, gained more and more support, while Dr. Gerson and similar researchers slowly became forgotten—until cancer overstepped the bounds of all epidemics ever recorded.

The protocols followed at the Gerson clinics are in essence the same as those of Dr. Gonzales. Because each patient's treatment is so highly individualized with respect to their needs and the requirements of their type and stage of cancer, the reader is referred to the excellent websites given below. The newly published The *Gerson Therapy* is highly recommended. Both approaches involve radical dietary changes, and both require the patient to be fully involved at every stage.

There are other equally rigorously science-based cancer treatment centers (see books by Moss and websites), and there are some great mavericks, such as Dr. Hulda Clark who works primarily with cancers caused by parasites, bacteria and viruses. Space does not permit discussion of that fabulous school of medicine that seems to be from another planet, namely Chinese medicine, which cures many cancers by methods the West is only beginning to understand. What they all have in common is *not* to cut, burn or poison, but to heal, build, and nourish. They focus on the biochemistry of the cancer and the healing processes the body can offer. Unlike the tradition-based therapies of standard medicine, most of which are not scientifically studied, but only statistically evaluated, biochemically based therapies are based on loads of verifiable research. An observation by Professor U. Abel of Heidelberg University's medical school in Germany points to the deep flaw in standard cancer care: "Arguing for the benefits of chemotherapy based on a few complete responses is like arguing in favor of gambling based on the profits of the winner."

Our irresponsibly poisoned environment has created battered organs and cells which we have the power to restore with gentle, nourishing persistence. Every cancer patient healed is testimony to the fact that the world can be healed also.

Sources and Resources

R.W. Moss, *Cancer Therapy: The Independent Consumer's Guide to Non-Toxic Treatment and Prevention*, Equinox, 1999

R.W. Moss, *Questioning Chemotherapy*, Equinox 2000

W.J. Diamond, MD, et al. *Cancer Diagnosis: What to do Next*, Alternative Medicine Guide, 2000

M. Gerson, MD, *A Cancer Therapy: Results of Fifty Cases*, Gerson Institute, (1958) 1999

C. Gerson & M. Walker, *The Gerson Therapy*, Kensington Publishing, 2001

H.R. Clark, *The Cure for All Advanced Cancers*, New Century Press, New Century Press, 1999

J. Gordon, MD, *Comprehensive Cancer Care: Integrating Alternative, Complementary and Conventional Therapies*, Perseus, 2000

L.M. Bower, *The Healthy Household*, Healthy House Institute, 1995

T.J. Moore, Simon & Schuster, 1998 *Prescription for Disaster*

J.S. Cohen MD, *Overdose: The Case Against the Drug Companies*, Tarcher Putnam, 2001

The following websites provide information on treatment, cost, prognosis, research basis, time involved etc:

www.dr-gonzales.com   takes you to Dr. Gonzales' clinic in New York

www.gerson.org   takes you to the Gerson Institute

www.cmbm.org   takes you to the Complementary Medicine department of the National Institutes of Health; downloading their conferences is free

www.preventcancer.com and **www.stopcancernow.com** best source for information on prevention and proof positive for the corruption in the cancer establishment (not to be confused with mega pharmaceutical and biowarfare producer Eli Lilly's **www.preventcancer.org** which is useless propaganda).

An excellent source for cell-based, non-toxic treatments is GET REAL. CANCER, call 714-842-1777.

Since mammography is potentially cancer triggering and not very useful, thermography is preferable because it is non-invasive and can detect many types of cancer early and reliably. Thermography clinics in Ontario are organized through the North York Thermography Center: 416-636-291

Healing–Not Drugging!" The Gerson Therapy for Cancer Sixty years of Proven Success

Vitality Magazine November 2004

You are in for an amazing treat: the keynote speaker of this year's Whole Life Expo is Charlotte Gerson, the daughter of Dr. Max Gerson who developed the cure for all cancers in the 1920s. All current non-toxic cancer therapies trace their way back to him. His daughter founded the Gerson Institute in California and the Gerson Cancer Clinic in Mexico. At 82 she speaks and writes with the fire of truth. I attended a workshop she was conducting in Toronto four years ago, when my own research into cancer had just begun. She made me sit bolt upright with shock when she said, in reference to standard oncology, "Unless they can show me that they can cure pancreatic cancer, I am not interested—because the Gerson therapy can." That is the fastest-killing cancer there is.

When I interviewed her for this article, I confided that I occasionally become very sad from my research into the criminality in modern medicine, the cancer industry probably being the worst. Knowing against what astounding political odds the Gerson therapy succeeded to offer successful and scientifically grounded therapy to cancer patients in many parts of the world today, I asked her, "What keeps you going?" She laughed heartily and said, "The patients! Seeing the patients recover! I see it happen all the time." That joy is, of course, denied to the doctors who have been duped into the standard paradigm (the cut-burn-poison doctrine of modern oncology), which over the past 50 years has advanced little, neither improved survival rates, nor quality of life, and certainly has not stopped the steady rise in cancer incidence.

Albert Schweitzer, who was a patient of Dr. Gerson's, said, "I see in Dr. Max Gerson one of the most eminent geniuses in the history of medicine." Historically, geniuses arise when they are most needed, but success tends to come generally after they are dead, and they tend to pay a heavy personal price for their determination to renovate the dominant view of their time. And so it was with Dr. Gerson also.

Dr. Gerson's tragic clash with the pharmaceutically oriented American Medical Association (AMA) and the corrupt American Cancer Society which had made toxic drugs, surgery and radiation the standard of practice, is a breathtaking story recorded—of all places—in the reports of the US Office of Technology Assessment which used to evaluate all forms of medical practice until recently. In the 1980s they made a determined effort to destroy alternative medicine—that is: treatments alternative to drugs. The *Journal of the American Medical Association* had in an astonishing change of heart published an article on January 25, 1980, suggesting that the AMA had staged a "Grand Conspiracy against the Cure of Cancer". The author, William Regelsen of the Medical College of Virginia, found that "inappropriate judgments have resulted in injury to good observations" and defended the results and the scientific basis of the Gerson therapy.

This was an alarming defection, so this government department contracted a known opponent to non-standard practices, Dr. Patricia Spain Ward of the University of Chicago, to investigate the Gerson therapy and provide a usefully negative report. When Dr. Ward had completed her investigation, she came to the unexpected conclusion that this was one of the greatest medical innovations in the history of cancer therapy. Every effort was made to stop her report from becoming public—it failed, and you can read the whole thing in all its marvelous detail on the Gerson Institute's website. It will make your heart sing and you will occasionally probably weep.

The suppression of the Gerson therapy almost succeeded. Dr. Gerson died in 1959, but his famous book remained, detailing the scientific evolution of this therapy and providing the case histories of patients with inoperable or too advanced forms of cancer who were cured; some are alive today. In a final attempt to stop non-toxic treatment of cancer, the FDA ordered the publisher of the book to stop marketing it. So, his daughter Charlotte wound up with several thousand copies in a warehouse. She decided to give some talks on it to small groups of interested people. On one such occasion, a doctor spoke up and suggested to start a clinic and offer this therapy to cancer patient again. After many battles with the American government this became a reality and is flourishing. Indeed, at the EXPO this November you will have the great pleasure of seeing a documentary film about Dr. Gerson. It won the 2004 *Palm D'Or*, the movie industry's highest award for documentaries.

At a time when antibiotics had not yet been developed, Dr. Gerson, who was trained in Germany's leading universities, enjoyed the support of the government and his colleagues, then the world leaders in medicine, when he began to develop highly successful nutritional treatments for that era's biggest killer, tuberculosis, for which no treatments existed then. Considering Gerson the foremost authority on nutrition and health, the German Ministry of Health asked him to help with soil rehabilitation, which already in the 1920s had become a serious problem causing measurable vitamin and mineral deficiencies. Dr. Gerson said: "The soil is our external metabolism." Foods grown in nutrient-depleted soil will invariably promote ill health in all its forms, so we become as sick as our inappropriate agricultural methods have made those very plants and animals.

At the very same time, the German philosopher Rudolf Steiner initiated the organic farming movement, and his concepts are still the basis of the modern organic agriculture. Charlotte adds, in a discussion of today's genetically engineered and pesticide-laden crops (Gerson Institute Healing Newsletter, March/April 2001) "Since people with degenerative diseases suffer nutrient deficiency and toxicity, it is obvious that they cannot be healed with deficient and toxic foods." She stresses that the only certain way to prevent cancer is to eat 100% organic food and avoid, as well as regularly detoxify from, the ubiquitous environmental toxins we are exposed to at work, at home, in our gardens, and in our bathrooms, laundry rooms, basements—and even in human breast milk and the amniotic fluid in which our babies float.

She continues in the same article, "In order for the body to heal, no matter what the imbalances, it has to release its toxic load and rebuild its nutrient status. When this occurs, the vitality arises and healing begins. The body's intelligence—not the brain—will determine which areas will be healed and in what order." Dr. Gerson used to call this process the work of the "the physician within". Indeed, the healing process even from metastasized cancer can be such that the scar tissue, too, dissolves.

It is a shock to read the following excerpt from the prestigious journal *Cancer* whose editor observe in 1927 (!) as follows: "We have lived so long on processed foods that we are in a state of unbalanced nutrition from birth. We have come to regard these processed foods as the hallmark of civilization, when it is a fact that these very foods set the stage for every sort of ill, including cancer." In the light of what has happened since 1927 in terms of food degradation and its attending burden of degenerative disease, including cancer, a famous statement by Winston Churchill comes to mind which Dr. Gerson was fond of quoting: "Men occasionally stumble over the truth, but most pick themselves up and hurry off as if nothing happened." When the Nazis took over Germany, Dr. Gerson went to the US where he worked for cancer patients for many years, presenting his astonishing results to Congress. Political lobbying from Big Business and the new nuclear power industry caused the US government to support research into radiation therapy instead of nutritional and environmental approaches to cancer. The result of that decision for public health can today be vividly seen in the astounding documentary "Supersize Me".

In the March/April 2002 newsletter, Charlotte reports a perfect example of cancer being the paradigmatic environmental disease, arising from a world poisoned by human activity that doesn't take organic vulnerability into account: "We saw two couples where both husband and wife suffered from lymphoma. In each case, these four people had worked many months to their build their own homes, therefore exposure to chemicals, glues, paints, solvents, phenols, wood preservatives and an unending list of toxins seemed to be main cause of their disease."

What makes these two cases medically so significant is the fact that all four people are not related to each other, so resorting to the standard cop-out of a genetic explanation of cancer is impossible. Of course, proof positive of cancer being an environmental disease was supplied some time ago (July 13, 2000) in the prestigious *New England Journal of Medicine*. It published the results of a huge epidemiological study involving the medical histories of 90,000 identical twins studied for 28 different types of cancer to determine whether genetics or the environment played the greater part in disease development. The conclusion was that "the environment has the principle role in causing cancer."

These findings do not seem to agree with the agenda of the American Cancer Society which two years later published on its website a warning article on the Gerson therapy in which they state the following: "The belief that poor diet and the build-up of toxins from foods, additives, and environmental pollution are the main causes of chronic disease is without scientific basis."

No wonder then, that Samuel Epstein, the famous cancer expert who was the moving force behind the ban on DDT in the 1970s and later on asbestos, observes that one of the most important ways to fight cancer is *not* to donate any money to the American Cancer Society. During the 1999 Cancer Conference in Hamilton he observed, that the same was true for its Canadian counterpart. In his book, *The Breast Cancer Prevention Program,* he details the corruption of this organization: lobbying to prevent the lucrative cancer drug Tamoxifen from being listed as carcinogen (it was listed as such anyway); when the Reagan and Bush administrations cancelled legislation pertaining to protecting against known industrial carcinogens, the ACS kept silent; they refused to support the US Clean Air Act and the Toxic Substance Control Act, and opposed the FDA's ban on the carcinogenic sweetener saccharin (they had accepted money from Coca-Cola which used it in their drinks). As Burton Goldberg observes, "Looking at the evidence, we wonder if ACS actually benefits from the promotion of cancer."

But there is a fresh wind blowing: the University of Pittsburgh has established a Cancer Institute (call 412-647-2811 for information). And this time it's the real thing, so to speak! Its goal is to examine how to *protect* individuals and the community from environmental factors that can cause cancer. The institute is run by Devra Lee Davis, one of America's leading environmental experts and epidemiologists. Her recent book, *When Smoke Ran Like Water*, is highly recommended.

Two thousand five hundred years ago, the father of Western scientific medicine, Hippocrates, taught "let food be your medicine and medicine be your food". Tradition has it, that he developed a special soup for cancer patients. In a charming historical twist, it was a patient in 1928 suffering from liver cancer, who had heard of Dr. Gerson's success with a nutritional approach to tuberculosis, and asked him to treat her with nutrition. She gave him an old German book on folk medicine in which this legendary recipe was recorded. When considering the biochemical assumptions underlying it, Dr. Gerson realized that here was something of great value. Indeed, the Gerson therapy now incorporates those nutritional principles. As he embarked upon this uncharted territory—the nutritional treatment of the worst possible systemic diseases –following Hippocrates literally, as it were, even Dr. Gerson was scared at first. He asked the patient to sign a statement that she would not hold him responsible for the outcome—and so the Gerson therapy began. He cured her within six months.

To learn how the Gerson therapy can work for all cancers, Multiple sclerosis, diabetes, Multiple Chemical Sensitivity and other chronic diseases, what the scientific basis for this approach is, how to do it yourself whenever possible, and especially to talk to Charlotte Gerson yourself—come to the Expo this November and partake in this celebration of medicine that works.

Sources & Resources
M. Gerson, MD, *A Cancer Therapy: Results of Fifty Cases*, Gerson Institute, (1958) 1999
C. Gerson & M. Walker, *The Gerson Therapy*, Kensington, 2001
(See also resources at the end of previous articles above)

The Role of the Earth in Cancer Prevention

Vitality Magazine September 2004

Billions of years ago, when the universe was born in unknown millions of galaxies, our planet eventually also appeared. The same star dust that became Earth, also created all life and maintains it every second of the day. Nobel laureate Christian de Duve writes, "All organic matter can be summarized by the formula CHNOPS, which stands for carbon, hydrogen, nitrogen, oxygen, phosphorus, and sulfur." If life was a symphony orchestra in which all instruments are equally important to the musical event, the players being vitamins, enzymes, proteins, hormones, and so on, it would be the minerals assuming the role of the first violinist who presents the correct key-note to enable the conductor to begin. Everything living and non-living is at every moment literally the earth as well as itself.

Andre Voisin, a French agricultural biochemist, observed in the 1950s in his magisterial book Soil, Grass and Cancer: "We should frequently meditate on the words of Ash Wednesday: Man, remember that you are dust and that you will return to dust. This great scientific truth should be engraved above the entrance of every faculty of medicine…[because] our cells are made up of mineral elements…the animal is a product of the soil, the biochemical photograph of the environment in which it lives, particularly of the soil which manufactured the nutrients for it." Voisin then outlined the "principles of protective medicine," which he believes is "the great medical science of the future" because what protects life is the earth itself. Minerals are the catalysts of all biological activity during which the boundary between organic and inorganic vanishes.

The Breast Cancer Research and Education Fund (**www.breastcancer ef.org**), held its annual conference on May 1 at Brock University in St. Catharines. Addressing the theme "Beyond Silent Spring: Striving for Optimal Personal and Environmental Health", the speakers included Dorothy Goldin-Rosenberg, the co-producer of the internationally famous documentary "Exposure" on the environmental causes of cancer (available through **when@web.ca)**, renowned activists James Brophy (on occupational links to cancer), Liz Armstrong (101 preventive measures), and Janet May (on successful actions against cosmetic pesticide use). I spoke on the politics of cancer.

One of the speakers was Mennonite farmer and homeopath, Murray Bast who runs Bio-AG, a consulting business "Working with Nature…Naturally" through which he offers farmers the biochemical knowledge to "produce quality crops and healthy livestock." Murray often cures through homeopathic therapies those who get sick from pesticides and herbicides. In the late 90s Murray read a *Vitality* article of mine on genetic engineering. He asked me to address the Mennonite farmers, most of whom knew nothing about GMO's soil-depleting, nutrient-reducing, and disease-promoting properties, nor did they know that pesticides and herbicides cause cancer; having no telephones or a modern scientific education, research through journals and internet was not an option. Following my workshop, many farmers returned to "working with Nature naturally."

Murray spoke about the effects of minerals on health and disease. When he put up an overhead with the following information, I stopped taking notes and sat through his lecture in a state of shock: in 1920—before the devil's brew of synthetic fertilizers, pesticides, herbicides, acid rain, and groundwater loaded with antibiotics and industrial chemicals—50 bushels of grain contained the protein that by 1968 required a 100 bushels. The vitamins found in 50 bushels then, by 1968 required 250 bushels. Worst of all, those 50 bushels in 1920 were chock-full of essential minerals, but by 1968 it required 500 bushels for the same amount of minerals.

Today it's even worse. U.S. Department of Agriculture food tables of March 2001 show that the calcium content in broccoli dropped 50% since 1975, iron in watercress is down by 88%, and vitamins in cauliflower by 40%. The vitamin C content in sweet peppers dropped from averages of 128 mg to 89 mg, potassium in all foods is down from 400 mg to 170 mg, and magnesium (the queen of minerals), is down from 57% to 9%. By the way, if your serum level of magnesium drops on any day by a mere 10%, you may have a heart attack — the less dramatic, everyday low levels merely set us up for one. (Full details on www.organicgardening.com.) Conventionally grown potatoes and apples now have very little or no vitamin C or potassium at all (*Nature*, April 19, 2001).

The *American Journal of Clinical Nutrition* warned in 1999 (L. Chasen-Taber, 70:509-16) that the currently low levels of selenium predispose everybody to cancer. On July 3 the *Toronto Star's* front-page headline read "Cancer crisis looming in GTA" and reported a 46% predicted increase over the next 10 years. Now, if we paid attention to the causes of cancer — all of which are known — we could reduce that incidence by at least that percentage in 10 years instead. A major cause of cancer is dead food that is unable to nourish our bodies, such as to make repair possible, and maintain biochemical defenses against carcinogens. It is at the level of the soil that our food is killed.

Even if you eat your three to five recommended servings of fruits and vegetables daily, you are not getting enough of the most essential nutrients, especially minerals. The U.S. National Academy of Sciences issued an alert this year, stating that we have to eat twice as many vegetables just to approximate the RDAs — which are already ridiculously low.

A world survey undertaken by The World Resources Institute in Washington DC, published March 2000, entitled "Underfed and Overfed," discussed the "global epidemic of malnutrition," showing that the poor do not receive the required nutrients because they lack the calories or food diversity, while the affluent are increasingly obese but are equally deprived of the same nutrients because our plentiful, instantly available and perfect-looking food is mostly dead. The fabulous documentary "Supersize Me," currently running in our theatres, is finally making millions aware of this creeping mass suicide.

Let's follow a 300-pound person through a downtown mall as he or she waddles along, huffing, puffing, sweating, depressed as hell. Maybe she is full of doughnuts, deep-fried foods, antibiotic-loaded chicken fingers, and a bag of trans-fatty-acid-laced chips — or maybe he thinks he is doing his best by avoiding sugar and drinking aspartame-sweetened pop instead, but that will really fry his nervous system and set him up for cancer (Ed: Aspartame is a known neurotoxin).

Or perhaps she is truly eating very little (like a fat friend of mine) and subsisting on bagels (made from dead flour), chicken breast (loaded with antibiotics, the toxicity of which causes the body to retain more water in a desperate attempt to stop the toxins from passing through the cell membrane), and some crispy salads laced with herbicides causing the immune system to shut down.

All these toxins, unopposed by mineral-dependent biochemical processes, prevent cell repair and the proper ratio of muscle to fat. In addition, these enormous starving bodies probably consume prescription drugs which further deplete whatever intrepid, lone nutrient might make it into that ground zero of a body.

So there they drag themselves full of false food, but really in a state of increasing starvation, towards a heart attack, cancer, diabetes, and arthritis —purchased at the local supermarket and supported in an unconscious suicide pact by Medicare. What might cause this oxymoronic state of obese starvation? Our perfect-looking produce and attractively-packaged supermarket foods likely lack all or most of the following:

boron (prevents osteoporosis by maintaining calcium), **calcium** (builds bones and teeth)

chromium (which regulates insulin and thereby appetite, protects against diabetes and cardiovascular disease)

copper (which ensures healthy blood, controls body temperature, fatigue, regulates fertility)

iron (required for cell repair, production of neurotransmitters, hormones, and enzymes)

magnesium (needed for everything from mental functioning to controlling blood pressure, protection against intestinal diseases and cancer, the food metabolism, and assignment of all nutrients to their proper functions, controls the entire energy system of the body, and enables plants to grow)

manganese (ensures corrects cholesterol levels, makes collagen, central for cell repair and more)

molybdenum (needed by the liver to do its detoxification job)—**nickel** (ensures proper iron absorption)—**phosphorus** (makes bones rigid and teeth healthy, maintains structure of cell membranes and essential fatty acids, enables DNA and RNA production)

potassium (needed for all cellular activity, nerve conduction, muscle contraction, and the beating of the heart)

selenium (in charge of all detoxification processes and immune functions)

silicon (required by bones and cardiovascular system)

sulfur (controls structure and function of all proteins)

vanadium (helps to prevent diabetes)

zinc (vital to proper immune, joint, and brain function, integrity of skin, hair, nails, and menstruation).

For complete information on all minerals and vitamins with their current scientific literature sources go to www.garynull. com and download for free.

All of these minerals are depleted by synthetic fertilizers, pesticides, herbicides, acid rain, and agricultural methods that have ceased to be in dialogue with the earth but only consider quantity, efficiency, and profit. The main effect of ignoring the earth is the depletion of those minerals which animals and people need in order to make catalase — the single most important enzyme needed to prevent incorrect cell duplication, or cancer.

Murray introduced me to Andre Voisin's 1959 book on soil and cancer. For anybody interested in nutrition it is pretty much the equivalent of a scientific religious experience. Voisin describes biochemical research into infectious disease, infertility, and cancer that appeared in the first half of the 20th century before it was successfully shelved (and almost forgotten) by those forces in society that worship at the altars of greed and efficiency, namely the producers of modern agriculture and drugs —bewitching us with the promise of fast-delivery of everything to everybody all the time.

An internationally celebrated scientist in his time, Voisin takes the reader through the biological activities of all minerals and shows how they protect, heal and maintain life. Rather than discuss cancer in the usual military terms we are used to, Voisin shows how mineral depletion causes cells to "adapt" by becoming cancerous, while nutrient replenishment can reverse that state.

Recently, worldwide epidemics such as AIDS and cancer and the total failure of the high-tech, super-synthetic approach to stem them, are forcing researchers back to examining the discoveries of earlier times. University of Victoria's medical geographer, Harold Foster, is a leader in the field. In his writings he discusses how, for example, Senegal with its naturally selenium-rich soils has almost no AIDS at all, even though the culture tolerates promiscuity, while certain parts of China are naturally selenium-depleted and virtually everybody has it. In industrialized countries, the AIDS rate is highest where foods are lowest in selenium due to processing and selenium-depleting agricultural methods.

Professor Foster just returned from South Africa where European nutraceutical companies conducted a study with AIDS patients by treating them with selenium and related nutrients — curing most of them at a fraction of the cost of drugs that merely extend life a little.

But the human mind can learn and indeed it does. Since January, when the truth about antidepressants hit the fan, doctors are faced with patients who "just say no." *The Medical Post* of July 6 reported in a front-page article that psychiatrists are in a panic because they have been trained as drug pushers and know next to nothing about nutritional biochemistry, environmental toxins and how those cause mental illness and depression.

Medical history has always advanced through non-compliant patients or the angry relatives of dead ones, so this will send doctors back to the libraries and the Internet. Similarly, since last year, when the scandal broke about HRT, consumption of those carcinogens is down by more than 60%.

Since March, when the Ontario College of Family Physicians published their report on the health effects of pesticides, insisting they be stopped and urging people to eat organic food, the chemically-addicted lawn is rapidly becoming history as people demand bylaws forbidding cosmetic pesticides. Soil rehabilitation projects are going on everywhere, with Prince Charles being the most prominent leader, and the organic food movement is curing the Earth and protecting us from degenerative disease at the same time.

Humanity evolved over five million years with planet Earth; we will make it "by the skin of our teeth," as Thornton Wilder's famous play on the subject put it. If we use our brains, the Earth will never forsake us We can stop Soil depletion, Herbicides, Insecticides, and Transgenics (figure out the acronym yourself) and save ourselves.

Sources and Resources

ANAMOL Laboratories, (905) 660-1225 or 1-888-254-4840 (for complete hair mineral analysis — $35)

J. Challem & L. Brown, *User's Guide to Vitamins and Minerals*, Basic Health Publications Inc., 2002

C. Dean, *The Miracle of Magnesium*, Random House, 2003 (also distributed by Kos Inc. (519) 927-1049)

C. DeDuve, *Vital Dust: Life as A Cosmic Imperative*, Basic Books, 1995

H. Foster, *What Really Causes AIDS*, Trafford, 2001

M. F. Holick, *The UV Advantage*, ibooks Inc., 2003

World Resources Institute Monograph 150: "Underfed and Overfed: The Global Epidemic of Malnutrition," March 2000

R. Pelton & J.B. LaValle, *The Nutritional Cost of Prescription Drugs*, Morton, 2000 (www.morton-pub./com)

A. Voisin, *Soil Grass and Cancer*, Crosby Lockwood Ltd., 1959 (out of print, for facsimile copies for $25 call Bio-Ag (519) 656-2460)

M.R. Werbach, *Textbook of Nutritional Medicine*, Third Line Press, 1999

4

Children

Reproductive Health Hazards

Vitality Magazine December 1999

The chemicals which we unwittingly use in our homes, and from which we are rarely protected at our workplaces, have the potential to initiate the extinction of humanity. They affect ovaries and sperm production and interfere with the development of our un born children. This chemical soup we live in supports the world's economy. We live in a war zone with chemical manufacturers creating ever more of these substances while striving to keep full knowledge of their effects from the public. Currently, each one of us may carry over 500 chemicals in our fat cells. None of these chemicals existed before World War I, nor where they tested for safety. A fetus is no match for an economic system that focuses on profit and deliberately ignores biological safety. Fetuses do not have a shareholder's vote.

But "there are worse things than extinction" even, as senior scientist of the World Wild Life Fund, Theo Colborn, observes in her landmark book, *Our Stolen Future* (1997). These chemicals, some 70,000 of which were developed after World War II, cause infertility and cancer, irreparably damage our immune system, and initiate faulty wiring in developing brains—thereby producing attention deficit disorder, retardation, and endocrine-mediated behavior problems.. Sperm counts throughout the industrial world are seriously low, and spontaneous abortion rates are way up. This century began with the search for effective methods of birth control and is closing with the real danger of humanity self-destructing—not with a nuclear bang, but a child's whimper.

United States Vice President, Al Gore, author of *Earth in the Balance* (1992) wrote in his foreword to Colborn's book that research such as hers influenced the Clinton administration to establish an expert panel at the national Academy of Sciences to assess this "invisible threat to humanity" and to "find ways to protect our children" because "we have the right to know the substances to which we and our children are being exposed."

The Reproductive Health Hazards conference held in Toronto in October (1999) focused on these threats, the right to know, and the right to protection. This event was sponsored by the Workers Health and Safety Center, Occupational Health Clinics for Ontario Workers, the Association of Occupational & Environmental Clinics, the Canadian Auto Workers, the Canadian Labour Congress, the Ontario Federation of Labour, and the United Steelworkers of America. The speakers were Canadian and US occupational health experts, toxicologists and epidemiologists, scientists from the World Health Organization and various universities, legal advisors to the provincial and national governments, and political analysts. Several outstanding videos were also screened.

Following this conference, I interviewed Theo Colborn, Dick Martin (president of the Inter-American Regional Labour Organization), Morag Simpson (formerly toxicologist for Greenpeace, now with Council of Canadians), Dr. Douglas Seba (US oceanographer and ecologist) and Canadian political journalist Linda McQuaig who was also one of the speakers at this event. As an amusing aside, it should be remembered that McQuaig's outspoken and insightful criticisms of the values informing current economic practices caused Canadian tycoon Conrad Black to say on CBC Radio's Gzowski Show that she "should be horsewhipped".

Swiss chemist Paul Muller unwittingly developed the first chemical endocrine disruptor, DDT. He won the 1948 Nobel Prize for this "miracle pesticide". Like the atom bomb, which produced long-term destructive radiation as a secondary effect, organochlorines are now known to do far worse than only kill agricultural pests or harden plastics.

"We have coated the world in these chemicals," (DDT, PCBs, dioxins, furans and many others) Dr. Colborn observed. By mimicking natural hormones they lock into the receptor sites of animal and human cells and alter the activity of natural hormones; they also damage the thyroid which results in immune impairment or dysfunction. Because our bodily enzymes cannot metabolize and excrete these chemicals, they accumulate, thereby magnifying their effects. Worst of all, Dr. Colborn said, "these endocrine disruptors are trans-generational", meaning that they cross the placenta, affecting fetal development in many different ways, ranging from retardation to autism and learning and behavioral problems. Endocrine disruptors also affect genetically mediated timetables, so that cancers or in fertility develop later in life.

U.S. oceanographer, Dr. Douglas Seba, who addressed the 34th annual conference of the American Academy of Environmental Medicine in Idaho held this year in October, told me that birth defects, infertility problems, and malformations of sex organs in wildlife have dramatically increased, primarily because of a potato pesticide, chlorothalonil. He described consensus-based research that correlates planetary wind and rain patterns (which transport these pesticides in the fall westwards) with the epidemiological patterns of thyroid problems, kidney failure, hypertension, and birth defects in humans and animals.

Rachel Carson wrote in her classic *Silent Spring* that "our fate is connected with the animals." Indeed, the extinction of frogs and birds, the malformation of sex organs in alligators and deer, are the signs of our own fate which has already begun. Dr. Frederick von Saal from the University of Missouri states in the documentary video on cancer, *They Speak in Whispers*, that the embryos of mice and humans are indistinguishable in their early developmental phases, and that the same enzymes are used throughout the living world during development. Therefore, all fetuses are equally vulnerable to these endocrine disruptors. Adult infertility, especially in men, is now thought to be triggered by these chemicals while they were still embryos themselves.

The prospective solvent study undertaken by Toronto's Hospital for Sick Children at their "Motherisk Clinic" showed that babies with birth defects are most numerous where mothers are occupationally exposed to industrial solvents: graphic designers, factory workers, print industry workers, chemists, painters (including artists), car and general cleaners, veterinary assistants, nurses, textile workers, photostat shop workers—all of whom can be exposed to aromatic hydrocarbons, phenols (derived from benzene found also in air fresheners, deodorants and most perfumes), dry cleaning fluids, xylene, vinyl chloride, aceton (also found in nail polish remover), etc. found in anything from typewriter correction fluids to plastics, glues and paints. These substances are also neurotoxic and/or carcinogenic to the mothers themselves. The US government estimates that 335 occupations are consistently exposed to reproductive hazards of this sort (i.e. 3 million women and 6 million men).

Scientific research on women's occupational health is virtually non-existent, as Karen Messing in her book *One-Eyed Science* shows. For example, waitresses have simply never been studied. Yet, they are likely to be exposed daily to second-hand smoke, neurotoxic propane and natural gas, carcinogenic fumes from detergents, harmful electromagnetic fields from microwave ovens, and stresses conducive to repetitive strain injuries. One also wonders if anything is known about the occupational hazards suffered by school teachers (such as carcinogenic benzene in markers, pesticides, neurotoxic mold in carpeting, solvents in paper glues etc.), or mal workers whose environments are saturated with carcinogenic benzene-laden air fresheners and formaldehyde from new clothing and furniture, or dental assistants exposed to neurotoxic mercury vapors, and home makers who are exposed to everything the supermarket, garden center and hardware store offer through much advertising but practically no useful information for health purposes. The amazing fact is, that in almost all instances these harmful substances are readily replaced with non-toxic alternatives—which has obvious negative implications for the profits of the industry that makes the toxic stuff.

However, possibly the most dangerous occupation is being a child, because children are most vulnerable to all these chemicals. Dr. Philip Landrigan, an occupational health expert at the Mount Sinai School of Medicine in New York, initiated a landmark study, published in 1995, which caused the US government to change legislation regarding the permissible concentrations of endocrine disrupting and carcinogenic chemicals to reflect the needs of children. Currently, the US chemical lobby is working overtime to water down this proposed legislation. Indeed, for oncologist Samuel Epstein "there is no such thing as a safe level of exposure". He flatly states, "If it's a carcinogen, replace it with a safe substance."

Notably, Quebec legislation has recognized the right of protection from dangerous environmental substances for the fetus, not just the mother. Canadian federal law in general pays (mostly unenforceable or unenforced) lip service to the mother's right for protection, but Quebec lawmakers understood the subtle and far-reaching distinction. If the fetus has environmental rights, the environment must conform to its requirements, which must take precedence over economic interests. Enforcing this enlightened view is, however, another matter.

Canada's Office of the Auditor General has just recently provided us with a financial interpretation of these issues: it is expected that health spending will reach $ 120 billion by the year 2011 and balloon to $ 200 billion by 2021. Since it is well known that the bulk of health care spending goes towards pesticide and radiation-triggered cancer, environmentally mediated chronic illness and so-called age-related diseases (e.g. heavy metal-induced Alzheimer's, pesticide and diesel fuel triggered asthma etc.) it is hardly unfair to ask which industries should be sent the nation's health care bill.

The video, *They Speak in Whispers*, features parents whose children died or are dying from the effects of chemical exposures acquired through their parents' occupations. One of the father's whose child died of a rare cancer, says that every time he mentioned the possibility of an environmental cause, "the doctors spoke in whispers. It's almost like a tabu subject." Some of these children developed cancer simply by playing in a field behind Stelco at Dofasco plants. Others may have got sick through endocrine disruptions that occurred in their parents at work before conception.

Canadian law has the Three R's: the right to participate in health and safety committees with management, the right to refuse dangerous work, and the right to know about health hazards in your work place. Its architect was a 1970s Saskatchewan Deputy Minister of Labour, Bob Sass. Because of the continued reluctance of governments to enforce these rights, many workshops at this conference focused on developing strategies to make government once again serve the people. The current World Trade Organization agreements are all designed to exclude public opinion or representation, and to free corporations from any accountability. In 1996 UNESCO reported that as a direct result of GATT, some of the world's biggest corporations locate themselves in Asia and "force children as young as 5 to work from 6 in the morning till 7 at night." We need to know these things so we can ask ourselves if we want to buy their products.

Dick Martin, formerly a miner in Manitoba and currently president of the Inter-American Regional Labour Organization, said that occupational health is still dealt with only "reactively instead of preventively". Therefore, workers and consumers alike have a right to demand a change, but says Martin "our governments have betrayed us." Deregulation gives license to pollute and exploit. In South America he watched pesticides, long outlawed in North America, being sprayed on export coffee without any concern for the world-wide systemic effects on health. He also watched Agent Orange being used to clear land for teak tree planting in Costa Rica, regardless of its devastating effects on the workers and their children; 90% of Cambodia's farmers are being poisoned because health warnings on pesticide containers are printed only in foreign languages. But he noted that the trade ministers are beginning to listen to international labour groups, and that consumers are responding intelligently. However, he also feels that the current threat posed by chemicals is of historically unprecedented danger due to its invisibility and delayed effects on the fetus.

Dr. Theo Colborn said that Canadians have one of the most precious ecological resources in the Great Lakes system. "I would urge Canadians to insist that their government return to the original mandate of the Great Lakes Water Quality Agreement, which was to clean up the lakes", and not just be content with partial restoration of the ecosystem.

Political journalist Linda McQuaig feels that every Canadian needs to work towards reclaiming our democratic right to participation. She is alarmed by the current attempt in *The National Post* to debunk as "junk science" everything that threatens the corporate interests. She was encouraged by the public's success in stopping the bank merger and the MAI (Multinational Agreement on Investment).

Indeed there are some signs that human values are returning. Nike has begun to change its unethical production policies in its offshore plants; General Motors is stopping the use of endocrine disruptors in its car manufacturing process; Baxter, the world's largest hospital equipment manufacturer, halted the use of toxic chemicals; Ford won an environmental award for its control of cyanide discharge in the Windsor plant; Greenpeace succeeded in its legal action against Petro Canada in 1995 by invoking environmental law successfully and the court-ordered clean-up has been completed.

What We Can Do

We can seek out available information. We can borrow the videos listed below and invite our friends and neighbors for discussion and action plans. We can write to corporations and demand to know under what conditions their products are made. We can boycott toxic coffee. We need not buy teak furniture. We can go to the "Motherisk Clinic" at the Hospital for Sick Children for accurate risk information and insist on protection at least during the critical first trimester of pregnancy. We can talk to school boards, teachers and bosses—after all, they too are people *with* endocrine systems and susceptibility to cancer. We can act on the knowledge that "the power of one" works, organize intelligent resistance, pester our MP's and MPP's and use our vote thoughtfully. The resources given below contain much of the knowledge that can help make us free.

Sources and Resources
M. Barlow, *The Fight of My Life*, 1998
CBC Health For Sale (2 part transcript) 1999
T. Colborn, *Our Stolen Future*, 1997
D. Fagin & M. Lavelle, *Toxic Deception*, 1999
A. Gore, *Earth in the Balance: Ecology and the Human Spirit*, 1992
J.A. Harr, *Civil Action*, 1996 (see also movie by the same title)
J. McMurtry, *Unequal Freedoms: The Global Market As An Ethical System*, 1998
L. McQuaig, *The Quick and the Dead: Brian Mulroney, Big Business and the Seduction of Canada*, 1992

L. McQuaig, *The Cult of Impotence: Seeing the Myth of Powerlessness in the Global Economy*, 1998

J. Ridgeway & J. St.Clair, *A Pocket Guide to The Environmental Bad Guys*, 1998

J.M.D. Sherman, *Chemical Exposure and Disease*, 1994

"Before Their Time" and "The Speak in Whispers" are videos available through—1-888-869-7950 or in libraries

"Everyday Carcinogens" features an international panel of scientists speaking about cancer. Contact **www.stopcancer.org**

"Exposure: Environmental Links to Breast Cancer" is an internationally acclaimed documentary and available through 416-928-0880

The ABC's of Healthy Children

Vitality Magazine December 2001

I am not sure if this is a proud boast or an embarrassed confession, but the truth is that my husband of 32 years and I raised 15 children: 3 home-made and 12 adopted from all over the world, seven of those with severe physician handicaps. Our regrets are few, but the perfection of hindsight mercilessly informs us of all we could have done better, so that is what this article is all about. Exploring how to have healthy children is a worthy Christmas meditation. Christmas celebrates children. Understood as a profound truth, rather than abstruse theological dogma, the story of the Virgin Mary's delivery of a divine child is what this poisoned planet needs more than ever. Children are not only literally our future, they are also the very incarnation of God's unfolding imagination. Paradoxically, it is up to us to protect and nurture this mystery, and indeed we can do it.

On November 19th internationally acclaimed ecologist Sandra Steingraber spoke in Toronto about her new book, *Having Faith*. It mixes science, poetry, the intimately personal, and the ecological majesty and environmental tragedy of the planet into a seamless masterpiece. It resonates deeply in the soul and strengthens one's resolve to help prevent the world from going to hell and being sacrificed to short-term economic greed.

Quoting a native American midwife, Katsi Cook, Steingraber observes that "a woman's body is the first environment." Describing her own pregnancy, Steingraber writes, "I am an ecologist, which means I spend a lot of time thinking about how living things interact with the environments they inhabit. When I became pregnant... I realized with amazement that I myself had become a habitat. My womb was an inland ocean with a population of one." That womb ocean is a part of planet earth's water and contains not only the vital nutrients the baby requires, but also all the pollutants which endanger fetal development, such as neurotoxic solvents which threaten brain development. Later, breast milk becomes an intolerable compromise between nature's best possible food and the worst possible environmental poisons all women's breast milk now contains. An expert on breast milk, Steingraber recently addressed the United Nations on that world wide escalating crisis and the need give priority to the human right of motherhood over the world's economic dependence on these poisons.

So, what can we do to give birth to and raise healthy children? The books listed at the end of this article are the ones I would have liked to have had when I raised mine. Fortunately, in the 1970s pesticides in food were a lot less than today, and having been raised in India and Europe, I raised my kids on fruit, vegetables and solid European bread. Today, a parent almost has to have a science degree to be able to make good choices when buying food or toys.

If you are planning a baby, the latest research indicates that both parents must avoid for at least 3 months contact with pesticides, solvents, chlorine, tobacco, and alcohol. The father's sperm is also compromised by these toxins such that his children have a measurably higher rate of cancer. The mother must also observe zero-tolerance exposure to neurotoxic heavy metals in pesticides (cadmium—causes birth defects), dentistry (mercury- damages the growing brain and immune system), drinking water (lead—compromises thyroid function and can cause retardation), aluminum (brain function), neurotoxic cosmetics of which nail polish and nail polish remover are the worst followed closely by dark hair dye, and any substances that contain chlorine. It is essential to avoid refined foods containing trans-fatty acids, cut out refined sugar and wheat completely, if possible, and reduce salt intake to avoid toxemia (pregnancy-related high blood pressure and kidney damage).

An article in the November 1999 issue of the *Journal for Integrative Medicine* summarizes what is needed to provide an excellent first environment. Of primary importance are supplementation with essential fatty acids such as Udo's Choice (my favorite) as well as cod liver oil or salmon oil (mercury-free brand). Folic acid supplementation is a must, as our foods—even when organically grown—do not contain enough for the high demands of pregnancy due to depleted soils. Folic acid the single most important supplement for the prevention of spina bifida; the highest rate of neural tube defects are in cultures that eat the least vegetables. Recent research shows that cerebral palsy and Downs' Syndrome, once thought to be genetic (the current cultural myth) are mediated by lack of vitamin C and magnesium, again insufficient in our diets due to soil degradation. The B and E vitamins are equally important, preferably all from natural sources, not synthetic so our cell receptors can absorb these nutrients fully. An organic diet is an absolute, non-negotiable must. Every pesticide is neurotoxic, many pesticides and all hormones found in factory-style grown meats are known to cause birth defects and, being endocrine disrupters, they can cause deformed genitalia, infertility, and many hormonal problems at puberty—all on the rise in the past 20 years.

To avoid low birth weight (implicated in later development of autoimmune diseases), post-partum depression, and toxemia, the mother needs lots of magnesium (citrate) and immediately following birth, some natural source supplementation of progesterone. During labor the blood level of progesterone goes from a maximum required for pregnancy to literally zero in a few hours—the major cause for post partum depression. A new baby does not need a mother so severely compromised.

Babies do not develop the famous blood-brain barrier, which protects the brain from the full impact of environmental toxins, until they are 6 months old. The immune system also grows slowly, triggered into action primarily through mother's milk. During the first year of life vulnerability is greatest to cancer (risen 200% in children since the 1980s) and asthma (risen by 92% since 1982 and directly linked to all petrochemical pollutants and household gas appliances). The growing immune system involves especially bone marrow development, and now we know that DDT also causes blood diseases. Our adopted daughter Arpana died at the age of 15 from such a blood disease. She was born to a family working in the DDT saturated fruit orchards of Goa, India, and was given up for adoption when she developed this blood-transfusion-dependent illness.

Last September a Global Forum on children's environmental health convened in Washington DC. Legislators are beginning to pay attention. Because children's metabolism is different and faster than in adults, they absorb a much larger load of environmental toxins from carpets, dry-cleaned materials chemically treated upholstery, air pollutants, and PCV containing toys which they tend to chew. Greenpeace spearheaded the campaign against PCV in toys. Europe banned PCV in 1998, in North America it is best to inquire from the manufacturer if toys are PCV free—none of the big toy companies are all safe as yet.

Baby mice wrapped in human chlorine-treated diapers die within 2 hours. Babies absorb chlorine through the skin also, but the neurological damage is slower to show, one being ADHD. Chlorine should never be used to wash baby clothes. A perfect home and garden with every sort of bug killer and pesticide is nothing less than the ground zero from which the chronic diseases of life emerge. The occasional cockroach won't harm your baby, but your perfect home and garden will—possibly irreparably.

The next challenge comes from vaccinations and dentistry. The books I am recommending are available in any large library—read and judge for yourself. The concept of vaccination is one of the greatest discoveries in the history of medicine, but then mass production required solving problems of spoilage. Mercury, the most toxic substance known on earth, began to be used as a preservative. Pumped into the still unfolding immune system of children, it has caused, among other horrors, autism to rise 1,500 % in the last 10 years. The largest class action suite ever in the US is currently ongoing against the FDA and vaccine manufacturers who knowingly allowed this "preservative" to be used in vaccines.

As for dentistry, silver/mercury amalgams are absolutely unacceptable. It is highly revealing to read Weston Price's great classic on how dental problems evolved throughout the world and through human evolutionary history. If your children do not receive any refined sugars at all and lots of raw fruits and vegetables, all those dental problems, from cavities to crooked teeth, simply do happen. And then there is fluoride—that byproduct of fertilizers some enterprising fellow persuaded the world we need. It is the major cause of autoimmune diseases. Read the books on fluoride and wake up. Whatever the Dental Association still parrots, fluoride has absolutely nothing to recommend it and does not belong into toothpaste or water. When EPA scientist Yiamouyiannis, presenting the horrid scientific facts about fluoride to the city council of Toronto, was asked what he recommended to be put into the drinking water instead, he fascetiously said "Arsenic, it's 80 times less toxic."

When it comes to children's nutrition, nothing beats Dr. Hoffer's book on the subject. It ought to be in every household. The books by nutritional scientist Simontacchi and investigative reporter Schlosser are as fascinating as a crime novel—except they are truth, not fiction. The scientific facts on the nutritional value of organic food (and the corresponding lack of it on the supermarket shelves) is beyond rational argument. You needn't endure the corporate irrational (PR) rhetoric, but are free to tune out. (For the full scientific information on organic food contact **info@-price-pottenger.org** or **www.price-pottenger.org**.) Yet, even with organic food, it will take a century or more before our soils are what they used to be before pesticides and mono-agriculture were invented. Therefore, kids do need vitamin C and E and mineral supplements (zinc, selenium, magnesium), and good old-fashioned cod liver oil as well.

Other potential minefields are dry-cleaned clothes, toxic laundry detergents and antibiotics. There are "green" dry-cleaners in Toronto now where neurotoxic chemicals are not used. I cured the psoriasis plagued children of my hair dresser by suggesting she stop using supermarket powdered laundry detergent and switch to a liquid plant based one, use hydrogen peroxide for bleach and vinegar as water softener. Her kids had been on cortisone creams all their lives—their skin cleared up in 2 weeks. Antibiotics are more problematic. Most of the time they are avoidable. Yet, my son Manu died at age 23, having had 4 open-heart operation in his short life due to heart damage from an untreated strep throat infection as a six year old orphan in the slums of Calcutta. That's the sort of situation where antibiotics would have prevented heart disease. Being too weary of them is causing a rise in strep throat infections (and subsequent preventable heart disease) that go untreated.

We now have the pleasure of watching three of my grandchildren grow up as they live in the same house with us. They are 5, 7 and 9 and thriving in this most difficult time. They have so far escaped the addiction treadmill of the fast-food world, the junk food routine, and the mind-numbing world of TV. They grew up breast-fed till age 3 and they eat only organic food. Miranda, aged 9 (going on 40 some days) observes about fast food stuffs, "How can people eat this crap!" They also never watch TV. Yes—never. They own about a hundred videos and many more books than that. Their imagination gathers up all that's in the house in an endless stream of entertainment. You never know what they are when you walk in the house: a witch, a dragon, a princess, Harry Potter, or a goblin. They are never bored, they make castles out of cardboard boxes, they draw dragons and princesses on my files if I don't interfere, and they abscond with my jewelry and kitchen utensils to enact their stories. Rivaling Henry VIII, the youngest has wedded and divorced to wed again her giant stuffed monkey, two teddy bears, one frog, and a panther in enormous ceremonies involving the whole household. Their idea of a treat is going shopping to the bookstore and on long walks with grandpa and the dogs when behind every tree is the entrance to a magic kingdom. They absolutely do not like Coca-Cola—it's no battle to keep the junk out of their diet.

Of course, they love ice cream, complete with toxic refined sugar. Five-year old Malhar informed me the other day, "A little bit of toscit (toxic) is good for you." This is a very dangerous world, but it is possible to live and thrive in. The terrible and the nurturing make up the totality of life. Merry Christmas!

Sources and Resources

L.M. Bower, *The Healthy Household: Complete Guide for Creating a Healthy Indoor Environment*, 1995, Healthy House Institute, 430 North Sewell Road, Bloomington, IN, 47408, USA

H. Coulter, *A Shot In The Dark: Why the P in the DPT vaccination may be hazardous to your child's health*, Avery, 1991

C. Dean, MD, *Complementary Natural Prescriptions for Common Ailments*, 1994, Keats

C. Diodati, *Immunization: History, Ethics, Law and Health*, Integral Aspects Inc. 1999

N. Hallaway & Z. Strauts, MD, *Turning Lead Into Gold: How Heavy Metal Poisoning Can Affect Your Child and How To Prevent and Treat It*, New Star Books 1995

Hoffer, MD, *Dr. Hoffer's ABC of Natural Nutrition for Children*, 1999, Quarry Health Books

M. R. Lyon, MD, *Healing the Hyperactive Brain*, 2000, Focused Publishing, Calgary

Rapp, MD, *Is This Your Child?*, 1999, Quill William Morrow, New York (national bestseller)

Rapp, MD, *Is This Your Child's World?*, 1996, Bantam, New York

Rona, *Natural Alternatives to Vaccination*, Alive Books, Burnaby BC, 2001

Sensible Life Products, **www.controlgerms.com**

Yiamouyiannis, *Fluoride: How to Recognize and Avoid the Devastating Effects of Fluoride*, Health Action Press, 1993

Walker, *Elements of Danger: Protect Yourself Against the Hazards of Modern Dentistry*, Hampton Roads 2000

Fallon, *Nourishing Traditions: The Cookbook that Challenges the Politically Correct Nutrition*, 1999, New Trends Publishing Inc., Washington DC (call 877-707-1776)

M. Katzen, *The Enchanted Broccoli Forest*, 1995, The Speed Press, Berkeley, California

Colborn, *Our Stolen Future*, 1997, Penguin

G. Gardner & B. Halweil, *Underfed and Overfed: The Global Epidemic of Malnutrition*, Worldwatch Paper No. 150, World Resources Institute, Washington DC, 2000

Price, *Nutrition and Physical Degeneration*, 50th anniversary edition, 1989, Keats

Randolph, MD, *An Alternative Approach to Allergies*, 1990, Harper Collins

D.G.Rosenberg, *Early Exposures: Children's Health and the Environment*, forthcoming video from Women's Healthy Environments Network, 416-928-0880, or when@web.ca

Schlosser, *Fast Food Nation: The Dark Side of the All-American Meal*, 2001, Houghton Mifflin (New York Times Bestseller)

Simontacchi, *The Crazy Makers: How the Food Industry is Destroying our Brains and Harming Our Children*, 2000, Tarcher Putnam

S. Steingraber, *Having Faith: An Ecologist's Journey Into Motherhood*, Perseus, 2001

C. Williams, *Terminus Brain: The Environmental Threats to Human Intelligence*, Cassell, 1997

A Primer on Kids' Health

Vitality Magazine December 2003

Time present and time past
Are both perhaps present in time future,
And time future contained in time past.

T.S. Eliot, *Burnt Norton*

At Christmas time we celebrate the birth of a Divine Child—who never grows up. If he did, the cycle of creation and the pageant of evolution would end. Contemplating the future of our children in the face of our current environmental problems, a crib in a manger two thousand years ago in Roman-occupied Israel seems like an excellent deal compared to the world into which children are born now.

Some years ago, at a conference, a scientist presented a computer model showing that if current trends of pollution continue, the human race would go extinct in about 500 years (about 1,500 generations). The process would be as in the currently threatened loon: the eggs can't hatch, and when they do, the creature is genetically compromised and can't survive long enough to reproduce. Indeed, in Europe about 25% of people under the age of 25 are infertile, and human sperm count is 50% down since the early 1960s—following which pesticides and synthetic chemicals began to saturate air, water, soil, food and medicines, almost always detrimentally.

Children comprise 30% of the world's population and 100% of humanity's future. The World Health Organization informs us that more than 40% of the total global burden of disease, known to be caused by environmental factors, is borne by the world's children under the age of five (**www.who.int** 2002 WHO fact sheet). This statistic does not include the effect of environmental toxins on the developing fetus and young children in determining the onset of chronic disease later in life. Studying this research curiously makes it hard to find the exact boundaries between past, present and future; they are inextricably intertwined, and causes and effects form a circle. This highlights the very essence of children.

Margaret Somerville of McGill University's Centre for Medicine, Ethics and Law observed in her famous book, *The Ethical Canary: Science, Society and the Human Spirit* (2001), that science, law, the economy, and social policy do not travel at the same speed because each has its own priorities which develop from different experiences. "Nature time" travels at speeds generally at odds with human concerns, but "nature time" is ultimately in charge. Nature moves at geological speeds of no personal relevance to human concerns, as well as at rapid biological speeds totally unpredictable and potentially disastrous when humans disregard ecological imperatives and genetic dynamics. "Business time" (which wants profits and growth in quarterly annual installments), "science time" (which wants no limits set to its curiosity), and "social policy time" (which always reacts after the fact) are all on a collision course with "nature time" which cares nothing for profit and theoretical curiosity and is unforgiving of tardy social policy. All it cares for is life itself. The Divine Child teaches us to adjust our priorities.

One can always startle doctors, politicians and the general public with the information that all diseases have a known history. The medical profession is astonished because this means there must have been a cause for everything and so-called "idiopathic" diseases are a myth. Politicians understand that rational public health policies are in theory possible. The anthropology of disease (my academic specialty before I climbed on this soap box of medical science writing) is the other side of a coin which reads "The Precautionary Principle".

This principle, first enunciated in the 1970s when it became part of Germany's environmental laws, asserts in its 1992 Earth Summit formulation: "Where there are threats of serious or irreversible damage, lack of full scientific certainty shall not be used as reason for postponing cost-effective measures to prevent environmental degradation." For ecologist Sandra Steingraber this is what "prompts us to buckle seat belts, get out of the pool when lightning flashes, and throw away mysterious leftovers discovered in the back of the refrigerator. It's why we keep plastic bags and book matches away from young children." Current knowledge of how disease is caused and physical degeneration evolves is so vast, we have all we need to justify the Precautionary Principle.

The classic 1989 study by Mark Nathan Cohen, *Health And The Rise of Civilization*, provides a magisterial survey of the evolution and origins of infectious disease to chronic illnesses. That history spans about 2 million years of unconscious behavior that had unknowable detrimental effects that remained with us until today. Some 100,000 years ago the Neanderthals had no way of knowing that their diet was the cause of the appearance of arthritis. The first experiments with agriculture 10,000 years ago reduced food diversity to reliance on just a few staples resulting in those foods becoming less nutritious through domestication and osteoporosis followed. The trend to living in villages, instead of roaming the earth, gave cancer and all infectious disease a chance to evolve.

The myth of the Garden of Eden is usefully turned on its head: we unknowingly have almost destroyed that garden, but we now know how to create it. For example, in the recent past we have the astounding results of three lines of research. First, the work of the dentist Weston A. Price in the 1930s compared the development of teeth and facial bone structure over several generations in peoples all over the world by looking at their diets. This study is generally considered the beginning of nutritional medicine as a science. Dr. Price's research identified for the first time what constitutes essential nutrients in the diets of those "primitives" who were totally healthy. He also showed (in the 1930s before pesticides!) that all those societies which had adopted the refined carbohydrate diet (today called SAD—Standard American Diet) showed high prevalence of bad teeth and those chronic illnesses which we now conveniently call "idiopathic", or worse: genetic. They never were part of the genetic program—now they are. We put them there.

The second study was begun in 1983 by Cornell University and lasted 25 years. It compared the disease burden of the Chinese and American peoples based on a large number of measures, most of them nutritional (**www.new-centurynutrition.com**). The results show that the "diseases of affluence" are cancer, leukemia, diabetes, and coronary disease—all based on nutrients refined out of the food. The "diseases of poverty" are infectious diseases, tuberculosis, and parasites due to malnutrition caused by over-all caloric and protein reduction. As in the earlier research of Dr. Price, the results also show that when food was adequate, health depends on the same set of essential nutrients, and disease is associated with our denatured SAD (see also monograph no. 150 from **www.worldwatch.org**).

Finally, we need to consider a conference held this May at the Mount Sinai School of Medicine in New York co-hosted by the US Environmental Protection Agency. Researchers examined the so-called "Barker Hypothesis" named after a British physician who noticed that "exposures and risk factors encountered early in life can predispose an individual to the development of disease later in life" chief among them Parkinson's, cancer and Alzheimer's (see **www.som.soton.ac.uk/research/foad/barker.asp**). These "are now thought to arise through a series of stages that require years and even decades to evolve." Just as toxicology now is based on the understanding that small, frequent amounts of a toxin will have large, unpredictable, often irreversible effects later on, so too developmental phases provide windows of opportunity for disease and genetic defects.

While normal aging involves some inevitable loss of brain cells, when a fetus or a young child is exposed to environmental neurotoxins (e.g. pesticides, solvents) "silent damage is inflicted" on the brain which during normal aging becomes expressed and much later causes overwhelming damage. The development of Parkinson's depends on "postnatal exposures to pesticides alone" which diminish the number of neurons (messenger molecules) that maintain appropriate levels of dopamine responsible for all fine-motor movement. If re-exposed later in life to even low levels of pesticides, the entire dopamine production runs down. Think about that the next time your toddler walks with you through a park or accompanies you while spraying the roses. Other presentations showed the same process at work in predisposing children to heart disease through the mother's exposure to various toxins in the environment and her diet. The overall conclusion was that environmental toxins "induce effects that can be trans-generational" because "exposure to environmental agents in the womb can alter gene expression in the developing fetus". (See **www.niehs.nih.gov/dert/home.htm**).

The power the past has over the present suggests that "a pill for every ill" is a totally inappropriate paradigm for the practice of medicine, as Dr. Stephen Davis, the editor of the *Journal of Nutritional and Environmental Medicine* (no. 5, 1995) observed. Health and disease are dependent upon time, and genetic expression is not a fixed pre-determined program, but is exquisitely dependent on the right protection and the right nutrients at the right time.

If there are to be children 500 years from now, the information medical science provides today demands action. The Sept. 12, 2003, article by Hauser et al in *Environmental Health Perspectives* shows that the chlorine's damaging effect starts with the sperm. Similarly, maternal exposure to DDT (banned in North America since the 1970s, but part of our diet through foods coming from Asia and Africa) continues its damaging effect across generations by causing neurological damage to the offspring of their daughters. A fetus exposed via the mother to plasticizers (phthalates) can due to its estrogenic effect shorten pregnancy, thereby priming the low-weight premature baby to various known health risks throughout life (*EHP* Nov. 14, 2003).

Commercial flame retardants used in electric appliances and building materials are highly carcinogenic and found in the breast milk of North American women at a 37% higher rate than anywhere else—thereby setting up the nursing child for cancer later in life (both from **www.ehpnet1. niehs.nih.gov/docs/2003**). Because children's immune systems mature over the first few years, exposure to all pesticides adversely affects that development and sets them up for all kinds of immune diseases later on (World Resources Institute study by R. Repetto, 2000).

What all of this does to the development of the brain is graphically illustrated by the drawings of children studied by Elizabeth Guillette over two decades. She observed the development of Mexican children born and raised in a village where pesticides were used liberally and compared them with children in a foothills area where no pesticides were ever used. The perceptual and mental skills of the valley children not only lagged dramatically behind those of the foothills children, but were beyond repair (EHP June 1998).

This study has staggering implications for the future of humanity, as Dr. Landrigan at the above-mentioned conference pointed out: even a 5 point shift in the average IQ of a population (via pre-natal exposure to pesticides) almost doubles the number of retarded children and cuts in half the number of gifted ones. But repair of such generational damage appears to be possible over time. Nature is stubbornly creative and produces excellence if we don't interfere: In a 10 year study on many generations of cats, Dr. Pottenger showed in the 1930s the following: healthy cats fed a diet similar to our SAD produced offspring with chronic illnesses in the second generation; the third generation was mostly infertile. However, those few who were able to reproduce, had perfectly healthy cats by the third generation—if all three generations had a nutrient-rich diet.

So what can we do? We have choices and we have the knowledge to make good ones. Consider the results of a National Institutes of Health study (EHP Oct. 31, 2002) showing that by just feeding children organic food, all those neurotoxic and carcinogenic pesticides were dramatically reduced in body fluids and tissues. "Honey, let me have that match box" should become "Honey, eat this organic apple and let's chuck that super market toxic one."

- If you are planning on having a baby, take plenty of folic acid, stay away from pesticides, eat organic. It prevents not only neural tube defects, but also childhood cancer by conferring protective developmental potential (*Medical Post* Nov. 4, 2003).
- Avoid carcinogenic benzene-containing perfumed toilet articles, and ensure that toothpaste does not contain neurotoxic and thyroid-damaging fluoride and phenols.
- Use cornstarch-based powders, vinegar in the laundry instead of artificial softeners and fresheners (all of which contain neurotoxic additives!).
- Baby food is now available made from organics, bottled in glass instead of plastic, fortified with essential fatty acids and B vitamins, devoid of hydrogenated vegetable oils—and keep that diet up for life.
- Protect against future diabetes by cutting out the colas and the refined sugars—as the World Health Organization guidelines of April 2003 urge.

- Make sure your dentist does not put carcinogenic and neurotoxic mercury amalgam into your child's mouth—have them removed if they are in there!
- Demand your doctor uses single-dose vaccines free of mercury and antibiotic preservatives. They are now available.
- Get radical: organize mothers into making the school environment safe from toxic chemicals (for practical tools see **www.epa.gov/iag/schools**).

Life survives our most enormous stupidities, misjudgments, and appalling acts of arrogance—at a horrendous cost, yet unstoppably so. We may take comfort in Nature's determined intelligence. The great 19th century religious poet Gerrard Manley Hopkins put it best: "And for all this, nature's never spent/ There lives the dearest freshness deep down in things…Because the Holy Ghost over the bent world broods with warm breast and ah! bright wings."

Sources and Resources

Alison, K. & Raymond, K. *How To Stay Healthy and Still Eat Chocolate*. Artemis, 2002
Breiner, M. DDS. *Whole Body Dentistry*, Quantum Health Press, 1999
Breggin, P. MD. *Talking Back to Ritalin*, Common Courage, 1998
Autism, neurological disorders and vaccines: **http://www.autismcanada.org/home.htm**
Nutrition: **www.PRICE-POTTENGER.org** or 619-462-7600
Doctors against junk-food: **http://www.pcrm.org**
To fight pesticide use: ECO PRAXIS: Research and Resources Center. 905-465-0667 or **epi@web.net**
On fluoride: **www.fluoride.org** for an information package to fight your local municipality with **www.hans.org** or call 604-435-0512

Autism—Causes Known and Preventable Possible Cures

Vitality Magazine May 2003

Some thirty years ago we had a foster child who was profoundly autistic. She came to us on an emergency basis from an orphanage in India. Her body was covered in scars that had been made by cigarettes. At that time, the famous Austrian psychiatrist Bruno Bettelheim had shown that it was sometimes possible to cure autistic children, provided the brain was not damaged. I took training at his famous Orthogenic School in Chicago in order to help her, but she had banged her head for years against cement floors, thereby causing too much brain damage. The view Bettelheim had, that autism is caused by extreme neglect or abuse at a very early age, seemed to make sense in Melanie's case. However, given the brain damage in her situation, the escalating anxiety in her was unstoppable, even with drugs, until the damage she did to herself was so terrible, only an institution could handle her.

It was a horrific, soul-numbing experience to observe autism at its worst unfold. It was then beyond imagining that the causes of, leave alone cures for, this horrible affliction could ever be known. Yet, this has come to pass: on June 21 and 22 the Autism Canada Foundation is hosting a conference for parents of autistic children in Toronto at which international experts on autism are offering real hope and real solutions.

History

Autism was first described in the 1940s. Often mental retardation is involved, but so-called "idiot savants" like Dustin Hoffman's character in *Rainman,* are also among them. Autistics cannot relate or communicate, are often self-destructive, suffer from night blindness, usually are extreme in their inability to pay attention or carry out a task, and are fixated on repetitive rituals. When these children were first observed, it was noted that most were born to educated and more affluent families which gave rise to then prevalent psychoanalytic views that these kids had become autistic due to emotional neglect (today, the more likely explanation is that those families were able to afford vaccines and mercury-amalgam dental care).

The terrible grain of truth came from the meticulously documented psychiatric information on victims of Nazi concentration camps. Child psychiatrist Dr. Bettelheim had observed as a prisoner in Auschwitz how severely abused people, who had given up all hope, became classic autistics. Today, we make sense out of this observation because medicine and psychiatry now knows that identical syndromes can be produced by emotional as well as chemical and biochemical causes; the one-disease-once-cause theory is antique.

When he later opened his practice in Chicago he researched case histories of institutionalized autistic children. Wherever he found serious neglect and physical abuse, he proceeded to remove them from their mental hospitals and treated them in a child-friendly environment with painstaking care. For some of them it worked dramatically. One of those kids lost on a backward of a mental institution, whom Dr. Bettelheim rescued, later became a psychiatrist and, for some years, the director of the Orthogenic School and helped restore many more such children.

Dr. Bettelheim's observation that autism can indeed stem from severe and prolonged emotional stress, today is part of psycho-neuroimmunology. The spectacular recovery of Barry Neil Kaufman's autistic son made through a program of intensive emotional support is documented in his wonderful book *Son Rise*. Equally astounding is the fabulous autobiography of the autistic Donna Williams, *Nobody Nowhere*; her treatment combined intensive psychotherapy to overcome her childhood abuse—with specific vitamins found to be lacking in her due to an apparently inborn inability to maintain sufficient levels.

Both cases show how treating mind and body can heal both, now that a great shift in medical theory has developed over the past 50 years, with the boundaries between body and mind no longer absolute, as they were thought to be since antiquity. Nothing is simple anymore in medicine. Just as a headache can be caused by a blow to the head, it can also come from a brain tumor, a drug reaction or emotional stress, and many more possible causes.

Causes

Today, autism is a catastrophic epidemic with an increase of 1,500% in the UK in the last decade. In California one in 150 children is autistic—a 54% increase in just 2001/2! The primary causes of autism known to come from vaccines, maternal overexposure to heavy metals and antibiotics, heavy metals from industry pollution of the air and water, and the chemicals used in the electronics industry. Significantly, the first cases of autism were described in the US shortly after the vaccines for whopping cough were introduced in the 1940s.

The sudden increase in the UK began with the introduction in 1990 of the triple vaccine MMR against mumps, measles and rubella. In California, the greatest increase is clustered in Silicon Valley where people are exposed to more than 700 chemicals, almost all of which are neurotoxic, especially to newborn babies with immature immune systems. (**www.secretsofsiliconva lley.org**)

At day 1 a child is automatically given a hepatitis B shot containing 12 micrograms of mercury—30 times the safe level set by the World Health Organization. By age four months, a second hepatitis B shot and the DPTP vaccination (against diphtheria, whooping cough, tetanus and polio) give your child 60 times the safe limit of mercury in addition to the first assault. The shot given at age six months contains mercury at 78 times the safe limit. By the time you get to the MMR vaccine, your child gets another 31 times the safe amount of mercury; if given as an intramuscular shot the toxicity of mercury is increased by an additional 30 times because it crosses the blood-brain barrier at once. By age 2 your child has been given at least 237 micrograms of mercury. The EPA recognizes as safe only a one-time exposure to 0.1 microgram! According to the best available evidence in the mainstream literature, autism becomes an extremely high risk at levels of merely 62 micrograms of mercury.

Unlike the *slow* assault of the developing fetus' brain through pesticides in the mother's blood stream and interstitial fluids, autism appears to be brought on by the *sudden* assault on the new baby by heavy metals—especially mercury, cadmium, and lead—used as preservatives in vaccines which then cause inflammation of the brain and dysregulate also gastro-intestinal and immune function and development. The preservative used in standard vaccines, thimerosal, contains mercury. Vaccine expert Dr. Neal Halsey at Johns Hopkins Medical School told the FDA and the public in January that this preservative was *accidentally tripled* when the vaccines for mumps, measles and rubella were made into a single combination (MMR). McGill University's epidemiologists Dr. Walter Spitzer and Dr. Victor Goldbloom urged the Quebec government to study this connection seriously, as now one in 300 children in Quebec is autistic (*Medical Post* April 17, 2001).

Genetic theories are of no help. Genes are always involved in every living process, but nothing is fixed in life. A BBC program of July 17, 2002, pointed out that with nine children per day being diagnosed as autistic, a genetic explanation becomes absurd. Epidemics are *always,* and by definition, environmentally mediated events. Conversely, genes are not only vulnerable to toxic insult, but also respond to curative intervention. Nothing is fixed in nature and that is the message of hope.

Autism expert Dr. Mary Norfleet Megson in testimony on April 6, 2000, before a US congressional committee explained how at least *one* genetic interaction with environmental toxins causes autism. When a baby is given the MMR vaccine at 15 months and the DPT at 18 months the mercury-based preservative "causes uncontrolled cell-growth differentiation of the G Alpha signals in the G proteins which upgrade and downgrade signals in sensory organs that regulate touch, taste, smell, hearing and vision"—all classic deficiencies in autism.

The child sees "only color and shape, except for a box in the middle of their visual field. Children try to make sense of the world by lining up toys, sorting by color. Their avoidance of eye contact is an attempt to get light to land off center in the retina where they have some normal visual function;

their mother's touch feels like sandpaper on their skin. Common sounds become like nails scraped on a blackboard."

Another well understood path to autism proceeds by mercury causing encephalitis and then general inflammation which becomes chronic and deregulates several bodily systems. Many autistic children also are found to have some fixated ("locked") cranial bones, presumably also due to developmental disruptions. These kids bang their heads with incredible force, causing outright brain damage, in an effort to loosen up the tension inside.

Politics

In 1998 one of the world's leading medical journals, Britain's *Lancet*, was the first to take seriously the vaccination connection in a study written by Dr. Andrew Wakefield of the medical school of London's Royal Free and University College. He proposed identifying autism as an autoimmune illness and implicated primarily vaccines as the cause (*Medical Post*, May 8, 2001). Harvard Medical School agreed, and by February of this year proposed, on the basis of their own research as well as Wakefield's, that treatment protocols should address autism as a brain-gut disease because, among other things, harmful gut bacteria such as *candida* literally thrive in a mercury-saturated environment and join forces with that heavy metal in escalating neurotoxicity.

That hit the pharmaceutical giants GlaxoSmithKline, Johnson & Johnson, Wyeth and Eli Lilly like a bad dream. Eli Lilly, also the world's leading producer of biological warfare materials, has the corner on vaccine production. In March 2002, when class-action suits by parents of children made autistic by vaccines, began to be registered throughout the US, the law firm Waters & Kraus introduced in court evidence showing that Eli Lilly knew since the 1930s, when vaccines began to be developed, that the use of mercury as a preservative was bad news especially for children.

It comes as no surprise, that Dr. Wakefield found himself suddenly fired because his "research was no longer in line with [his employers'] strategy"— understandably so, as that university is heavily financially supported by those pharmaceutical giants. However, higher powers must have been looking out for autistic children, and Dr. Wakefield was immediately hired by Dr. Jeff Bradstreet at the International Child Development Resource Center in Florida. You can meet and hear Dr. Bradstreet, parent to an autistic child himself, this June. It is Wakefield's, Bradstreet's and other researchers whose successful treatment of autism you can learn about directly at this conference designed for parents.

Unable to stop the research community from pursing the vaccine connection, Eli Lilly's CEO, a personal friend of President George W. Bush,
decided a bigger gun was needed. Calculations had shown that if even a small
number of the currently registered class action suits succeeded, the payments
then ordered could actually exceed Lilly's current net worth. President Bush
obligingly tacked on to the first Homeland Security Act—a bill supposedly
focused on protection from terrorism—a little clause which immunized
(pardon the pun) Lilly from any payouts exceeding $ 250,000. Republican
congressman Dan Burton is the grandfather of a child made autistic by
MMR vaccine. He had chaired the hearings at which Dr. Wakefield and Dr.
Megson had testified. Burton noticed the trick and all hell broke loose. The
tacked-on rider went down in flames.

A twist to the politics of medicine came from Prime Minister Tony Blair.
In February 2002 he exhorted his fellow Brits not to turn away from "lifesaving vaccines"—as is the case by now in unprecedented numbers. When
asked if he had permitted his 20-months old son to be vaccinated, Blair
refused to answer, citing the need for privacy.

The ongoing usual skullduggery includes vaccine manufacturers refusing
to share raw data with medical scientists investigating their products, protocols doctored by obliging industry scientists to achieve results contradicting
Wakefield's studies, and the usual conflict of interest scene: the US government's Center for Disease Control is both charged with promoting vaccine
use as well as evaluating their safety. (*Medical Post,* May 8, 2001). However,
some of the CDC scientists leaked the secret report on the relationship
between vaccines and autism to the public. Visit **www.mercola.com**. This
report shows, that not only is the mercury preservative part of the problem,
but vaccination itself may be equally serious an assault on a baby's immature
immune system, even without any preservatives.

The latest typical (to my mind criminal) example of medical politics
comes from the fact that a study involving some 6,000 children supposedly
showed that there is no risk of autism from vaccines—it was financed (you
guessed it) by the industry. The media reported this widely. However, a joint
European study (a Danish university and UK's Cambridge University)
involving more than half a million children showed that the risk of vaccines
increased the chances of autism by a whopping 850%. That was not industry-funded and not reported. Read all about it on the excellent website
www.wddty.co.uk.

Prevention and Cure

Prevention is easy. Only vaccinate your child if absolutely necessary, do so only when your child is older (over the age of 2), and insist on *single-dose preservative-free* vaccines—they exist! Phone Health Canada and tell them what you want. The law guarantees you the right to informed consent and safety from harm. The notion is absurd that we need to vaccinate the population till the end of time against the 19th century diseases modern hygiene more than vaccination programs brought under control.

The tests needed to treat autism have been developed and are exceedingly refined. They allow the doctor to assess toxicity levels, identify the toxins involved, and what the nutritional imbalances are as a result of this assault. Hair analysis provides long-term information; biological terrain and mineralization assessments, as well as fecal, blood and urine analyses, show current processes in your child's body. The PH balance tests show how alkaline or acidic the body is and allow one to determine which foods to avoid or increase. Additionally, due to the fact that autism is a gut-brain illness, many allergies need to be identified; these allergies developed due to the assault on the immature immune system by the mercury preservative.

Treatment requires removal of the toxins which have accumulated and can never be metabolized, while at the same time doing the needful to protect the organs of elimination (kidneys especially) as the toxins begin to be eliminated. International protocols have been worked out for these procedures, such as the DAN protocol ("Defeat Autism Now"). In most cases the use of the hormone secretin is essential to achieve improvement and outright cures at the level of about 50%. All of this is available through Canadian labs and physicians. How I wish I could turn back time and give Melanie what this conference is sure to offer.

Sources and Resources

Dr. J. Krop's, 2003 book *Healing The Planet One Patient At A Time* contains the detoxification protocols which you can take to your doctor to enable him or her to treat an autistic child; available through Kos Publications 519-927-1049 or any book store.

Most useful website: **www.wddty.co.uk** (stands for "what doctors don't tell you")

Autism Canada Foundation, P.O. Box 1998, Burlington, Ontario, L7R 4L8, 905-332-4766, or 905-331-4480 and at **www.autismcanada.org** : for audiotapes of the conference held on June 21-22, 2003. Dr. J. Bradstreet's institute can be reached via **www.icdrc.org** Also visit **www.autismresearchinstitute.com**

DG Medical Corporation in London, Ontario, carries an excellent oral detox system for heavy metals. Call: 1-866-560-3834

International Center for Metabolic Testing in Ottawa provides the nutritional status, toxic load and urine peptide tests for doctors treating autistic children according to the protocols discussed in this article. Call for info and names of doctors 1-888-591-4124

For doctors trained to work with autistic children in Canada and the USA call American Academy of Environmental Medicine 316-684-5500, visit **www.AAEM.com**

The Holistic Alternative provides access to oral detox methods and especially all the tests discussed in this article: 416-318-8871

For up-to-date information on vaccine damage visit **www.909shot.com** and join the free e-mail list of the National Vaccine Information Center **News@909shot.com**

Best source for comprehensive overview of all issues relating to autism is **www.mercola.com**

Bettelheim, B., *Surviving*, Vintage Books, 1980

Coulter, H.L. & Fisher, B.L., *A Shot In The Dark*, Avery, 1991

Cave, S., MD, *What Your Doctor May Not Tell You About Children's Vaccinations*, Warner, 2001

DeVita, C., "Attention Deficit Disorders, Autism, and Heavy Metal Toxicity", *Whole Life Expo* lecture Nov. 2002; order through Audiotree 905-665-9000

Kaufman, B.N., *Son Rise*, Warner Books, 1976

Williams, D., *Nobody Nowhere: Autobiography of an Autistic*, Doubleday, 1992

Update October 2004: *On April 8th the **United States Senate** voted unanimously to instruct the Department of Health to seek ways and means immediately to stop the use of mercury or any other potentially harmful preservatives from being used in vaccines. The Senators who initiated this bill have children who became autistic when given their MMR vaccinations. **California**'s Governor Arnold Schwarzenegger signed a bill in September 2004 which orders the elimination of all heavy metals and other neurotoxic substances from vaccines, and both President Bush and Democratic candidate John Kerry have come out against mercury-preserved vaccines. The **British Government** has initiated a major university-based scientific investigation into the autism-vaccine connection involving tens of thousands of children. Consult the websites given below for updates on all of the above. A large international scientific conference on autism and its causes and treatment options is taking place in Toronto November 10— 12 this year. The proceedings can be obtained on audio cassette or CD ROM through 416-504-4500.*

5

The Public Interest

Who is in Charge of Modern Medicine?

Vitality September 2002

The International Conference of Medical Regulators took place in Toronto June 15-18, and those charged with maintaining medical standards throughout the world attended in large numbers. While most of the participants appeared to be stereotypical administrators—low-key, burdened, mildly bored—their presentations were shocking to the point of making my pulse race. This was a post mortem on medicine and a collective funeral dirge for what was once known as values: ethics, trust, professional honor, integrity, altruism—all that upon which the science and practice of medicine depend. I was the fly on the wall hearing what none of them want shouted from the rooftops.

My request for a media pass came with the comment that this was the first time the press would be allowed in. As it turned out, I was the only media person. No press releases had been sent out. This crowd (about whose Canadian members' crimes against patients and doctors I have written frequently—see *Glasnost Report* in this section below) does not like publicity. I suppose, they didn't want to get caught saying no to a journalist who *asked* for a pass, but they sure weren't about to invite them *all* in! Since none of the presenters knew a reporter was present, they held their dismal wake without restraint and let it all hang out.

The themes of the conference sessions were *Secrecy* and its resultant betrayal of the public interest; *Continuing Medical Education*, the lack thereof as doctors go on automatic pilot when leaving medical school; *Corruption* through conflicts of interest with the corporate sector and government interests, also bound to corporate priorities; *Research Misconduct* such as ignoring human rights of patients and fudging data; and finally: Who Regulates the Regulators? Apparently nobody, which is why everybody complained that nobody trusts the regulatory system anymore. These were the *actual* session headings and are not my nasty interpretation of them. The last speaker, MPP

Thomas Mulcair from Quebec urged the regulators to deal with all of the above with integrity "*before* the TV cameras of W5 and the microphone of investigative journalists are in your faces".

We ought to be thankful regulators admit, when they are amongst themselves, that they have made a royal mess. By contrast, their publications are insufferable spin. The College of Physicians and Surgeon of Ontario (the conference's host), for example, publish their bi-monthly glossy *Members' Dialogue* referred to by many members as "Member's Monologue" and "Members' Pravda", because of its similarity to the former Soviet Union's national newspaper.

Speaking of secrecy—the first day of the event I arrived exactly on time only to be informed that all of Day 1 was held "in camera" and I was only allowed to attend the following days' events. That first day's presentations were "Regional Reports on Current Issues and Trends in Medical Regulation" and constituted a survey of Canada, USA, Europe, Africa, Asia/Pacific and the Middle East. The revelations of the next three days, which I was permitted to attend, were such that I sincerely hope the first day's educational session did them a world of good.

History

The attempt to regulate medical practice goes back to the earliest known laws, the Code of Hammurabi, written on stone tablets in cuneiform script some 4,000 years ago in ancient Mesopotamia, now Iraq. It prescribes nasty penalties for doctors whose patients had bad outcomes—not very encouraging for research, so unsurprisingly the Middle East remained a medical backwater for thousands of years. On the other hand, in ancient Egypt and Greece, were medicine had divine status and doctors were bound by religious ideals, medical science made the greatest strides from which we are still learning today. The same is true for China.

In the west, legislative regulation and administration became serious in 1511 when England's parliament passed the first regulatory laws and founded the Royal College of Physicians in 1518. In our hemisphere, the College of Physicians of Upper Canada came about in the 1850s, and Texas was the first in the US to have a medical regulatory body in 1873. The US Supreme Court in 1888 ruled that doctors had to have uniform, specified qualifications before they could be let loose on people. Today, self-regulation of the medical profession is legally a privilege granted by the government but also anchored in law.

The need for verifiable, standardized qualifications became necessary as scientific medicine and surgery were emerging alongside superstition of the most deadly kind as well as ancient medicine with a proven track record of millennia. However, when order is imposed, power politics takes over as well. For example, in Canada, medical regulation has always been associated with a policy of "restricted entry", as Canadian historian Hamowy observes. In Ontario Jews and Eastern Europeans were unable to join the CPSO until the 1960s. (Today doctors risk excommunicated by disciplinary trial if they "fail to meet the standard" because they cure people without drugs.) By the late 1960s the drug companies joined the regulatory process—first with genuine wonder drugs like antibiotics, then with the toxic brew designed to control symptoms as well as a huge slice of the world economy. Dr. Philip Hebert of the Clinical Ethics Center at Toronto's Sunnybrook Hospital put it bluntly in his conference presentation by sadly pointing out that now we have a "new ethos" for which "altruism is a thing of the past" and "medicine has become just another money-making enterprise" as business and politics "de-professionalizes" them.

The Current Mess

There are three main areas in which medical regulation has failed to live up to its mandate: 1. Protecting bad apples, i.e. doctors who are important to insurance and drug companies or are just plain incompetent and get away literally with murder. 2. Witch hunts against innovative doctors or those who don't get their information from drug company reps, but through primary biological research, and who have developed replicable and biochemically based cures, not management strategies, for cancer, asthma, and chronic diseases. 3. Turning a blind eye to rotten science and conflicts of interests. The difference between the first area mentioned and this third one is, that the first one is active participation in corruption, while the third one is just ordinary neglect. All three areas surfaced at the conference as topics of discussion in excellent presentations by Drs. Richard and Sylvia Cruess of McGill University, the UK's Dr. Kerry Breen of Australia.

Medical regulators all over the world are reeling from the impact of huge disasters. One UK speaker wondered how one could start preventing "medical Enrons". What profoundly disturbed me was that though these facts were acknowledged, they were discussed in the dispassionate manner of meteorologists enumerating the tornadoes of the last thirty years. These were not "acts of god", as the insurance industry calls natural disasters. These are acts of people, quite ungodly and wholly preventable. I worry, though, that for most attendees it was going to be business as usual. I hope I am wrong.

The UK's Dr. Shipman, now confirmed to have murdered 215 of his patients (after having most of them rewrite their wills in his favor) nearly escaped unnoticed because he was a member in good standing—in spite of the disproportionate number of death certificates this one country doc was signing. Canada's Dr. Nealey did his worst in British Columbia, then in Ontario, went on to the UK and was finally caught—by a patient's relative. All those dead babies in Bristol and Winnipeg wound up being victims of a system that focuses on paper and no longer relates to flesh and blood reality.

Other international scandals involve doctors aiding totalitarian regimes in torture, their unchecked commerce in poor countries with "donor" kidneys and eyes, and in affluent countries (including Canada) involving their patients in drug trials without their knowledge—all of which the regulatory bodies seem not to confront. In some places regulation has become virtually incapacitated. In India, patients' relatives were reported recently to have vented their rage against this rampant corruption in a New Delhi hospital such that a slug fest ensued and everybody wound up as patients in the emergency department, doctors included. For the details on the Canadian regulatory failure, the best sources are the Toronto Star series, "Medical Secrets" available on their web site, and the harrowing accounts collected by Susan B. McIver, a BC coroner, in her recently published *Medical Nightmares—The Human Face of Errors*. For the Canadian Colleges see **www.co llegeofphysicianswatchdog.com**. Its "Glasnost Report", was prepared by 3 medical associations and 6 patient advocacy groups.

In the area of patient relations, the problems range from the lackluster support of the World Health Organization's effort to stop female genital mutilation to actively blocking patients' treatment choice. In Ontario, the CPSO fought to the last moment to stop the December 2000 health freedom legislation, the Kwinter Bill. Inadvertant comic relief was provided by the French. A senior French medical regulator (not present at the conference) was asked by an American medical journalist, how French regulators handle sexual misconduct. The French official asked, "What do you mean?" The reporter said, "Sex with patients." The reply, "For us that's a private matter between the doctor and the patient."

The world's most prestigious science journal, *Nature* (March 28), ran an article entitled "Can you believe what you read?" showing how the editors of the most respected medical journals have had to engage in some fundamental housecleaning because research data too often reflect corporate interests instead of reporting observed facts. It announced two international conferences held this year on conflicts of interest in medicine (Atlanta and Warsaw). On June 27th Nature reported that even medical bioethicists are now "being offered stock board positions, consulting contracts, research grants, and even stock options" by pharmaceutical companies—and they accept these goodies! The former editor of the *New England Journal of Medicine*, Marcia Angell, justly famous for her fearless scrutiny of conflicts of interest in medicine, now works closely with the Center for Science in the Public Interest (**www.csip.org**).

An example of the third area of concern happened here in the 1990s. When Health Canada's scientists, led by Dr. Shiv Chopra, asked for input from the Canadian Colleges on what they thought about the impact of bovine growth hormone on human health, they responded, it was fine. Their response was based on no scientific data whatsoever, and when Dr. Chopra and colleagues, following a Senate inquiry, succeeded in banning BGH, the Colleges remained unconcerned at having rubber stamped a carcinogen and endocrine disrupter, now also forbidden in Europe.

Why would regulators suppress good medicine? Perhaps because their council's non-elected members not only represent the pharmaceutical and insurance industries as "stake holders", but also sit the discipline committee where they can select their perceived enemies? Or because even the elected members and the executive are, through their university jobs and research grants, may serve agendas other than patients' needs? More than 80% of all Canadian doctors have financial ties to the industry. Such interests are not served by doctors whose diagnoses implicate that industry's products as causes (e.g. cancer-causing pesticides are made by pharmaceutical companies). The treatments of these doctors, scientifically based on biochemistry, are bad for business, being a direct attack on the merely symptom-controlling and mostly toxic pharmaceutical products which they render obsolete.

The zeal with which North American medical regulators prosecute good doctors has inspired Canadian and US lawyers to specialize in protecting them. In Texas, a whole law firm is dedicated to this field: Brown & Fortunato works throughout the US. Its Health Care Group chairman recently told me that some of their lawyers are especially well qualified because they hold degrees in law as well as in those offered now by universities in legal medicine focused exclusively protecting medical innovation against medical regulators. Thankfully, if Truth and Justice are forsaken in one area, they have a way of finding instruments elsewhere in society.

Just how bad things have become can be measured by the fact that on

February 5 of this year the prestigious journal, *Annals of Internal Medicine* (vol. 136, no. 3) published simultaneously with the UK's famous Lancet (same date) the "Physicians Charter" (**www.professionalism.org**). The charter asserts that it is time doctors get back to the basics and reads like the Hippocratic Oath of 2,500 years ago in modern English. The message is simple: don't screw your patients financially or sexually, don't hurt them, let them chose among available treatments, and treat them properly even if they are black, Jews, poor, retarded, dying, just plain old, or don't have any money, and don't blab about them to others without their consent. (Canada's Privacy Commissioner, George Radwanski spoke at the conference and handed out the government's fat report on this last issue: **www.privcom.gc.ca** .) Most of all, don't lie when you do research because somebody offers to pay you for it. Wow! Hippocrates is groaning in his grave. This document, prepared by an international team of medical ethicists for the "Medical Professionalism Project" was handed out to all conference participants. It states at the outset: "We share the view that medicine's commitment to the patient is being challenged by external forces of change" which "the tempt physicians to forsake their traditional commitment to the primacy of patients' interests."

The best presentation was that by Dr. Solomon Benatar of South African, currently teaching bioethics at U of T (**http://dante.med.utoronto.ca/ethics**, and **http://icarus.med.utoronto.ca/ethics**). His was a breath taking tour through the suffering of humanity and the profit that can be made from it: 86% of annual global expenditure on health care goes to 16% of the world's population, and 90% of all health care research goes to 10% of the actual disease burden of the world, focusing on impotence, hair loss and blood pressure control, because the really sick people are "superfluous to the market as they cannot produce or consume." Medical regulators should stop this trend of "erosion of professionalism" he said. He concluded that doctors, researchers, regulators, governments and patients must "move away from a military and market metaphor and embrace an ecological metaphor" and focus on "population health as well as individual health".

Most immediately, though, what can you do to protect yourself while medicine sheds its old skin and struggles to be reborn? Read the books suggested below, especially Susan McIver's excellent book—tough to read, but great on advice on how to empower yourself as patient, how to avoid getting killed inadvertently, and how to get decent medical care, how to learn when to trust and when to be defensive. McIver's book might save your life. Remember, only informed patients will transform rotten regulatory systems and help create good medicine.

Sources and Resources

K. Ausubel, *When Healing Becomes a Crime*, Healing Arts Press, 2000

J.S. Cohen, *Overdose: The Case Against the Drug Companies*, Tarcher-Putnam, 2001

M. L. Culbert, *Medical Armageddon*, rev. edition,, C & C Communications, 1997

R. Hamowy, *Canadian Medicine: A Study in Restricted Entry*, Fraser Institute, 1984

S.B. McIver *Medical Nightmares*, S.B. McIver, Chestnut Publishing Inc., 2001

Jeffrey Robinson, *Prescription Games*, McClelland & Stewart, 2001

The Olivieri Report, Canadian Association of University Teachers, James Lorimer & Co.2001

Complementary Medicine Under Siege

Vitality Magazine April 2003

It is the fate of every Old Boys' Club to be forced to acknowledge changing realities, eventually. One of these is the College of Physicians and Surgeons of Ontario (CPSO), the medical regulatory body that controls the licenses of 40% of Canada's doctors. The CPSO erects fences and creates prohibitions against whatever bright new idea they happen not to like, so that all but the most heroic doctors are effectively deterred from incorporating these new ideas into their practices; they become CPSO targets for discipline of one sort or another, ranging from disciplinary trials to "Quality Assurance" reviews, neither of which have the safeguards against abuse a common criminal can expect in court. Indeed, one of the compelling reasons that prompted such physicians to form the Ontario Medical Association's Section on Complementary Medicine was because they were fed up with being persecuted by the CPSO who didn't give a damn for excellent treatment results, patient demand, and international research favoring a new medical paradigm.

What the CPSO doesn't tend to like shares certain characteristics: treatments that are low-tech, natural, don't require drugs, use drugs in novel ways—and diagnoses that implicate as causes the deadly side-effects of drugs and our pesticide-loaded food, polluted air and water in chronic illness. The internationally accepted warnings against smoking and high-fat diets, valid as they are, nevertheless belong into the "blame-the-patient" category that, ultimately, does not impact on the sickness industry. However, since it is environmental pollution, not sinful behavior, that causes most cancer and chronic disease, the blame lies squarely with those industries that create the cancer-causing agents—primarily the drug and pesticide manufacturers.

Instead of actively encouraging doctors who work to rid our bodies of disease-causing toxins and who teach us how to make our environments safe, this country's largest medical regulatory agency uses its formidable powers and resources to discredit medicine that addresses the most important health issues of our time and to harass physicians who want to help us. One of the instruments of control the CPSO uses to ensure everything stays the same (high-tech, toxic, symptom-control-oriented, and lucrative) is the "Complementary Medicine Policy". It is up for internal review this year. This is an opportunity for action.

The CPSO is used to exercising control over medical standards unchallenged by virtue of their authority as a self-governing body protected by 19th century administrative law. In 1997 the wide-spread public protest over the then ongoing disciplinary case against environmental medicine expert Dr. Jozef Krop forced them into a public relations effort. The infamous Complementary Medicine (CAM) Policy was hatched. It was supposed to make the CPSO look tolerant and progressive, but in fact it is a holdall for everything the CPSO has a history of trying to discredit. That CAM policy makes it possible to keep the drugs-as-usual scene in place and curb the availability of some of the greatest medical discoveries of the last 50 years: in nutrition, detoxification methods for environmental toxins, mind-body therapies, new approaches to cancer and degenerative disease, recognition of new diseases (like Multiple Chemical Sensitivity), effective novel treatments of old diseases like chronic pain—all summarized as "magic" or lacking in "evidence" (as defined by themselves).

One lawyer specializing in legal medicine refers to this policy as "pernicious", described in the dictionary as "having a harmful effect, especially in a gradual or subtle way." The only ones on whom this policy does not have a pernicious effect are the drug companies and the insurance companies to which so many of the CPSO council members are connected.

"What about the Kwinter Bill?" those of you will ask who fought long and hard to help make it law. It was passed with unanimous legislative consent in 2000 even though the CPSO fought it literally to the last day. Now a guiding principle of the *Medicine Act*, it states that a doctor "shall not be found guilty of professional misconduct or of incompetence under section 51 or 52 of the *Health Professions Procedural Code* solely on the basis that [he/she] practices a therapy that is non-traditional or that departs from the prevailing medical practice, unless there is evidence that proves that the therapy poses greater risk to a patient's health than the traditional or prevailing practice." MPP (Lib.) Monte Kwinter famously observed in one of his addresses to the legislature that "at the CPSO the attitude tends to be, that if it ain't invented here it ain't invented."

What we have today is legislation that protects medical innovation and the consensual doctor-patient relationship, which the medical regulatory agency chooses to ignore by maintaining a policy that stands in contradiction to the law. What's more, in interviews with *Charter* and criminal lawyers, I was told that the CPSO's CAM policy could be challenged in court as being contrary to natural justice and in contravention of at least one section of the *Charter*.

Interestingly, the view that the CPSO is out of touch with reality is supported by an Ontario government-sponsored report produced by KPMG in July 2000. Over 52 pages it details how this medical regulatory body has no idea what responsibility it has to the public. Yet, the very legislative mandate on which the CPSO's powers are founded, the *Regulated Health Professions Act* (RHPA), states that it is their "duty to serve and protect the public interest" (Schedule II, Section 3/2). Kwinter put it well when he observed, after his famous bill became law, "It will take a lot more than my bill to bring the CPSO under control."

In 2000, several medical associations and patient groups got together and in 2001 produced the *Glasnost Report* which meticulously documents the CPSO's abuses of the law and, thereby, of patients and innovative doctors. The CAM policy figures prominently in that abuse of power. (Available on **www.collegeofphysicianswatchdog.com**). That same group is now supporting the demand made on February 21 by the doctors of the Ontario Medical Association's Section on Complementary Medicine that "this CAM policy be brought in line with current thinking" and the law.

The CAM policy was introduced by the CPSO in 1997 while the trial of Dr. Krop was in progress. The PR exercise included public hearings for two days and many presentations, most by CAM physicians. The CPSO's committee responsible for the final product was perfectly stacked: not one practicing complementary physician on it. Not surprisingly, the final version does not reflect what the CAM medical community had actually presented or what the public had asked for. And in the case of Dr. J. Krop, this very policy has already been used as an instrument of control: he was ordered to adjust his practice to this policy or risk losing his license altogether. In 2000 the policy came up for internal review, and discussion was quickly swept under the carpet, so it remained in force. Now it is up for internal review again. The complementary doctors, supported by other medical groups, have written a letter to every council member identifying this policy's legal and medical iniquities.

The CAM Policy

When the policy became public, the press release issued in 1997 opined sanctimoniously that "there is no alternative to good medicine" and paid lip-service to our legally enshrined right to the medical care of our choice by stating, "patients have every right to seek whatever kind of therapy they want." The real meat of the press release is found, however, in the final observation that "physicians are not only accountable to their patients, but also to the college"—and guess which of the two is really in control...

- Dr. X. was brought into discipline for offering chelation therapy for cardiovascular disease instead of the usual cholesterol-lowering drugs which mainstream research now recognizes do not work (*Journal of the American Medical Association*, Dec. 18, 2002). The trial has not started yet.
- Several doctors lost their licenses for using nutritional regimes in conjunction with standard cancer therapies, e.g. Dr. Jerry Green of Toronto, even though the cancer associations highly recommend such protocols now.
- Dr. Y., a nutritional researcher as well as a practicing physician, followed the latest information on the connection between infantile autism and gastrointestinal disease (recently confirmed by studies at Harvard Medical School), for which he wound up being taken into discipline as well; the case is still unresolved.
- Many doctors are involved in the fight between the nutritional approach to ADHD versus Ritalin therapy with its serious side effects. The drug has a chemistry similar to cocaine and causes addiction, reduced blood flow to the brain's frontal lobes, and personality changes.
- As for Multiple Chemical Sensitivity, the College convicted Dr. J. Krop of diagnosing it and sentenced him for this offence the same month that MCS was officially recognized by the National Institutes of Health in the US; they published the international consensus statement in June 1999.

A short and harmless-looking version of the CAM policy is available on the CPSO's web site **www.cpso.on.ca** . It does not include the devilish details, the worst being a phrase that allows the CPSO to bypass legal obligations to fundamental fairness and retain arbitrary control the process. The policy states: "a fair review [of a CAM practitioner] can be achieved independent of the particular expertise of the assessor. In other words, if the CPSO chooses to look into the practice of a CAM physician, they can send in anybody they please who doesn't have a ghost of a notion about CAM. I have sat through the trials of several such physicians. In the trials of environmental medicine physician Dr. Krop and asthma and allergy expert Dr. Kooner, the College-appointed assessors admitted in cross-examination that they knew nothing about either physician's type of work. The College's expert witnesses in the Krop trial all admitted the same. Worse, these "experts" asserted that they wouldn't be caught dead even going to a CAM medical conference and swore they had never read any of their journals. This is taking prejudice to a level of a fine art—sponsored and endorsed by the CPSO.

The apparently tolerant and encouraging language of the policy notwithstanding, the full text of the policy is permeated with the notion that complementary medicine is, by definition, "unproven", "not generally validated", "magical", "of less proven value", etc. Adding insult to injury, the policy implies that CAM physicians do not want complementary medicine "to be exposed to scientific scrutiny before being provided to the patient". The policy then sanctimoniously refuses patients to be exposed to such risks. However, CAM physicians want no such thing. That implication is pure fantasy. Instead, historically, the evidence available from many discipline decisions proves that the CPSO is determined to disregard and discreet whatever it decides is CAM. For example, Dr. Krop, Dr. Kooner and many other physicians produced hundreds of then current studies from mainstream medical research publications—only to have all simply ignored—without explanation. Indeed, world-class defense witnesses were simply not even mentioned as having appeared in the final trial decisions! (See physician case histories in the *Glasnost Report*.)

As for the patients, the policy assumes that a CAM doctor is trying to pull the wool over their eyes. Much paternalistic fuss is made in the CAM policy about informed consent. To ensure the patient is protected against these assumed quacks, the doctor is expected to inform the patient of all conventional therapies first, and must even "arrive at a conventional diagnosis" first—never mind you have already seen a dozen doctors who didn't know how to fit your symptoms into the traditional boxes available, and never mind you are not willing to continue with cortisone, antidepressants or take chemotherapy.

What You Can Do

To understand the enormous importance of this policy to your good health, read the 2001 *Glasnost Report* (*a small extract pertaining to some of the persecuted doctors is provided in this section below; the whole report can be downloaded for free from* **www.kospublishing.com**), browse the College web site, and inform yourself as fully as you can. Write a letter demanding the CPSO review this CAM policy with full public input (*as of October 2004, with this book going into press, it still hasn't been reviewed, even though this is legally mandatory every 3 years!*). State that you are disturbed by the unfairness in the assessment process (*has not changed either!*), that you would like the wording of the Kwinter Bill (now in the *Medicine Act*) included in the revised CAM policy, and that you would like a legal analysis to be made by an **independent** (not College in-house lawyer) expert in *Charter* or medical law to ensure that the final version is in line with the law. Then fax or e-mail your letter to 1) the CPSO, 2) the Minister of Health, 3) the Health Critics of the Opposition Parties, and 4) your MPP.

Remember, freedom of medicine depends on citizens who demand freedom. The courageous CAM doctors need your help so they can continue to help you when you need them.

The following books are on some of the areas of medicine that have been the subject of CPSO persecution (see details in *Glasnost Report*):

P. Breggin MD, *Talking Back to Ritalin*, Common Courage Press, 1998
E.M. Cranton MD, *Bypassing Bypass Surgery*, Hampton Roads 2001
R.N. Firshein ND, *Reversing Asthma*, Warner, 1996
C. Gerson & M. Walker, *The Gerson Therapy*, 2001, Kensington
Hoffer MD, *Hoffer's Laws of Natural Nutrition*, 2001, Quarry
J. Krop MD, *Healing the Planet One Patient At A Time*, Kos Inc. (519-927-1049)
W.B. Parsons MD, *Cholesterol Control Without Diet:The Niacin Solution*, Lilac Press,1999
U. Reiss MD, *Natural Hormone Balance for Women*, 2001, Pocket Books
S. Rogers MD, *Detoxify or Die*, 2002, Sand Key Co., 1-800-846-6687
D. Haley, *The Politics of Healing*, 2000, Potomac Valley Press

The Kafkaesque Conviction of Dr. J. KROP

This article appeared in CONSUMERS HEALTH OF CANADA January 1999, FRASER FORUM March 1999, VITALITY MAGAZINE Fall 1999, in various US-based magazines and in expanded form in THE TOWNSEND LETTER FOR DOCTORS AND PATIENTS in March 2000.

After 9 years of investigation and 37 days of hearings, spread out over 4 years, the Ontario College of Physicians and Surgeons handed down their Decision on Environmental Medicine physician Dr. Jozef Krop of Mississauga. At the end of their 64-page Decision, the committee states that Dr. Krop fails "to meet the standard of practice in the Province of Ontario." Hallelujah! It is a great blessing for Ontario residents to have among them a doctor who refuses steadfastly to sink to that antideluvian standard of medicine which the CPSO tries to enforce and which its disciplinary committee so eloquently presented in their Decision on Dr. Krop.

The first curious fact is that, although the actual Sentencing Hearing is yet to come, when the punishment will be pronounced, the CPSO was apparently so thrilled with its efforts, they could not wait to let the world know about it. So, on January 6th Dr. Krop received a call from a Toronto Star reporter, asking for a comment on the CPSO's decision on his case. He replied, that he was still awaiting one. The reporter then informed him that she had a copy of it in her hands, dated December 23, 1998. Newspapers all over Ontario had received a copy, presumably from the CPSO directly, on January 5th. Dr. Krop himself did not receive his copy of the Decision on his case until the afternoon of the 7th.

Exactly 10 years earlier, on January 5th 1989, this investigation began. Unlike any common criminal, Dr. Krop does not know to this day on what basis it all started who accused him of what, and what necessitated the invocation of the Health Disciplines Act. Every effort by his lawyers to obtain the legally mandated disclosure was stonewalled, and finally, in cross examination CPSO investigator Leah Tunney explained that all the files pertaining to the commencement of this case had been "shredded, as is the practice" of the CPSO.

Next, the mandatory investigative report on Dr. Krop's practice composed by a CPSO appointed doctor was not sufficiently negative, so it was withdrawn by the CPSO, but the process continued without the benefit of a known accuser and the legally required report. Dr. Krop was ordered by Deputy Registrar Dr. John Carlisle to provide scientific evidence for his diagnostic and treatment methods, and he complied by handing in several pounds of documentation. In cross-examination, Dr. Carlisle stated, that he never read any of it, nor had he considered it necessary to give it to anybody else to read. This attitude flows logically from the CPSO's stated decision in September 1989 when Dr. Carlisle wrote in an internal memo his superior, Registrar Dr. M. Dixon, "This may be a costly and lengthy process, but may be the only way of finally, once and for all, dealing with these clinical ecologist." Indeed, Dr. Dixon confirmed this in cross-examination; asked by the defense lawyer if indeed the objective was to "deal with clinical ecology once and for all", he replied "Yes."

The formal charges against Dr. Krop are truly baroque: he is charged with suggesting a patient drink pure water, get an air purifier, avoid hydro towers, undergo acupuncture therapy, and eat organically grown foods. He is charged with diagnosing Multiple Chemical Sensitivity and failing to refer such people to a psychiatrist. He is charged with diagnosing food allergies, Sick Building Syndrome, systemic Candidiasis, and poisoning by neurotoxic and lung damaging solvents listed in all industrial toxicology manuals. He is charged with prescribing vitamin C, calcium, magnesium, evening primrose oil, and antifungal medication.

These accusations are upheld by the CPSO Disciplinary Committee in the face of the fact that the Canada Health Act for the past 11 years has a special section protecting all alternative medical practices as specified by the Helsinki Accord on human rights which Canada signed in 1988; even though for the past 11 years Canadian tax law provides a specific section for tax relief for chemically injured individuals; in spite of the fact that the Canada Mortgage and Housing Corporation was the world's first government organizations to develop housing safe for people suffering from chemical sensitivities. Ironically, 14 years ago the *Thomson Report* on Environmental Hypersensitivity Disorders, commissioned by the government of Ontario, provided the world-wide impetus for the first international, government sponsored medical conferences on this issue. The publications of the researchers in top medical centers cite this report as the watershed event that opened up the whole field of environmental medical science. The irony is enriched by the fact that Judge Thomson used Dr. Krop's practice as one of the primary sources for his committee's study!

Although the committee repeatedly observes throughout their Decision that no evidence of any harm was found, they even added a few more items to prove that Dr. Krop "fell below the standard of medical practice". These are 1) the suggestion that a chemically injured patient exposed to neurotoxic solvents undergo sauna therapy and 2) the observation that a particular drug, not available in Canada, would perhaps be helpful, (it was not used). Finally, 3) the Committee opined that the use of intravenous vitamin C at any time just "may be" harmful, and therefore is unacceptable in Ontario. Not a shred of evidence was cited in support of this statement, of course, since none exists. I know, I did a literature search and received the absolute latest scientific information on the subject from the Linus Pauling Institute in Oregon, the premier Vitamin C research centre in the world.

In summarizing just how Dr. Krop doesn't meet the standard of medicine in Ontario, the Committee painstakingly lists virtually every diagnostic and therapeutic procedure used by environmental physicians everywhere all based on the work of universities the world over, gained from international peer reviewed journals, and for epidemiological problems identified by the World Health Organization in their many reports.

Well, all one needs to do is look at the list of expert witnesses called by the CPSO and compare them to those called by Dr. Krop's defense to get a feel for which camp had the bright lights. The CPSO had the American allergist Dr. J. Anderson, a professional witness who does not practice medicine, whose business it is to provide his standard denial of the validity of environmental medicine in whatever forum pays him, while simultaneously admitting without a blush that he is totally unfamiliar with the relevant literature. Then there was the CPSO's Professor G. Sussman of the University of Toronto. As the defense proved, he served as the chairman of the advisory board for the drug company giants Pfizer and Merrell Dow; his opinion was considered valid in the case of a doctor whose treatments are designed to avoid the products of those companies and others. Another of the CPSO witnesses, Dr. Moot, admitted to receiving during the period of 1985 1995 more than $ 1.3 million from pharmaceutical giants Sandoz, Upjohn, Fison, Schering, Astra, Ciba Geigy, Janssen, Glaxo Wellcome, and Abbott; he also provided lectures to family physicians on behalf of Fison, Sandoz, and Parke Davis to introduce them to those companies' latest drugs.

By contrast, the expert witnesses for Dr. Krop were professors from Stanford University, Johns Hopkins Medical School (the world's Mecca of medical science), the University of Saskatchewan, and Nova Scotia's Dalhousie University which has the world's first (Canadian) government funded environmental health clinic. One witness was Dr. W. Rae, the author of the 4 volume standard medical textbook on chemical sensitivity conditions.

Curiously, the CPSO Decision describes each of these allegedly non-existent "occult diseases" and "unscientific treatments" by providing their definitions and purposes using Dr. Krop's own writings. Thus the CPSO has composed a tight little catalogue of all the latest and the best advances modern medical science has given us to protect our health and our frequently challenged immune systems and chemically assaulted organs in this our increasingly degraded environment. Yet, in the end, like the captains of a medical Titanic, the Committee firmly declares, that No, there is no iceberg anywhere! Anybody who says otherwise, is best chucked overboard... Mark Helprin wrote some time ago in *The Wall Street Journal,* "The truth, which is indestructible, has a way of accumulating against pride and arrogance, and then sweeping them from their path." The scientific observations and medical advances so arrogantly denied in this CPSO Decision will yet haunt their authors.

Having ignored or circumvented a host of legal requirements in order to proceed regardless, they were compelled to provide at least the appearance of grounds for their judgment. This was achieved by rejecting all scientific literature past 1990, simply declaring it all as "lacking in authority of acceptable scientific evidence". The sum total of the defense's evidence and Dr. Krop's own published double-blind studies were simply rejected and for good reason, since the CPSO's purpose would have been totally undermined by accepting them; this field of research exploded in the 1990s and has become a major focus in virtually every medical school; the conditions Dr. Krop treats successfully have since been recognized by government and most professional bodies (a few dinosaurs lurk about here and there to amuse us and they are kept well fed by those who stand to gain by keeping us sick). The Committee also has the temerity to cite the *Thomson Report* of 1985 repeatedly as the basis for their opinions, even though the co-author of that report, Dr. J. Gerrard, testified *for* Dr. Krop, making it explicit that this report was never intended to be used for the conviction of a doctor, since its primary purpose was to stimulate research. But for the CPSO nothing whatever has been stimulated in the last 14 years.

Among the many stunning examples of procedural abuse is an accusation concerning a drug potentially harmful to the liver. Not until the 1998 edition does the CPS (Canada's pharmaceutical compendium) include an observation concerning this. The patient in question was treated ten years earlier. Yet, D. Krop's own standard of practice was to routinely monitor patients with liver function tests whenever using this drug more than a decade before the standard practitioner became aware of the need for this safety measure.

In Kafka's famous 1920s novel, The Trial, the hero is told, "You can't defend yourself against this court, all you can do is confess." The hero replies, "A single hangman could replace this entire court." The CPSO does not reign supreme in Ontario as The Court did in Kafka's great parable. Dr. Krop does not intend to accept this verdict, but will continue to meet this surrealistic disciplinary process with the unwavering demand for rationality on behalf of patients in Ontario, and indeed everywhere.

Healing the Planet—One Patient at a Time

Vitality Magazine, October 2002

The five thousand year old Chinese oracle text known as the *I Ching* advises in Hexagram 18 that "work on what has been spoiled has supreme success", adding that people of real worth "stir up the people and strengthen their spirit." We live in a time in which the physical environment, on which our survival depends, is seriously spoiled by toxicants, and the human spirit very badly needs strengthening by having our courage and healthy rebellion stirred up. Dr. Jozef Krop, the environmental medicine physician from Mississauga, a medical rebel of skill and worth, takes this challenge to work on our spoiled world very seriously. His book, *Healing the Planet—One Patient At A Time: A Primer on Environmental Medicine* will appear on October 18th.

For years Dr. Krop used a small booklet he had compiled for his patients, the *Ecology Guide*, to teach them how to make their homes, gardens and workplaces safe, how to avoid environmental toxins, and what to do to become healthy again in partnership with their doctor. Starting in 1988, Dr. Krop became the subject of the longest known disciplinary investigation initiated by the College of Physicians and Surgeons of Ontario (CPSO), the medical regulatory body that licenses doctors. Dr. Krop was charged with prescribing clean water, air filters, using vitamins and mineral supplements in his treatment of multiple chemical sensitivity (MCS) and Candidiasis—which the CPSO charged him with diagnosing.

The CPSO used the *Ecology Guide*, along with the charts of especially successful patient cases, as the basis for finding him guilty in 1999 of diagnosing MCS and systemic candidiasis—both conditions which the CPSO insists have no basis in fact. He was also found guilty of using the standard treatments of environmental medicine for the treatment of pesticide poisoning and food sensitivities. He was not found guilty of having done any harm. The very patients, whose charts were used to convict him, took the stand and testified to the fact that their lives had been profoundly changed for the better through environmental medicine.

Dr. Krop is practicing as before, as his case is in the appeal's process, but his license is conditional on amending his consent forms so as to state the CPSO's view that none of these diagnoses and treatments have any scientific validity. During this trial the defence lawyers tabled hundreds of medical studies from the peer-reviewed literature in support of these treatments and diagnoses—the CPSO offered none to support their condemnation of them.

(The great Linus Pauling used to say that "when somebody isn't up on something, they will be down on it".) In September Dr. Krop's lawyers filed an appeal with the Supreme Court of Canada to hear this bizarre indictment on the grounds that rectifying such nonsense is of national importance.

Trying to cope with the terrific stress of this long defence of environmental medicine and his license, Dr. Krop found it personally helpful when he began to turn that *Ecology Guide* into a book. Working on the spoiled world and encouraging people is what a doctor is supposed to do, for the word "doctor" comes from the Latin verb "to teach", and all teaching stirs up healthy rebellion, which Dr. Krop states is the purpose of this book. It is organized so that the reader can understand the biochemical basis for environmentally induced illness (roughly 2/3 of whatever ails humanity). It informs us how triggers work in molds, inhalants, fungi, chemicals and heavy metals in our everyday world, pesticide-laden foods and chemically contaminated furniture and clothing. It deals with food sensitivities, genetic engineering versus organic produce. It has entire sections of special interest such as ways to handle and treat autism, attention deficit disorder, hormone- and dental amalgam-related illnesses, menopause questions, premenstrual syndrome and much more. The bibliography will seriously challenge the prejudices of even the most conservative doctor. It also contains up-to-date sources from books, journals and the Internet for the lay reader and desperate patient. Here is an excerpt from the introduction:

"When you decide to take charge of your health you stop functioning on automatic pilot. You no longer blindly trust your doctor because you suspect he or she can't know everything either; you doubt the government's assurances on health matters because it is the nature of power to be in conflicts of interest; you question the advertisements on drugs because you realize that their aim is to sell drugs not cure you and loose a customer. You listen to your body because it knows best; you are not a statistic or a population average but a unique person with an individual genetic endowment and a very personal health history requiring personalized attention. The health care industry, being geared to mass production as the car industry, understandably finds that an inconvenience. Living things are characterized by diversity; even our sufferings are not created equal.

Without the birth of fundamental doubt and the growth of critical thinking health is not possible, nor is advance in medicine. Doubt is the beginning of the cure. Trusting your self is the first step on the road to recovery. I would consider the effort of producing this book well worth it if it causes you to check out for yourself the basis for the claims the health industry and doctors make (including myself!).

We need to know that human beings on planet earth are like fish in a tank of finite dimensions. As the Greek master physician, Hippocrates taught 2,500 years ago, our health is determined by the air we breathe, the food we eat, the soil in which we grow it, the water we drink, and the way we feel and behave towards others. All illness and all health are ultimately a function of our physical and emotional environment. Even most genetically mediated illnesses are triggered by unhealthy environments and ultimately preventable.

Second, modern medicine, ecology and biochemistry have provided us with the answers to the prevention of illness. Medical science has gone well beyond telling you not to smoke. We now know that we have to break the lethal dependence on toxic chemicals not only in ourselves, but also for our lawns, our agricultural practices, and our industrial economy. We can prevent cancer, heart disease, diabetes, arthritis, and many more illnesses …

When you no longer blindly follow advice, but engage in a critical search for verifiable and workable solutions, you also begin the task of saving planet earth and human life. Like a stone thrown into a pool, the stone is small but the ripples go on and on covering immense distances for a very long time. In fact, what you actually do is to become politically engaged on behalf of life itself when you assume responsibility for what you eat and drink, what you permit to be in your surroundings, and what you will expose others to. You begin to make choices that have an effect on everything around you: your supermarket, your pharmacy, your local school, your garbage disposal, the way you furnish your home, the recreations you pursue, the car you buy, the information you spread through your friends and relatives.

Of course you will always act on incomplete information (we all do, all of the time), but if you are in charge and engage your doctor in a critical dialogue and partnership, the result will always be better than whatever you got on automatic pilot. The truth does make us free."

Dr. Krop tells the story of his medical training in and escape from Communist Poland to Canada, his training under Dr. Abraham Hoffer in Saskatchewan in the early 1970s, and attending his first conference at the American Academy of Environmental Medicine in 1979. At that conference he went through a dramatic personal shift in understanding medicine when Dr. Doris Rapp showed a video of her work with "the impossible child" suffering from what is now labeled as ADHD:

"Dr. Rapp was testing a child for food sensitivities, and when she tested for oats the child had a dramatic reaction. This food actually had a neurotoxic effect and the child began to scream and thrash about. When Dr. Rapp finally established and administered the neutralizing dose, the child rapidly and totally recovered. Then Dr. Rapp asked the patient, "Do you remember anything that happened during the past two hours?" The child, genuinely bewildered, said, "No, I don't."

Well, at that point I got goose bumps all over and I knew, deep down and without any doubt, that this was the medicine I had to practice. Whatever I had learned in standard medicine did not even consider the neurotoxicity of ordinary foods! I was only taught about IgE mediated allergies (regular hay fever and the like). What I had just seen was something completely different, and even if the biological pathways were not yet fully understood (as is the case in IgE-mediated allergies), here was the opportunity to understand and treat conditions otherwise simply discarded as "psychiatric"—unfair to psychiatry and brutally neglectful of the patient's real needs. The notion that such reactions could be treated with neutralizing doses of the offending substance, rather than with symptom-controlling drugs, was revolutionary. What's more, the same approach, I learned, could be taken in treating the toxic effects of environmental chemicals. The key point was that the offending cause could be found and treated. Standard medicine teaches how to classify symptoms, what drugs to use to control them, and how to use them cautiously to prevent their toxicity from killing the patient.

I realized that I would be striking out in a 180 degree opposite direction to where all my colleagues were going. [The father of environmental medicine] Dr. Thereon Randolph used to warn young doctors, eager to learn the techniques of environmental medicine, saying,"You realize this is a one-way street. There is no turning back." Not that the training I had had so far was useless—standard bacterial infection and trauma is perfectly treated by the standard medicine I had learned. But everything else—chronic disease which has become the subject of most of medicine—only talks about symptom control, not finding causes and trying for a cure. I was devastated and actually rather scared.

It was an intense—but not a very long war—that I waged within myself. It was the patients that decided it in the end. Whenever I looked at them with the search frame of standard medicine, and then again with that of environmental medicine I quickly knew what I had to do. The patient's environmental exposure and nutritional history generally explained the causes of the observed signs and symptoms often quite elegantly and rationally.

Symptom-control became intolerably boring. So, I took every available course, including one intense one with Dr. Thereon Randolph himself. I am still taking courses every year; none of my treatment protocols remain the same for very long: there is so much happening in this field of medicine."

Now, that Dr. Krop has been through more than a decade of the current version of the Inquisition, he has no illusions about the politics of medicine:

"After all, identifying pesticides, petrochemicals, many symptom-controlling drugs, and processed foods (to name just a few serious health hazards) as the causes of cancer and chronic diseases is not going to make a doctor very popular with the captains of industry. The findings of environmental medicine, and the demonstration that avoiding all these toxic substances can restore people's health, constitute a most formidable critique of our modern world and its commercial values.

Medical regulatory bodies are also as conflicted in their interests as they were 150 years ago when bacteria were the heresy of the day and washing one's hands, before examining a patient or performing surgery, was an affront to professional pride... [and] symptom-control is a multi-billion dollar business and not likely to take the back seat without a fight. Symptom-control is the market, and wealth is measured in this market, as in any other, by growth not by the diminishing returns cures would generate.

Speaking the truth about what we see in our patients on a daily basis— carcinogens and neurotoxins in their blood, pesticides in their fat biopsies, heavy metals in their urine and stools—is nothing less than a total indictment of governments that have ceased to be regulators and protectors of society and become publicly funded butlers serving the big corporations."

This book should be in everybody's life because the quality of our lives depends on having information—the right information from somebody whose experience one trusts.

Dr. Krop's book (second, expanded edition, 2003) can be ordered from KOS PUBLICATIONS INC. :1997 Beechgrove Rd., Alton, ON, L0N 1A0, by FAX: 519-927-9542, or e-mail: **helke@inetsonic.com** *Cost: $ 25.00 plus 7% GST and shipping and handling. It is also available through any book store. (It is currently being translated into Polish and Japanese.)*

The following preface was written by me, the publisher, for the second edition (November 2003) of *Healing The Planet* in order to bring readers up-to-date on how the case against Dr. Jozef Krop has ended

Publisher's Preface to the Second Printing

The first printing of this book, November 2002, was quickly sold out, making a second printing necessary eight months later. It is a matter of special satisfaction to me personally, that while sold in major bookstores everywhere, most were sold in doctors' offices. This means that this book is primarily in the hands of patients whose doctors work *with* them.

For more than two decades, Dr. Krop's name has been associated in North America with the politics of medicine. He is best known for his role in helping to launch the popularly known "Kwinter Bill" (after Ontario's Liberal MPP Monte Kwinter), which enshrined patient's freedom of choice in the Medicine Act of Ontario in 2000 (see Ontario *Hansard* of August 28, 1991). Dr. Krop also contributed, in the early 1980s to the World Commission on the Environment (the *Brundtland Report*), and his practice was used by the Ontario government to begin the process of establishing guidelines for dealing with environmental causes of illness (the 1985 *Thomson Report*). He also participated in various university and federal government –sponsored efforts to raise awareness of the environment's impact on population health. In the 1980s he was a co-founder, and for many years served as the secretary of the Canadian Society for Environmental Medicine.

As is the fate of many pioneers, he spent more than a decade defending environmental medicine in a disciplinary trial initiated against him by the Ontario medical licensing authority, the *College of Physicians and Surgeons of Ontario*. The CPSO based their prosecution not on patient complaints (there were none), adverse treatment outcome (they admitted all files studied showed the patients had improved), but alleged that practicing environmental medicine "lacked acceptable scientific evidence" [1]. The CPSO then ensured that such scientific evidence appeared indeed to be missing by totally ignoring its existence when handing down their final 1999 Decision. Many of those hundreds of scientific articles, all from the mainstream medical journals, provided by the defense lawyers during the trial, are now part of the reference section in this book. Of course, this throwback to medieval doctrinal wars and its legal instrument, the Inquisition, begins to make some sense when one realizes that the majority of CPSO council members are either directly or indirectly connected to the pharmaceutical and pesticide industry.

Dr. Krop's trial is legally, politically, and medically one of the great scandals in medical history. His patients and supporters fortunately believed in this cause and footed most of the defense bill which, over that long decade of the trial, reached almost Can. $ 2 million. However, due this immense effort and the involvement of so many first class lawyers, the legal profession became sensitized to the abuse of process and law the CPSO and other regulatory bodies committed without ever being checked. Today there are many lawyers working for many more innovative doctors and defending medicine properly. Before the Krop case few lawyers and judges knew just how deep the rot ran. Those who want to know more about this story and the worldwide battle for Environmental Medicine, may want to read **Malice in Medicine**—*The 14-Year Trial of Environmental Medicine Physician Dr. Jozef Krop* due to be published in 2005

This book is a primer in environmental medicine. It is unique among the many excellent books currently available on many aspects of health and environment because this one is meant for *both* patients and doctors. Knowing that patients are intelligent people who can understand anything in medicine if the courtesy of full explanation is offered, Dr. Krop includes in this book the complete treatment protocols which the reader can take to his or her doctor to study. These protocols are supported by an exhaustive medical bibliography intended especially for those Doubting Thomases who are willing to examine widely-held prejudices against environmental medicine and are willing to consider seriously its claim to be able to help those many illnesses standard medicine calls idiopathic, i.e. cause unknown. Every year more and more research is published showing; that what was once considered an idiopathic illness is now well understood as environmentally and nutritionally mediated. Water, air and soil polluted with neuro-toxins and carcinogens, and nutrient-deficient processed food laced with endocrine disrupters and pesticides cause or trigger virtually all modern epidemics, such as asthma, chronic fatigue, most neurological diseases, Parkinson's, Alzheimer's, allergies, osteoporosis, attention deficit disorder and many psychiatric conditions, cardiovascular disease, depression, and the greatest scourge of our time—cancer.[2]

Since *Healing The Planet Once Patient At A Time* appeared last year, Dr. Krop was reprimanded in September 2003 for practicing medicine lacking scientific proof—as interpreted by Ontario's medical licensing authorities. Dr. Krop is free to practice; the CPSO's "victory" is more of an embarrassment than a triumph and will serve to help spread the word about environmental medicine rather than deter its practice. For purposes of comparison, the reader may be interested in how the CPSO's monumental ignorance and arrogance measure up to current developments in environmental and nutritional medicine. This is merely a sample—a complete list is beyond the scope of this preface. Indeed, a great shift in understanding is taking place in medicine, which will, no doubt, eventually leave the corporately contaminated regulatory authorities and medical practitioners in the dust.

- The December 2000 health-freedom amendment to the Ontario Medicine Act sponsored by Liberal MPP Monte Kwinter and whose wording he took from the 1988 international Helsinki Accord on Human Rights, has taken on a lifer of its own. Similar bills are now being sponsored by provincial legislators in Saskatchewan, Manitoba, and Quebec. It already exists in British Columbia; Alberta was the first to make it law.

- Following the Canadian Supreme Court's Hudson Decision of 2002 on the right to pass local by-laws against pesticide use, an immense public campaign brought about in March this year the passage of an anti-pesticide law for the whole Province of Quebec where its cosmetic use will be phased out completely. Within a decade we may have epidemiological evidence that in Quebec population health has markedly improved, compared to the rest of Canada.

- The World Health Organization recently published a consensus report on the need to reduce drastically the use of refined sugar, remove vending pop machines from school cafeterias, and reduce the amount of sugar in processed foods. The sugar industry was infuriated and demanded from the WHO's Director General, Gro Brundtland, that this report be withdrawn, threatening that otherwise the industry would see to it that the WHO's annual financial contribution from the United States government would be withheld. Dr. Brundtland responded by publishing both the report and the threats. [3] Incidentally, in 1993 the CPSO reprimanded Toronto's Dr. Carolyn Dean for warning against the intake of too much sugar while being interviewed on the Dini Petty television show—the warning was specific to diabetic patients and warned also against high sugar intake as causing diabetes. A complaint by Canada's Sugar Institute had initiated this disciplinary investigation on the grounds that there was "no scientific basis" for such a claim against refined sugar. This casts an interesting light on where the CPSO gets its scientific advice. [4] (For information on Dr. Dean's and many other such physicians' cases before the CPSO visit: **www.collegeofphysicianswatchdog.com**

- Commencing in April of 2002, the Canadian Medical Association's official journal, the CMAJ, published a six-part series on environment and health covering the proper way to take an exposure history (April 16), the effects of outdoor pollution (April 30), recognizing and treating lead exposure (May 14), management and prevention regarding pesticides (May 28), the health effects of persistent organic pollutants (June 11), and understanding carbon monoxide poisoning (June 25). The authors are leading experts in those areas and teach at Canada's medical school. Most noteworthy is the fact that the references and research sources provided in those articles were almost all also those Dr. Krop's defense lawyers had given to the CPSO during his trial. [5]

- In October 2003 the Ontario College of Family Physicians hosted its first medical conference on Environmental Medicine and participating physicians received full continuing study credits from the Ontario Medical Association.

- At the beginning of this year, Canada's Ministry of Human Resources responded to requests for help from advocacy groups working with victims of Multiple Chemical Sensitivity (MCS). RAINET (Research, Advocacy.) approached the Minister, the Hon. Jane Stewart and provided case histories of individuals who were totally disabled by exposure to certain toxic chemicals, but were denied CPP and other applicable benefits solely on the basis of an MCS diagnosis. A review was initiated and MCS is now in the process of being included for CPP benefits. The core problem in the case of Dr. Krop before the CPSO was the diagnosis of MCS which was rejected as being "scientifically invalid" the same month, June 1999, when the international consensus statement on MCS as a valid diagnosis was published by the National Institutes of Health in the USA. [6]

- One of the treatments for which the CPSO condemned Dr. Krop is a desensitization procedure for environmental and food allergies through the use of sub-lingual drops. (See footnote no. 1 for Internet access to the CPSO decision). In April 2002, 4 months after the CPSO verdict, the World Health Organization published a report, based on the review by 34 internationally recruited allergists, stating that this treatment should be considered the treatment of choice. [7]

- The Ontario Human Rights Commission wrote in April of this year to Ontario's Minister of Health, the Hon. Tony Clement, instructing him that in the event of spraying for West Nile Virus being considered, the Minister has the obligation to protect people with chemical sensitivities and to ensure they receive medical care if affected by the spraying. The federal government made a similar statement. [8]

- A few years ago, the American Preventive Medical Association (APMA) sued the United Stated Food and Drug Administration (FDA) because of that agency's persecution of anybody making any health claims for vitamins and other neutraceuticals. The case was decided in favor of the APMA, but in clear defiance of the court order, the FDA continued to harass doctors and neutraceutical companies. This year in May, another court case was decided once again in favor of the APMA, and now the FDA obeyed the court. Health claims for all antioxidants (such as Vitamins C and E), Folic Acid, various fiber supplements and Saw Palmetto are now appearing on supplement bottles.

- In an abrupt turn-around only comparable to a conversion experience, one of the world's leading experts in nutrition and health, Bruce Ames of the University of California at Berkeley published a comprehensive review article in April 2002 in which he asserts that Linus Pauling was right all along. Coming from Bruce Ames, that's a bit like the leader of the Alliance Party joining the NDP. Shortly thereafter, the Journal of the American Medical Association published in June 2002 two articles, which conclude that everybody needs to take vitamin and mineral supplements to prevent chronic disease, and that no diet provides enough of the nutrients needed for basic good health and to prevent chronic illness later in life. [9]

- One of the sections in Dr. Krop's book deals with autism, its causes and treatment for which he provides the appropriate protocols. Due to the efforts of Congressman Dan Burton in the USA, whose grandson became autistic after being vaccinated for Mumps Measles and Rubella, the vaccine industry has been forced this spring to remove the offending mercury used as a preservative in vaccines. [10]

All these developments in such a short period of time led Dr. Krop to observe jokingly, "If we wait long enough, they'll make intravenous vitamin C the standard of treatment for SARS."

While all these shifts in understanding are very encouraging indeed, this is not the time for complacency. Nutritional and environmental medicine is still under attack because its claims, research and success are a fundamental threat to the pharmaceutical and pesticide industry. As Cornell University's ecologist and cancer expert Sandra Steingraber has pointed out, the world's economy is "chemically addicted", [11] and that the health of the world is endangered by nothing as much as by that "toxic trespass"[12] committed without our knowledge, and often against our will, by a chemical industry in conscious disregard of the biological requirements and biochemical integrity of humanity. Similarly, the drug industry's products are now, due to their serious adverse "side"-effects, considered to be the second most frequent cause of death [13]. Clearly, we have a long way to go before doctors and patients become free from quick-fix delusions and understand that health is a matter of prevention, proper nutrition, and therapies that work *with* nature.

The fact that a book such as this one sells well and that all of the above (and much more) is published by the mainstream medical journals, and supported by standard national and international medical organizations, indicates that a big change is happening. People are taking charge and thinking critically. Fortunately, the Internet ensures that information cannot be buried as it used to be and high-speed communication has created something of a level playing field for health activists.

Yet, there are many actions still ongoing which are of grave importance and require our determined support. For example, the international battle being waged against CODEX, the international regulatory body controlled by the pharmaceutical companies; it seeks to make all neutraceuticals available by prescription only. Another important and parallel cause is that championed by Canadian federal MPP Dr. J. Lunney's and his courageous and timely effort (Bill C 420) which seeks to prevent Health Canada from gaining control over food supplements; in view of Health Canada's track record with regard to drug approval and its efforts to prevent information on food safety from becoming publicly known, they certainly don't need to control neutraceuticals as well. [14]

In antiquity it was believed that the source of medical knowledge was divine and that the ability to practice medicine was a gift granted by the god of medicine himself, Asklepios. By definition gods are immortal, and divine truth cannot be destroyed and, therefore, will once again make us free.

ENDNOTES

[1] CPSO Decision on Dr. Krop, December 23, 1998, available on their website: **www.cpso.on.ca**

[2] One of the best sources for information on the environmental component or cause of any disease is found in *Environmental Health Perspectives*, a medical journal published monthly by the National Institutes of Health and Harvard University's School of Public Health; available on-line.

[3] *The Medical Post*, May 13, 2003.

[4] The College of Physicians and Surgeons of Ontario reprimanded Dr. Carolyn Dean on April 29, 1993, based on a complaint filed by Sandra Marsden of the Sugar Institute of Canada; the complaint was filed, as stated in the admonishment document, because Dr. Dean had spoken about the *dangers of refined sugar intake by diabetics on a television show aired on December 11, 1990. The reprimand states: "The respondent made inaccurate and misleading statements addressing health issues related to sugar and sugar substitutes...which tended to potentially arouse concern in the viewing public . The Committee believes the respondent expressed opinions which appeared to be exaggerated with respect to the relationship between sugar and diabetes, infection, osteoporosis, hyperactivity and addiction."* This amazing nonsense, unsupported by any published medical evidence, was signed by Dr. D.M.C. Walker, then the CPSO president and now the Dean of medicine at Queen's

University in Kingston, Ontario. In her defence, prior to this admonishment, Dr. C. Dean had submitted more than 200 citations from the then current, standard, peer-reviewed medical literature on sugar and sugar substitutes upon which her remark on television had been based. This material is not even mentioned in the admonishment.

[5] CMAJ, Vol. 166, April 16 through June 25, 2002

[6] *Archives of Environmental Health*, vol. 54, No. 3, pp. 147-149, June 1999

[7] See summary in *Scientific American*, April 2002, p. 26, "Drink Your Shots" by B. Goodman

[8] Letter from the Ontario Human Rights Commission, dated April 16, 2003, signed by Chief Commissioner Keith C. Norton, addressed to the Hon. Tony Clement, Ontario's Minister of Health; the legal basis cited is the *Ontario Human Rights Code*, Section 29 and the Policy *and Guidelines on Disability and the Duty to Accommodate*

[9] The *American Journal of Clinical Nutrition*, April 2002 and *Journal of the American Medical Association*, June 19, 2002

[10] For a copy of my article on autism contact Vitality magazine at 416-964-0528; it provides the historical, legal and treatment information. See also Autism Canada Foundation, P.O. Box 1998, Burlington, Ontario, L7R 4L8, call 905-332-4766 or 905-331-4480, visit **www.autismcanada.org**. Dr. J. Bradstreet's institute can be reached via **www.icdrc.org** and **www.autismresearchinstitute.com**

[11] S. Steingraber, Living *Downstream*: An Ecologist Looks at Cancer, 2nd ed. 1999

[12] S. Steingraber in the upcoming documentary, *If You Love Our Children*, sponsored by The National Film Board of Canada.

[13] J.S. Cohen, *Overdose: The Case Against the Drug Companies*, Tarcher-Putnam, 2001. J. Robinson, *Prescription Games*, McLelland & Stewart, Toronto, 2001. T.J. Moore, *Prescription for Disaster*, Simon & Schuster, 1998. J. Glenmullen, *Prozac Backlash*, Touchstone Books, 2000. Canadian Association of University teachers, *The Olivieri Report,* Lorimer, 20021.

[14] To help stop the international efforts under the United nations' CODEX ALIMENTARIUS to restrict the availability of vitamins and supplements, contact the worldwide effort being coordinated by Dr. Matthias Rath in Germany at **www.4.dr-rath-foundation.org**. In Canada, Dr. James Lunney introduced Bill C 420 for the same purpose, to maintain freedom of choice for Canadians. The bill is available on **www.parl.gc.ca/37/2parlbus/chambus/house/bills/private/C-420I/C-420cover-E.html** and you can contact your own MP and express your support for this bill.

The Case Against Dr. S.S. Kooner

The Scoop, Windsor, Ontario, October 2001

There is a terrible injustice in danger of happening in Windsor, Ontario. A highly trained doctor with extraordinary success in treating one of the great scourges of humanity, asthma, may lose his license to practice on November 14th. His patients love Dr. S.S. Kooner, but the body that licenses and oversees doctors in Ontario (the College of Physicians and Surgeons, CPSO) wants to strip him of his license. No patient was harmed, no medical practice rule broken. Hundreds of patients have written to the Premier, the Ministry of Health, the CPSO, and the MPPs of Dr. Kooner's catchment's area protesting the unwarranted CPSO prosecution of their doctor. One character witness stated on the stand at the CPSO hearing, "I am deeply offended by these proceedings." Dr. Kooner has treated him and his family.

Part of the problem seems to be that the good doctor, who hails from India and was trained in Canada and by the American Academy of Environmental Medicine and the Pan American Allergy Association, is especially good at treating asthma and allergies such that the conventional (patented and expensive) drugs become unnecessary. The fact that most of his patients had their health restored seems to be uninteresting to the OPSO. The lawyer for the CPSO, Donald Posluns, instructed the Discipline Panel during the hearings, "You have never heard of the Pan American Allergy Association, therefore you have to find him guilty." They took that to heart. Their July 9 Decisions states: "The Committee finds Dr. Kooner guilty of professional misconduct by failing to maintain the standard of practice of the profession ....he is unfit to continue in practice ...."

That "restriction" part of the Decision refers to Dr. Kooner's treatment of asthma, his specialty. Several times during this long investigation begun in 1996, the CPSO offered to stop the proceedings, provided he stops treating asthma patients. This equivalent to blackmail was based on no patient harm or evidence in Dr. Kooner's practice or in the medical literature pertaining to even potential dangers. Even though Dr. Kooner was under the gun, his professional conscience never wavered and he refused to abandon his asthma patients. They have since formed a patient support group (Chair: Dean LaBute 519-944-5504) which lobbies on his behalf. Dr. Kooner also enjoys the support of the Sikh Temple community to which he, hailing from India's Punjab Province, belongs.

This Decision was handed down seven months *after* the Ontario *Medicine Act* was amended to stop precisely such absurd decisions by many of which CPSO history is tainted. One is forced to conclude that the CPSO either does not take notice of amendments to the health care legislation they are supposed to supervise, or they don't understand that they, too, must obey the law. Evidence of the CPSO's gross disregard for patients and incompetence in handling serious and well founded patient complaints has been widely publicized in the *Toronto Daily Star* series since May 5th and is still ongoing (see **www.thestar.com** –go to " medical secrets").

A government initiated investigation of the CPSO done by international management consultants KPMG concluded in 1999 that the CPSO's discipline and complaints processes were lacking in accountability, transparency and were devoid of an appreciation of public concerns and ethical considerations. They declared the CPSO to be out of touch with reality. (For the report see *Glasnost Report* of which an excerpt is given below in this section).

One of Canada's top criminal lawyers, Michael Code, spent a year investigating the cases of a dozen doctors brought before the CPSO in the same manner as Dr. Kooner. Mr. Code came to the conclusion that in all cases he studied there was clear abuse of power and process and, in one case, possibly, outright criminal obstruction of justice committed in the CPSO disciplinary process. Mr. Code felt strongly enough about his findings that he discussed them in a press conference held at Queen's Park on May 20, 2000.

This summer, the Minister of Health, the Hon. Tony Clement, had a couple of showdowns with the CPSO which made it clear that the Minister (which means the people who elected him) is in charge of medicine, and that "the old boys' club" can't do whatever it pleases. (See story on the *Toronto Star's* web site.) As a result, the Registrar, Dr. J. Bonn was fired July 2. The by-laws require the Deputy Registrar, Dr. John Carlisle, to be interim Registrar. That is a case of falling from the frying pan into the fire because Dr. Carlisle has been in charge of discipline for the better part of his almost 30 year tenure and is responsible for the majority of the abuses, including those in the case of Dr. Kooner.

There is a history to all of this. On December 17th last year, a fabulous Christmas present was given to the residents of Ontario in a graceful display of statesmanship by the Harris government. Putting party politics aside, it was unanimously agreed that it was high time to pass an important amendment to the *Medicine Act.* Although only a private member's bill, it was unanimously supported in all three readings and became law in time for Christmas. Private member's bills almost never make it into law, but this one had such loud support from so many people, it was impossible to ignore. Taken from the medical clause of the international human rights treaty, the *Helsinki Accord* (which Canada signed in 1988) and sponsored MPP M. Kwinter (Lib), it is "is sublime in its wording but profound in its impact" (Ontario Legislature, *Hansard* of April 27, 2000). It states:

> "A [doctor] shall not be found guilty of professional misconduct or of incompetence under the Health Professions Procedural Code solely on the basis that the doctor practices a therapy that is non-traditional or that departs from the

prevailing medical practice, unless there is evidence that proves that the therapy poses greater risk to a patient's health than the traditional or prevailing practice."

Alberta, Nova Scotia and B.C. have similar legislation, and several other provinces are working on it. That members of all parties in government agreed proves that deep down we are all on the same wavelength on what really matters. Of course, the CPSO fought this legislation to the last. During the government debate on the "Kwinter Bill", Monte Kwinter, addressing the great need for his bill, observed, "There are people at the College of Physicians and Surgeons with the attitude, 'If it ain't invented here, it ain't invented'... and as a result they are not prepared to support any treatments that don't fall into what they consider good medicine." (*Hansard* Dec. 11, 2000). MPP Brad Clark (PC) supported Kwinter but warned, "If this bill does pass, I don't want it to be perceived by the public that this is going to be the big fixer...of all that ails the CPSO." He then pointed out that existing CPSO regulations already protect innovative medicine, but the government supported this amendment because the CPSO seems not to follow its own regulations. A bigger hammer was needed.

Nothing seems more reasonable than the notion that doctors, often faced with very difficult situations, would need to be free to find new solutions in cooperative agreement with the patient. No progress could take place in medicine—that most practical and experience-based of all the sciences—if patients are not free to decide what works for them, and if doctors are not allowed to try something new. Yet, the fact is, that over the past twenty years, many doctors who departed "from the prevailing medical practice" in this province have been brought to trial by the CPSO in spite of the public protest of their patients and in the absence of negative evidence in medical research. These doctors lost their licenses, had them severely restricted, or fought expensive appeals to have their licenses restored. The CPSO trials have been described by witnesses as outright kangaroo courts blatantly ignoring the rules of conduct which regular courts obey.

Dr. F. Ravikovich, also highly successful with asthma treatment, had his license restricted without a single patient being harmed. Twice the CBC's *Fifth Estate* featured the story and the hundreds of protesting asthma patients in 1993.

Environmental medicine expert, Dr. J. Krop, was on trial for almost ten years. The evidence in favor of his medical practice was so overwhelming, the discipline panel backed down to a mere reprimand which he is appealing before the Divisional Court in December because of the gross legal improprieties in his trial.

Dr. Carolyn Dean, a doctor specializing in nutritional medicine and author of many books, lost her license in 1993 following her appearance on the Dini Petty show. She spoke about the dangers of sugar for diabetics. The Sugar Institute of Canada complained to the CPSO about her "inflammatory and unscientific statements" for which Dr. Dean was "admonished" and then, eventually taken to discipline. Incongruously, this decision was made a few doors down from the building in which Drs. Banting and Best did their world famous research into diabetes. They won the Nobel prize for their discovery of insulin and for establishing the dangers of sugar for diabetics. Dr. Dean now practices in the USA.

World-renowned pain expert, Dr. F. Adams was featured in the media continuously for the past year and a half. Without patient harm, but outstanding successes with the most intractable chronic pain patients, the CPSO restricted his license so severely, he had no choice but to go to the USA in March. There he can practice according to international pain management guidelines, which he happened to have co-authored for the American Federation of Medical Licensing Boards and the World Health Organization. Ontario's CPSO chooses not to follow international guidelines, even though the Canadian Colleges are officially affiliated with the American medical boards, which entails that they recognize each other's medical guidelines.

Currently, the case against nutritional expert, Dr. Tom Barnard, has begun at the CPSO. He offended the status quo by daring to attempt treatment with autistic children, a condition for which standard medicine has nothing to offer. (*Update 2004: he got off and is working freely.*)

Dr. Kooner came to the attention of the CPSO because he properly registered an anaphylactic reaction of a patient who was being tested for allergies. This is so common an event in allergy medicine, that doctors are instructed in a specific protocol published by the Ministry of Health. The patient revived in minutes and went to school the next morning. Thousands of such events occur every year in Ontario. None of them are the substance of disciplinary proceedings—except with Dr. Kooner. Why? And why years after the event? This is a mystery.

The CPSO Decision shows they worry about anything except good medicine. This is ironic in view of the revelations published over the past months in the *Star*, that when truly terrible things happen, nothing is done. Yet, Dr. Kooner's treatments, as the evidence supplied by the defense showed, are far safer than the traditional treatments the CPSO insists must remain standard—no matter how outdated and unsupported by current medical research. Yet, corticosteroids cause osteoporosis and depression, and in children with asthma they stunt growth; they also loose their effectiveness after prolonged use. It appears the Discipline Panel did not read the evidence.

Last year, the World Health Organization declared asthma on the rise to epidemic levels. In July the OMA issued a damning report on air quality in Ontario and the related health effects such as the dramatic rise in asthma. Environmental improvements will take time to achieve, and meanwhile doctors successfully treating these conditions, remain unprotected against such arbitrary prosecutions, simply because the CPSO can't get its head out of the sand—or is unable to comprehend that the people of Ontario have given themselves a law that protects good medicine which the CPSO is supposed to follow. Given the recent show-downs between the Ministry of Health and the CPSO, it is to be hoped that the Hon. Tony Clement will exercise the powers invested in him by the people of this province to ensure that Dr. Kooner's patients will not be deprived of the breath of life.

Update October 2004: *Dr. Kooner lost his license and on appealing to the Ontario Provincial Court, the CPSO was ordered to return it to him, but the CPSO appealed that court decision—twice more, each time without success. This left asthma and allergy patients in the Windsor area without Dr. Kooner's services for close to two years. The Court understood the issues involved very well and even ordered certain fundamental safeguards to be observed in any future proceedings the CPSO might wish to undertake against Dr. S.S. Kooner, thereby establishing also a benchmark for all future prosecutions of any other doctor on medical standards issues. Ironically, those safeguards require appropriate expert witnesses and enunciate other basic legal principles even any common criminal can expect when charged with a crime. Dr. Kooner is practicing again in Windsor, Ontario. Yet, many more cases were initiated against doctors without patient complaints or medical mishaps. Most were resolved, and the architect of most of these cases, Deputy Registrar Dr. John Carlisle, left the CPSO in November 2003 when his contract was not renewed. Many doctors have now taken out insurance with MARSH, an international company specifically dedicated to protecting physicians and dentists against their own regulatory bodies. Most significantly, the roster of lawyers working for MARSH share one important characteristic: none have pharmaceutical and insurance industry clients.*

The Case of Dr. Felix Ravikovich

Another asthma expert, **Dr. Felix Ravikovich** of Toronto, was prosecuted in the early1990s for using histamine therapy instead of cortisone. His case his summarized in the *Glasnost Report* of 2001, which is reproduced in part below. The CPSO ordered Dr. Ravikovich never to use histamine or any other substance containing histamine in the treatment of asthma and allergy—without providing a shred of scientific evidence to support this order, nor any evidence showing that histamine is harmful. As a Google search on the Internet will reveal, histamine has been the subject of international medical research for about a century and even has entire medical organizations dedicated to its investigation. Its curative role in asthma and allergy is documented scientifically throughout the world literature—see also the international medical science website **Medline/PubMed**.

Here follows an excerpt from my introduction to his 2003 book, *The Plot Against Asthma And Allergy Patients* in which he describes the mainstream scientific research into asthma therapy and the betrayal of such patients by standard medicine with its lucrative addiction to cortisone therapy which controls symptoms, but certainly cannot cure. The book is being translated into Russian. Its original English edition is available through Kos Publishing Inc. 519-927-1049.

Renovating Medicine

"Practicing medicine without knowledge of biochemistry and physiology is merely pop-gun pharmacy."　　　　　　　　　—Sir William Osler 1890[1]

"Far too large a section of the treatment of disease is today controlled by the big manufacturing pharmacists, who have enslaved us in a plausible pseudo-science."　　　　　　　　　—Sir William Osler 1909

To make medicine once again patient-centered, not patent-centered, and to free medical research from corporate priorities, is the task of our time as surely as it was the task in the 18th century to remove political power from kings and put it into the hands of the people.

Indeed, the most profound insight I have experienced first as a medical science writer, and now as a publisher of "Books on Medicine that Works", is the discovery that in virtually all areas of medicine the basic scientific breakthroughs achieved in the leading research institutions are *rarely* communicated to people, are very often *not even taught* to medical students, and are *not readily available* to practicing doctors.

What IS readily available to everybody is information on yet another supposedly miraculous drug which promises to alleviate the symptoms of any known disease. Pick up any recent edition of *Macleans Magazine*, for example, and attached to its outside you will find, courtesy of GlaxoSmithKline, in dramatically colored red, white, and black a folder stating: "IMPORTANT INFORMATION FOR PEOPLE WITH ASTHMA ENCLOSED." A handy little quiz inside allows the reader to be sure in seconds that he or she may suffer from asthma more seriously than previously thought and that their "asthma is not under control." This message comes to you courtesy of GlaxoSmithKline, the world's largest producer of steroid puffers.

You are holding in your hands a book that, unlike the above advertisement, really does contain important information for people suffering from asthma. Dr. Ravikovich is fully familiar with the worldwide basic science research on allergic diseases, successfully used a cure and reported on his results at international conferences. He also tells you why that cure is not generally known or available. Here is the story of a doctor who fought for his patients.

This book provides the reader with a political revelation, a medical tour de force, and a scientific detective story. It will take you into the world of the immune system and its biochemistry and you will become thoroughly familiar with the world's leading medical journals and the elegant medical research into the bio-chemistry of the causes of asthma and allergic disease.

But this is also a shocking detective story: you will learn how those very same medical researchers, who to this day are celebrated leaders in the community of immunologists, mysteriously disavowed their own findings and effectively betrayed patients worldwide as they bowed to corporate agendas—for reasons best known to themselves. Although this seems unbelievable at first, it is not without precedent.

Today, the sell-out of medical practice to agendas that have nothing to do with curing the sick, is nearly total. Patients are now referred to as "consumers" who are encouraged to believe that they have "choices" of treatment offered in that enormous market of modern medicine run as a business. It is as if illness has become an accepted life-style choice—right after the car industry. After all, Pfizer is not only the world's largest pharmaceutical corporation, but also the world's second largest corporation. The representatives of the drug companies are accepted as "stake-holders" in medicine to the point where they are part of determining standards of practice, sit on the councils of the medical licensing authorities, virtually control all medical research in the absence of publicly funded research (but not in most of continental Europe), and act as policy and fundraising staff for our political leaders.[2]

As for the business mantra of "consumer choice", for the asthma and allergy patient it's basically steroids or steroids or steroids: mint flavored syrups for kids, or laced with antibiotics (to cover all bases), or as shots, as creams, and usually as the ever present puffer shaped as a toy for kids, handy and pretty like a lipstick for the ladies. As for the cure, "profits can only be harvested from chronic disease" a CEO of a pharmaceutical giant observed in a recent shareholder's meeting.[3]

But whose responsibility is it to fix this situation? Consider this then: The world's most prestigious science journal, *Nature* (March 28, 2002), ran an article entitled "Can you believe what you read?" showing how the editors of the most respected medical journals have begun to do some radical house-cleaning when it became overwhelmingly apparent that published research too often reflects corporate interests o the point of distorting the observed facts. On June 27th 2002 *Nature* reported that even medical bio-ethicists are now "being offered stock board positions, consulting contracts, research grants, and even stock options" by pharmaceutical companies—and they accept these goodies! Two international conferences were held in 2002 on conflicts of interest in medicine (Atlanta and Warsaw). The former editor of the *New England Journal of Medicine*, Marcia Angell, justly famous for her fearless scrutiny of corruption in medicine, now works closely with the *Center for Science in the Public Interest* (**www.csip.org**), a watchdog exposing unethical behavior of doctors selling out to industry and industry's false or self-servingly incomplete product claims.

This book is not simple. But neither is living with asthma, hives, irritable bowel syndrome, chronic fatigue, constantly itchy skin, the annual round of hay fever, or potentially fatal food allergies. The information in it is not "alternative"—the research is entirely mainstream. Here you will learn why you are sick, why your standard treatments don't work very well and make you sicker through so-called side effects, how you could become healthy, or at the very least greatly improved and get off drugs, and what you can do to help make this healing treatment available.

This is no ordinary self-help book—indeed I wish it was. This book is a crash course in asthma and allergy medicine designed to empower you with knowledge and hopefully inspire you with a holy rage and the determination to help bring out these facts so they become generally known to doctors and patients alike.

The Epilogue is something of a bombshell because it describes the most recent publication on allergy research that came out only two weeks before this book was submitted in its manuscript form to me. This research paper fully validates everything you read in this book and returns to the research that was more and more successfully hidden over the past two decades. The politically significant fact of this development is that this was published by the Swiss government's research institution funded by tax money, not drug companies. The equally important medical historical facts are that now "the truth which was denied entrance through the door has forced its way in by the window"—as the Russian proverb puts it and as Dr. Ravikovich is fond of reminding us.

Treating asthma, allergy and related diseases successfully, at a fraction of the current cost of mere limited symptom control, is an art and a science easily learned by any interested doctor. There is currently a great deal of interest in therapies that cure and are not merely symptom control methods generally employed by the majority of physicians. What suffering patients often don't realize is how terrible the frustration of doctors is who wish to help but often are prevented by the regulatory systems from employing new methods.

Note: Marcia Angell, after twenty years as the editor of arguably one of the most important medical journals of the world, The New England Journal of Medicine, *published a book in August 2004 en titled* The Truth About The Drug Companies; How They Deceive Us And What To Do About It, Random House. *Highly recommended because it not only explains how such a travesty as the Ravikovich case is possible, but what also appears to motivate the medical regulatory bodies, such as the CPSO.*

The Case of Dr. Frank Adams

Vitality Magazine September 2000

Pain is a country to which the whole human race holds a passport from our first to our last breath. And though the very house of medicine is built upon the universal fact of pain, it is not a recognized medical specialty. The annual cost of pain is greater than that of heart disease and AIDS combined. The consensus at this year's World Congress of Anesthesiologists was that the lack of pain control is "one of the biggest medical failures of the 20th century." One of the participants, Dr. Ellen Thompson of the University of Ottawa, added, "pain is one of the last frontiers in medicine"—sadly, primarily because of the underlying outdated attitudes to pain and murky medical politics.

Professor M. Somerville, one of McGill University's medical ethicist, who has been an advisor to the World Health Organization, set an international standard with her often cited statement that leaving "a person in avoidable pain and suffering should be regarded as a serious breach of fundamental human rights."

Senator Sharon Carstairs' committee released a report in June 2000 entitled "Quality End-of-Life Care: The Right of Every Canadian," showing that the lack of pain management for the dying is an avoidable and unnecessary disgrace in this country. While the Carstairs Report focuses primarily on palliative care, it is only the tip of the iceberg—the management of *chronic* pain is an equally serious disgrace in Canada, a fact she hopes to highlight over the next two years.

Canada happens to have several internationally acclaimed experts in pain research and therapy. For example, definitions of pain in medical textbooks were first penned by psychiatrist Dr. Harold Merskey, founder of the Canadian Pain Society and editor of its acclaimed journal, one of the leaders in medical publications. He is also a co-founder of the *International Society for the Study of Pain*, a 7,000-member organization begun in 1975 by a Sicilian-born anesthetist, John Bonica, who put himself through medical school in the U.S. with professional wrestling. The chronic pain he sustained from wrestling injuries, and his later medical experience during World War II, focused his interest on pain relief. The ISSP put pain onto a scientific basis worldwide.

Dr. Frank Adams of Kingston is an internationally renowned expert in brain injury-related chronic pain. Of the dozen or so internationally utilized neurological pain tests available to practitioners, Dr. Adams developed two thirds of them. He was instrumental in framing the recent pain management guidelines for the U.S. through the National Institute of Health which defined pain as equivalent to "a major pathogen" that is as dangerous to health as a virus or bacteria. The federation of medical licensing boards accepted this definition and U.S. laws have been brought in line accordingly. Pain is now the "fifth vital sign" that it is compulsory to treat to the fullest extent, just like blood pressure etc. These guidelines were accepted by the World Health Organization and, in Canada, have so far only been accepted by Nova Scotia, from where the rest of Canada will hopefully take its lead. *(Update: All Canadian Provinces have accepted these guidelines, but Ontario's CPSO does not encourage pain doctors to follow them.)*

In the opinion of Dr. Merskey, Dr. Adams is one of the top pain experts in the world. Yet, in July, the College of Physicians and Surgeons of Ontario (CPSO) tried to suspend his license because they found it "abhorrent" that he involves pain patients in the decision on how much pain medication is required for relief. The College's position was, once again, as so many times before, that patient outcome is not relevant. Not surprisingly, a flood of thousands of protests delayed the CPSO's decision on Dr. Adams.

Dr. Peter Rothbart is the chairperson of the Ontario Medical Association's Section on Chronic Pain, which he founded—the first of its kind in Canada. The rest of the provincial medical associations and the national CMA do not have such sections. He has organized several international pain conferences and researched especially chronic pain stemming from head and neck injuries.

The CPSO tried to go after him and several of his colleagues at the Rothbart Pain Clinic for the same reasons as they did in pursuing Dr. Adams which included charges of having "excessive amounts" of pain killers on hand—in a pain clinic! What did they expect? He and Dr. Thompson, who specializes in whiplash and lower back pain, developed new nerve-block treatments which are highly effective. They also treat fibromyalgia with the respect it deserves, showing through sophisticated tests that such patients (as indeed all pain patients) have objectively measurable changes in their spinal fluid, unique to their condition, proving the reality of their complaint.

Angered by the antiquated and harmful attitude of the CPSO, Dr. Thompson ran for office with this licensing authority and became an outspoken council member, insisting on the need to rely on clinical experience and basic science. "Above all you must believe the patient!" she says. That didn't go over too well with the CPSO. When she publicly supported Dr. Adams at a press conference in Queen's Park, the CPSO Registrar called her into his office for a regular dressing-down and ordered her to "be a team player".

Pain management in Canada is a mess for many reasons. There is the usual federal-provincial turf war, with public health being a federal responsibility and hospitals being in the provincial turf; universities are in the middle of the same war. Medical schools don't teach pain management, but focus on high-tech research. The exercise of compassion is, quite logically, a dead end for careers and for research grant money. Dying people aren't valued for their vote, so health care systems do not provide pain management as a core service (except in the Netherlands). Thus the care of the dying and the chronically ill is primarily family and volunteer work.

Not surprisingly, the data consistently show that chronic pain patients have the highest rate of suicide and, among *all* types of suicide attempts, they are the most successful ones on the first try; these patients really mean it.

Finally, there is what Dr. Merskey calls the "opiate phobia". Historically, the power and prestige of the medical profession, he explained, evolved over two centuries largely from the fact that doctors took on the sole responsibility for controlling opium as a public service to fight addiction. Since then, of course, we know that the potential for opiate addiction in the general, as well as in patient populations, is very small.

Dr. Adams' research showed that chronic pain patients metabolize opiates completely differently than do persons without pain. The pain patient's brain *clears* and he or she becomes functional again, while in the addict opiates create drowsiness. In pain-free people the drug floods the brain in addition to the naturally existing metabolic pain managers, the endorphins. In patients with chronic pain these endorphins have been exhausted and the introduction of opiates presents an equivalent to insulin being given to a diabetic: it restores brain function and thereby also the immune and endocrine systems which are controlled largely by the brain. Without effective and complete pain relief, Dr. Adams explained, people die, as all systems become exhausted.

Yet, the antiquated prejudice against opiates remains in place. McMaster University's Dr. Alejandro Jadad searched the pain literature and found 40,000 citations of which only three (!) dealt with opiates. Interestingly, all these doctors told me that patients *prefer* treatments that do not involve opiates. Therefore, the specter of a horde of addicts beating down doctors' doors is a wild 19th century fantasy.

Dr. Thompson told the story of a young man who had had his arm torn off in an industrial accident resulting in debilitating, chronic pain including phantom pain, where the pain of the missing limb continues to be signaled in the brain. Opiates rarely work in such cases, as the body's cells have only one receptor site capable of interacting with opiates. Demerol, which can interact with many receptors, worked for him. However, current (but outdated) guidelines prohibit the use of Demerol on a long-term basis because of potential for seizures.

When Dr. Thompson wanted to explore this case for a research project, she tried to find the patient (who had been returned to his area physician). She was informed that he had committed suicide because the subsequent physician stopped the Demerol, in accordance with guidelines on long-term use. Devastated, Dr. Thompson presented this case for purposes of policy revision to the CPSO council, saying, "A possible seizure I can treat, but death I cannot treat." She was informed by the council that this death was unfortunate, but that the guidelines take precedence.

Drs. Rothbart and Merskey feel that the major attitude problem is a holdover from the British "stiff-upper-lip" tradition that brands chronic pain as wimpish. "God forbid that people might get a lift and feel good!" is how Dr. Rothbart caricatured this mind-set.

While acute pain from injury or surgery is usually treated well, doing so has no implications for insurance companies and university research grants, because that sort of pain goes away, as does the patient—unlike chronic pain patients. They remain the thorns in the sides of the insurance companies because they don't want to pay for long-term pain management. On the surface it appears that ignorance is officially sanctioned, an interdisciplinary approach is discouraged, current basic research in neurology and brain sciences is rarely consulted by doctors, but really it is money that has a lot to do with it. At the CPSO, for example, at the time of the Adams case, council members included persons who were directly employed by the insurance industry, one of them being a lawyer for the industry who even sat on discipline panels. Obviously, the interests of the patient are not the CPSO's primary concern when "stake holders" of this type are admitted into the medical regulatory system as active "partners". Indeed, it was an insurance agent who informed one of Dr. Adams' patients that he better get a new doctor, since Adams was going to lose his license. This took place before Dr. Adams had any idea that the CPSO was going to prosecute him—the insurance company knew what the CPSO was planning before Dr. Adams knew and what the outcome was going to be before the trial had even taken place.

Dr. Dean Ornish, the famous U.S. heart specialist, who proved that heart disease can be reversed without surgery and drugs, can be our guide here in Canada, too, on the issue of insurance companies: "The insurance industry is really the major determinant of health care—not science and clinical experience," he said on Bill Moyers' 1993 PBS television show.

Of course, this war between insurance and pain patients costs millions—all unnecessarily so, observed Dr. Thompson, since genetics has shown that only 15% of the population is genetically predisposed to develop chronic pain following injury.

Drs. Rothbart and Thompson lodged a formal complaint with the CPSO about doctors who make huge incomes *solely* by writing negative reports on chronic pain patients for insurance companies. They even take courses, which teach how to discredit a patient's testimony and medical documentation.

One of the improperly prosecuted pain doctors, Dr. George Gale (details of his case are in the 2001 *Glasnost Report*) decided to take those courses himself, so he could learn how to counteract the pernicious influence of these assessors later in court and to protect his chronic pain patients.

These insurance doctors, against whom Drs. Rothbart and Thompson complained on ethical grounds, belong to an organization called the *Association of Independent Assessors* which serves the insurance industry only. The then Deputy Registrar, Dr. John Carlisle, whose primary responsibility was all these prosecutions, including Dr. Adams' case, was also a member of that association at the same time as he was serving on the CPSO. Drs. Rothbart and Thompson pointed out the obvious and shocking conflict of interest involved and asked the CPSO's ethics committee to investigate. The irony is rich in the subsequent reply they received, which was this: that the CPSO doesn't have an ethics committee.

The battle for enlightened medicine continues, but Senator Carstairs expressed guarded optimism about the future of at least cancer pain management because public support has been enormous. Meanwhile, the problem of chronic pain remains. The answer is to become informed about the many existing options and to support both mainstream doctors and complementary pain medicine. This empowers the patient. It is also important not to let the CPSO get away with their systemic conflicts of interest.

The choices in complementary and alternative pain relief therapies are many and varied. They include acupuncture, biofeedback, therapeutic touch, meditation, orthomolecular medicine, massage, osteopathy, chiropractic, homeopathy, herbal medicine, and prayer. Every one of these has rigorous scientific information to back it (even prayer), published in mainstream journals, generally of that famous "basic science" variety that is struggling to inform medical practice and to remove the cobwebs of prejudice and antiquated attitudes.

To find what works best for you is a journey of exploration and frequently of hope fulfilled. One thing is certain: the quick fix is an illusion in medicine. The bio-individuality of the patient is the only solid reality. Even more amazing is the realization in medical science that any *one* intervention can positively affect the entire system; everything is interconnected. Furthermore, the failure of one approach is no reason to despair, but an invitation to try something else. And something new is being discovered all the time, as are unexpected applications.

Consider the problem of phantom pain, one of the greatest challenges to pain doctors. EMDR (eye movement desensitization and reprocessing), the fairly new therapy for post-traumatic stress disorder, can also cure chronic pain in certain cases. At this years' Pacific Northwestern EMDR conference, Robert H. Tinker and Sandra A. Wilson, both EMDR therapists specializing in post-traumatic stress problems, discovered to their own surprise that this psychotherapeutic method produced a lasting cure for chronic phantom pain.

Chronic lower back pain from a serious sports injury can be successfully treated with a variety of approaches, such as sophisticated nerve block techniques, acupuncture, meditation, massage and therapeutic (i.e. large) doses of magnesium and vitamins E and C. Arthritis pain, usually treated with steroids with serious side-effects, can often be controlled totally with essential fatty acid supplementation, glucosamine sulphate and MSM. Migraine headaches can be cured with osteopathy as well as (in women) with progesterone (which set me free after 20 years of debilitating migraines) and sometimes merely dietary changes. Diabetic neuropathy can be reversed by chelation therapy, therapeutic doses of vitamin E, as well as opiates. Many forms of pain, as has been demonstrated at Harvard Medical School, can be controlled with meditation.

Since inflammation is the common denominator for many pain conditions as well as heart disease, high blood pressure, cancer, diabetes, PMS, irritable bowl syndrome, and asthma, it is often drastically reduced by essential fatty acids, coenzyme Q_{10}, various vitamins, and a pesticide free diet (i.e. organic food).

One of the most astonishing instances of pain control I witnessed last fall. One of my sons sustained a terrible injury to his left hand at work. The injury became seriously infected. Fancy hand surgery was required, intravenous antibiotics were lifesaving. Due to the presence of so many nerve endings in one's hands, post-op pain medication is given very liberally. Knowing about the healing power of vitamin C, the pain-relieving effect of calcium, and the anti-inflammatory properties of vitamin E, I smuggled it into the hospital, leaving the choice up to my son—after all, it was his hand. My son took the supplements and, after the first day following surgery, no opiates at all. The surgeon, amazed at seeing him sitting in bed and reading comfortably, asked several times why he wasn't taking the shots. Finally, my son told him. Unfortunately, this brilliant surgeon was unable to shed his blinkers. He refused to believe it.

The sources supplied below were chosen to provide the reader with information backed by rigorous scientific research—the kind that forces the attention of even the most conservative mind. The body's dynamic biochemistry and continuously adaptive strategies with their personal environment have provided for many gates of entry through which help can be administered in many different ways.

Sources and Resources

L. Bucci, Pain-Free: *The Definitive Guide to Healing Arthritis, Low-Back Pain, and Sports Injuries through Nutrition*, by Summit; 1995

Encyclopedia of Natural Healing, ALIVE books; 1997

J. Heimlich, *What Your Doctor Won't Tell You*, Harper Collins; 1990

R. Firshein, *The Nutraceutical Revolution*, Penguin;1998

W. Jonas & J.Levin, *Essentials of Complementary and Alternative Medicine*, by Lippincott; 1999

J. Kabat-Zinn, *Full Catastrophe Living*, Delta; 1990

B. Moyers, *Healing and the Mind*, Doubleday, 1993

F. Shapiro & M. Forrest,*EMDR The Breakthrough Therapy*, Basic Books; 1997

M. Walker, *The Chelation Answer*, Second Opinion; 1994

Association for Applied Psychophysiology and Biofeedback, 303-422-8436, e-mail: **aapb@resourcenter.com**

Transcendental Meditation: **www.tm.org**

Chelation and orthomolecular medicine: American College for Advancement in Medicine, 1-800-LEAD-OUT, **www.acam.org**

The Rothbart Pain Clinic, Toronto 416-512-6407

The Rapson Pain Clinic (acupuncture), Toronto 416-968-1366

Ontario Medical Association's Sections on Pain and Complementary Medicine via OMA, Toronto, 416-599-2580

To find an EMDR therapist: **www.EMDRA.org** or 512-451-5200

The Glasnost Report 2001

Following is a short excerpt of the *Glasnost Report* which was provided to the government of Ontario in September 2001 by a group of medical organizations and patient groups. The aim was to make public the abuses of power committed by the CPSO, the medical regulatory body of the Province of Ontario, and to suggest in concrete detail how the *Regulated Health Professions Act* should be amended so that such abuses could not happen again. Its centerpiece is a legal opinion by Michael Code of Sack Goldblatt & Mitchell, Toronto.

Only the Executive Summary and a few case histories of improperly prosecuted doctors are provided here to supplement my articles for the general public on them. The entire report with all its recommendations for legislative change is available for downloading on the website of Kos Publishing Inc: **www.kospublishing.com** .This report contains highly interesting information from CPSO whistleblowers, *Toronto Star* investigative reports, a government-ordered investigation of the CPSO's complaints process, and much more. Anybody who ever intends to complain about a doctor or who wishes to protect a doctor against improper prosecution needs to know what stone walls they are up against and how to deal with these obstacles.

Subsequently, during 2002 and 2003, various meetings between the authors of this report and the CPSO took place, and the Ministry of Health became involved and was most supportive. By the end of 2003, the chief architect of most of these abuses and the improper disciplinary investigations, Deputy Registrar Dr. John Carlisle, did not have his contract with the CPSO renewed and has left that position. He worked at the CPSO for almost 30 years. The doctors, whose cases are summarized here are all working now, after years of interference which was traumatic for them and their patients, and in some cases were financially devastating to the doctors' families.

Almost all of the "doctors from hell", so many of whom the CPSO shielded against floods of complaints from injured patients or their relatives, have been properly prosecuted since 2001 as well, mostly due to the *Toronto Star's* relentless investigative pursuit of their victims. The *Glasnost Report* includes their stories also as well as provides suggestions on how to stop the CPSO from shielding such doctors.

The courts, in most cases, came through and served the public interest as well as setting legal precedents the CPSO can no longer ignore. Amusingly, in what most have been his last address to the CPSO council, Dr. John Carlisle in November 2003 told council members that the most important task for the coming year 2004 would be to concentrate on the courts—to "educate them about the CPSO's role" and duties, because, he complained, the courts had not been at all supportive. Really now.

The legislative reform advocated in this report has not happened yet.

EXECUTIVE SUMMARY

Several physician and patient groups as well as concerned individuals joined forces and have pooled their information bases in order to inform the government and the people of Ontario of their concerns about the manner in which doctors and patients are treated by the *College of Physicians and Surgeons of Ontario* (CPSO). The consensus is that the CPSO may be violating the human rights of both doctors and patients through the arbitrary interpretation and misuse of the existing legislation governing medical practice in this province. It is agreed also that the manner in which the CPSO conducts its complaints and disciplinary processes to a large extent serves to retard medical progress in Ontario, discussed in Section VI. We provide our view of the current crisis in the CPSO's handling of the complaint process in Section IV.

This consensus is supported by the findings of the KPMG Report of July 2000, commissioned by the Ontario Ministry of Health in 1998 and by the legal opinion of criminal and *Charter* expert Mr. Michael Code of Sack Goldblatt and Mitchell, Toronto. His analysis was requested by a group of doctors, patients and concerned individuals called *The Committee for the Investigation of the College* which was founded in 1998. Mr. Code analyzed several physicians' discipline cases, some of which were the subject of many media reports; they are summarized and presented in Section V. Mr. Code concluded in 1999 that

> In at least one case "there was *prima facie* evidence that CPSO officials may have committed the criminal offence of obstructing justice by repeatedly misleading the Executive Committee as to the true state of the evidence in this case". In the remaining cases Mr. Code found "evidence of abuse and misuse of power", "systemic unfairness and repeated abuse and misuse of power", and "a consistent pattern of unfairness".

In addition to the presentation of these discipline cases studied by Mr. Code, this report also provides information and documentation received from "whistleblowers" from amongst the CPSO staff on aspects of the problems identified with the CPSO's handling of complaints and discipline. We also rely upon exhaustive interviews with many physicians affected by the disciplinary process, and the records of aggrieved patients; some of them had their stories covered in the investigative reports on the CPSO commenced in *The Toronto Star* in May of 2001.

A focus of this report is on the submission made by the CPSO in December 1999 to the HPRAC Review. In their submission, the CPSO requests changes to the existing legislation which, in the opinion of the authors of this report, are insupportable because they demand an unacceptable increase in powers and open up even more opportunity for violations of human rights. An analysis of the CPSO submission—their "wish list"—

to HPRAC follows in this report in Section VIII and our specific recommendations for the inclusion of safeguards against future abuses of power and process are found in Section X. It is our belief that the existing legislation lacks adequate safeguards. We also comment on the HPRAC Report, "Adjusting the Balance".

Our recommendations deal with

1) general recommendations,

2) a suggested test for public accountability in all CPSO handling of complaints and discipline, and

3) specific recommendations for changes (safeguards) to the *Regulated Health Professions Act* and the *Medicine Act*.

Abuse of College-driven discipline cases: Sections 75 and 59 of RHPA

In 1998 a group of deeply concerned doctors, health care advocacy groups, one lawyer, and one investigative medical journalist decided to form a group called *Committee for the Investigation of the College*. The Committee retained Mr. Michael Code of *Sack, Goldblatt & Mitchell* and provided him with all the available documentary information on a group of 9 Ontario physicians 7 of whom had been subject to disciplinary proceedings under Section 75 and one under Section 59. Over the course of a year, Mr. Code provided his considered opinion on each case. The executive summary of this opinion is to be found in the Appendix as item No. 1. (The full text of this document is

being provided to Premier Harris, the Minister of Health, the Attorney General, and the official Health Critics; it is available to any reader upon request from the Committee whose contact information is given at the end of this report.)

Mr. Code found

1. That in the case of Dr. M. Smith of Almont "there was *prima facie* evidence that CPSO officials may have committed the criminal offence of obstructing justice by repeatedly misleading the Executive Committee as to the true state of the evidence in this case". In the remaining cases Mr. Code found
2. "evidence of abuse and misuse of power"
3. "systemic unfairness and repeated abuse and misuse of power" and
4. "a consistent pattern of unfairness"

As Mr. Code had no prior experience with the CPSO or with doctors' cases, he came to this task unbiased and viewed the evidence from the point of view of criminal law. He was sufficiently disturbed and concerned about his findings that he spoke at a press conference held in Queen's Park on May 30th, 2000, where he described in more general terms the cases he had examined. The transcript of that statement is item No. 2 in the Appendix.

Dr. F. RAVIKOVICH

Dr. Ravikovich, a graduate of the Leningrad Medical Institute, worked for many years at a teaching hospital in the former Soviet Union. He earned his specialization degrees in allergy and internal medicine. He came to Canada as refugees in the early 1980s. During the Cold War, medical science progressed in different directions on either side of the Iron Curtain. Most notably, the development of pharmaceuticals was prevented by the Communist regimes of the east block, which resulted in medical research focusing on what we would call "alternative" ways of treating disease—often with extraordinary success. Hence, Dr. Ravikovich brought with him knowledge and research into the treatment of allergy, and especially asthma, which had been validated in medical science and clinical application in the former Soviet Union. He lectured widely, including at the annual International Congress of Allergy and Immunology and attracted the attention of researchers at Stanford University in the US. In 1992 the University of Tel Aviv, Israel, asked Dr. Ravikovich to join an Israeli research team at Hadassa University in a large double-blind study of histamine treatment for asthma. He had to abandon that project because he was brought into discipline by the CPSO—on what basis is **still unknown.**

> No patient complaint is on record against Dr. Ravikovich. Yet, to this day the CPSO web site states that the action taken against this physician is based on five patient complaints. Numerous efforts at correction, even by Dr. Ravikovich's lawyers, have been unsuccessful.

Initially, the CPSO asked questions in 1988 about his practice, which Dr. Ravikovich misunderstood to be **interest** in a new and effective asthma treatment with which he had a vast experience. He has reported in the international literature the results of histamine treatment with some 1,500 patients. Naively and enthusiastically, Dr. Ravikovich provided the CPSO with 200 files voluntarily for purposes of discussion. He quickly learned that, instead, he was the subject of a Peer Assessment. While he continued to be under the impression that he was to be peer assessed, Mr. Code's analysis shows the following had actually happened:

"The initial s.64 Order against Dr. Ravikovich was made by the Executive Committee on December 12 and 13, 1989. The appointment of inspectors under s.64 did not occur until September 13, 1990 [i.e. 9 months later]. In between these two dates, Dr. Carlisle, the Deputy Registrar, wrote to Dr. Ravikovich, by letter dated February 6, 1990, and elicited information about Dr. Ravikovich's use of histamine therapy. Dr. Carlisle did not inform Dr. Ravikovich that the Executive Committee had already made a s.64 Order against him two months earlier. Indeed, Dr. Carlisle's letter is positively misleading on this subject, as he states: The *Executive Committee has not reached any conclusion on this matter, but invites your comment.* This letter should have been written before the s. 64 Order was made. It was unfair and less than frank to write such a misleading letter after the s.64 Order had been made. The conduct of CPSO officials, in this aspect of the matter, provides further evidence of a number of themes that we have seen in the other cases."

Mr. Code concluded that "this case does support and confirm the pattern of abuse and misuse of its disciplinary powers by CPSO officials." This abuse is further compounded by the fact that it is completely improper to transmute a Quality Assurance case into a disciplinary one—leave alone without telling the physician that the second is already approved while pretending that it is the first that is in progress.

The s. 64 Order against Dr. Ravikovich is based on a "histamine challenge test" which the CPSO Executive correctly identified as being obsolete for at least 30 years. (See item 7 in Appendix) Dr. Ravikovich never used this test which, incidentally, requires equipment no longer available. He invited the CPSO inspectors to see his office and confirm his statement. The disciplinary process ended in June 1995. This original stem allegation, which it was incumbent upon the CPSO to prove, was never mentioned again, no arguments were made, no witnesses called, and Dr. Ravikovich's assertion that he never used such a test was not dealt with in any way whatsoever. Indeed, the basis of the entire disciplinary action against Dr. Ravikovich mysteriously transformed itself on

September 13, 1990, when the allegations against him changed from the original alleged use of the "histamine challenge test" to the use of histamine as a therapeutic agent. Proof that the Executive Committee had, in fact, approved this change of direction, was never provided despite Dr. Ravikovich's lawyers asking for it repeatedly.

No patient complaints existed either, instead the proceedings became focused on whether or not Dr. Ravikovich's work was "scientifically valid". The CPSO provided only **one** published medical paper in the prosecution's support which was an article published by the *British Society of Allergy and Immunology*. This article asserted that the basis for clinical work should be a) double blind studies and b) clinical experience and personal judgment. The CPSO prosecution did not mention point b in their legal arguments and in the exhibit cited only point a. When the defense drew attention to this selective quoting, the prosecution withdrew its one and only piece of supporting evidence completely. The case proceeded without expert witnesses, without discussion of patient files, and without consideration of the 200 (!) scientific papers provided by the defense, and without discussion of the stem allegation in the Notice of Hearing. Originally, the CPSO sought revocation of license, but the near total lack of any material on which to base anything at all, may have forced the Discipline Panel into changing the penalty to a reprimand— and a most peculiar restriction on his license.

The Sentence of June 23, 1995 provides for the following penalty: "1. Dr. Ravikovich is to be reprimanded and the fact of the reprimand is to be recorded on the Register. 2. A restriction on Dr. Ravikovich's Certificate of Registration is to be imposed for an indefinite period, prohibiting Dr. Ravikovich from employing histamine for purposes of diagnosis or therapy.... Dr. Ravikovich is not to employ any biological material which contains histamine." The Penalty concludes:" The Committee believes that the public is protected by the Order it made, in that it prohibits Dr. Ravikovich... from using histamine as a diagnostic or therapeutic tool when there is no scientific or medical validity to use it."

The irony of this Penalty is that histamine is a substance that does not require a doctor's prescription and is required to be on hand in every allergist's practice for various emergency situations or as a control substance.

A significant procedural impropriety occurred in this case as well: item 8 in the Appendix is the copy of a scientific paper published by Dr.

Ravikovich in which he reproduced a table of facts concerning the biological activities and effects known to science about histamine. It is derived from publications of a world-renowned expert on histamine, S. Holgate. Additionally, a similar table from the then current textbook on allergy (used also at the University of Toronto medical school, while this case was being pursued at the CPSO) was appended to Dr. Ravikovich's article. That textbook then was *Allergy*, edited by A. Kaplan, 1985. Both these tables were central to the defense's documentation because they provided the summary of the internationally accepted basis for the medical use of histamine. These two tables were missing in the files provided to the Discipline Committee. Repeatedly attention was drawn to the importance of these documents and the demand was made to correct the error—but it was not corrected.

> In sum, the case has an unknown origin, was initiated secretly on the basis of an erroneous allegation concerning an antiquated testing process, proceeded as an argument about scientific validity without the benefit of the published science involved, and was concluded without supporting scientific or patient-outcome evidence. The prosecuting CPSO failed to prove anything, but asserted that they were protecting the public from potential harm, which was neither discussed nor proven. The Ravikovich case has the characteristics of a phantom.

Item 9 in the Appendix is a letter dated November 8, 1992, by Dr. Ravikovich to Deputy Registrar Dr. J. Carlisle asking him what to do with his desperate asthma patients. No reply was ever received. Asthma, especially in children, has increased four fold in the last decade and is identified by the World Health Organization as one of the most serious health problems. Far from experiencing themselves as the protected public, hundreds of these desperate asthma patients went public, resulting in a *Fifth Estate* TV program aired March 16, 1993, the transcript of which is provided in item 10 in the Appendix.

An important question is raised here: does the passage of the Kwinter Bill renders this absurd CPSO decision against Dr. Ravikovich's asthma treatment obsolete? Many asthma patients in Ontario are waiting for an answer breathlessly.

Dr. J. KROP

This case is possibly the longest running discipline case in medical history. It began in 1988, the investigation itself commenced in 1991, and the Notice of Hearing went out in 1994. A total of 37 hearing days took place between 1995 and 1998 with a hiatus of no activity or hearings in 1996. This hiatus is one of the many mysteries of this case. Presumably a disciplinary hearing is supposed to serve the public interest and such a delay requires explanation. The delay was caused by the CPSO, not the defense. The case cost over $ 1 million to defend, most of it raised by public donations through the efforts of the *Environmental Health Group* which is a sponsor of this submission. The cost to the CPSO was likely close to double that. Deputy Registrar, Dr. J. Carlisle observed in an internal memo of September 1988 to the executive committee: **"This will be a costly and lengthy process, but may be the only way of finally, once and for all, dealing with these clinical ecologists".**

The CPSO's then legal counsel, Mr. Richard Steinecke, recommended in a memo of September 17, 1993, **not to proceed** on the grounds that "such cases [note the plural] cannot succeed unless one has either 1) an angry, exploited patient, or 2) actual harm to a patient." He went on to say, "In order to succeed, we will have to prove that his defense experts are not reputable or credible. In my view the College does not have a solid case at this point, and the matter should not be referred to a hearing. As you know, there are additional reasons for caution as this case has a high publicity potential." But the case went forward with another lawyer, Mr. Robert Armstrong of Tory & Tory.

Every effort was made to find a patient who would side with the prosecution. An internal e-mail memo from an investigator to the then chief of investigations, Mr. Ed Singleton, of March 3, 1994 is seen in item 11 in the Appendix. It states that **"interviews have been conducted with potential witnesses. All of whom are very supportive of Dr. Krop. We have been unable to locate others and attempts are continuing in this regard."** This memo is signed **"thanks, Ed [Singleton who was chief of prosecutions then]".** An estimated 200 patients of Dr. Krop's were sought out for interviews by the CPSO inspectors—without success.

One person was persuaded to testify against Dr. Krop. This former patient did not file a formal complaint. During cross-examination this patient's testimony fell apart and had to be withdrawn by the prosecution. This case is briefly referred to a "complaint" in Mr. Code's opinion given below where the context of his remarks is that moment in time where the prosecuting CPSO attempted to make this patient into a complainant. Interestingly, just prior to coming on the stand, this person claimed disability for repetitive motion injury after having worked in a flower shop for three weeks. She received this pension shortly after, following her testimony before the CPSO, during which she referred to the CPSO lawyer, Mr. Robert Armstrong, always as "Bob". The details are in the transcripts and available upon request.

The procedural improprieties and peculiarities in this case are so numerous, that only a few can be mentioned here. For example, during a disclosure meeting at the CPSO offices, Mr. Armstrong slammed a wooden gavel on the table and exclaimed, **"You are not entitled to disclosure, your only aim is to destroy the College."**

Furthermore, the charges were formulated **after** the inspectors had taken patient charts and commenced the investigation. Dr. Krop also did not know why and by whom he was accused of what. In response to Dr. Krop's lawyer insisting on knowing why an investigation was being initiated, Deputy Registrar Dr. John Carlisle replied on February 19, 1989,"**We understand that Dr. Krop is presently participating in a research project proposal at the University of Toronto, and it is partly in response to that knowledge that we believe these preliminary inquiries are necessary."**

Since this reasoning parallels the approach taken with Dr. Ravikovich, one gets the impression that the discipline process is used to establish medical standards such as to prevent medical developments from occurring.

The hearings proceeded without a mandatory report on Dr. Krop's practice presumably because the original report, provided by Dr. McFadden, even after several re-writes, was so unacceptably full of errors, the CPSO prosecution could not use it. Instead, a report by Dr. McCourtie (who had also done a report on Dr. Ravikovich) was circulated among the members of the Discipline Panel, but Dr. McCourtie had never set foot in Dr. Krop's practice and had not had the opportunity to review the files taken by the inspectors. Because of his stated bias against environmental medicine, Dr. McCourtie's report also had to be withdrawn when the hearings finally began.

The record shows that the prosecution's expert witnesses all admitted in their testimony that they were unfamiliar with environmental medicine. The extensive peer review done by the *American Academy of Environmental Medicine* (AAEM), an international medical association that trains physicians in environmental medicine, was not considered by the CPSO: Deputy Registrar Dr. John Carlisle stated in a memo to the Registrar, on this issue, that allowing the opinion of a peer would be **"like sending the fox to guard the hen house."** The American Medical Association recognizes the AAEM, of which Dr. Krop is a fellow. AAEM courses are accredited in the USA, and a considerable number of their members also hold university positions at medical schools in the US, Canada, and Europe. Germany has since 1995 incorporated environmental medicine into the curriculum of every medical school in the country.

Virtually all medical literature (much of it double-blind and placebo-controlled studies from around the world) published after 1990 was simply ignored by the CPSO in their deliberations and final Decision. The Notice of Hearing was served in 1994. Ignoring the material available in the international literature between 1990 and 1994 suggests deliberate bias. This means, that the explosion of scientific information from universities around the world dealing with the impact of environmental agents on health was effectively ruled out. The CPSO's discipline panel observed in their 1998 Decision with the sophistry of a latter day revival of the Spanish Inquisition, that all the evidence submitted by the defense was found **"lacking in the authority of acceptable scientific evidence".** The Decision handed down in 1998 stated that **"the central issue has to do with the use of an unscientific hypothesis"** concerning various environmentally induced conditions and various treatment modalities.

Patient outcome was of no consequence. In the transcripts, the then Registrar, Dr. Michael Dixon, stated in cross-examination in December 1995: **"that fact that patients are benefited is not necessarily information that's terribly helpful".** Being asked at this time also whether he agreed with Dr. Carlisle's assertion that this disciplinary investigation was intended to be an example to all doctors practicing environmental medicine (clinical ecology), so that it would "deal, once and for all, with these clinical ecologists", he replied **"Yes."**

> Seeking originally revocation of license, for some mysterious reason, the CPSO downgraded the penalty to a reprimand. The Sentence stated that Dr. Krop was free to continue all those very therapies which the decision had judged to be sub-standard. Dr. Krop was asked to accept a reprimand because his diagnoses and therapies were "lacking in scientific validity". In addition, a Byzantine amendment to the consent forms was ordered: Dr. Krop is to tell his patients that whatever he is diagnosing and whatever treatment he offers is based only on his "personal opinions and beliefs, not scientifically substantiated medicine". Dr. Krop is appealing because he is not willing to allow his patients to be treated as fools and to be party to untruthful assertions. The numerous legal improprieties also demand an appeal.

Mr. Code studied the Krop case and focused on the many legal improprieties of which only a couple are discussed here.

In his June 9,1999, analysis of the Krop case, Mr. Code observes further: "The allegations against Dr. Krop, from beginning to end, involved the simple assertion that he was practicing an experimental form of medicine (known as Environmental Medicine), whose practices and premises have not yet been rigorously tested.... Nevertheless, the core of this form of medicine appears to be the rather unremarkable proposition that environmental toxins influence our health." Mr. Code points out that after ten years of investigation, "the Discipline Committee concluded that Dr. Krop's experimental medicine practices 'did not harm them [his patients] in any physical sense."

Mr. Code is especially shocked by the following impropriety: "The only records we have, as to whether senior CPSO officials formed these requisite beliefs [about whether reasonable and probable grounds for an investigation actually existed] is the September 27, 1989 memo from Dr. Carlisle to [Registrar] Dr. Dixon, and the October 6, 1989, Minutes from the Executive Committee. Neither document appears to reflect any real attempt by Dr. Carlisle or Dr. Dixon to direct their minds to the proper statutory test. Dr. Carlisle's memo states: 'In all the circumstances, the Department is of the opinion that Dr. Krop's practice should be subjected to an investigation under s.64 <u>and if anything is needed to form a basis for that, the complaint of Mrs. C. will do.</u> All the other complaints may be seen as in aid of this'. [Emphasis added by Mr. Code.]"

Mr. Code then observes," Dr. Carlisle's memo to Dr. Dixon is particularly shocking, in my opinion. It reveals a very casual, almost cavalier, approach to the very serious task of formulating reasonable and probable grounds. His statement *if anything is needed the C. complaint will do*, suggests outright contempt for the strict process enshrined in statute. At a minimum he has failed to direct his mind to the requisite test in law, as set out above, namely, an objective basis for a belief in probable guilt."

Mr. Code discussed the various documents in which Deputy Registrar Dr. Carlisle and Registrar Dr. Dixon express deep bias against virtually anything connected with clinical ecology and Dr. Krop's practice. The most serious evidence of bias appeared in their not reading the material provided by the defense and submitted by the defense at the request of the prosecution, specifically by Deputy Registrar Dr. J. Carlisle himself in his correspondence with Dr. Krop's lawyers. The full details are found in the cross-examination of Dr. Carlisle in item 12 of the Appendix. The full cross-examination is provided so none of the context is lost in the reading.

Mr. Code stated: "In my opinion, Dr. Carlisle and Dr. Dixon could not fairly and impartially carry out their statutory duties under s. 64 in this case without reading and considering the materials submitted by Dr. Krop.... **When a judge decides a case without considering evidence tendered by the defense that is relevant to a material issue, we say that there has been a miscarriage of justice because the decision 'is not based exclusively on the evidence and is not a true verdict'. This what happened in Dr. Krop's case, in my opinion.**" (Emphasis ours.)

Mr. Code was especially disturbed by the following quote from a letter by Deputy Registrar Dr. John Carlisle to Dr. Krop's lawyer: "**We are, with respect to Dr. Krop and his patients, not interested in receiving affidavits from patients who are satisfied nor any other form of testimonial...We do not for a moment mean to suggest that these parties are not telling the truth or are exaggerating their statements, but merely that testimonials are of no value in establishing scientific principles.** (Emphasis added by Mr. Code.)."

> In conclusion, Mr. Code observes: "The proceedings against Dr. Krop would, therefore, appear to involve the *Alice in Wonderland* proposition that doctors are to be disciplined on the basis of some pure scientific principle that has no regard for actual harm and no regard for the satisfaction or dissatisfaction of the patients. That CPSO would spend ten long years, from 1988-1998, pursuing this kind of enormous expense through endless disciplinary processes would seem, at a minimum, show inappropriate judgment and over-zealousness."

Dr. Krop has appealed the CPSO Decision because, in addition to the procedural abuse he experienced, he rejects the reprimand which is based on arbitrary assertions about science and requires, through the consent procedures, that patients agree with the arbitrary CPSO view. Thus the Decision essentially condemns a number of diseases recognized internationally, researched at the world's top medical schools, and recognized by the *World Health Organization*. It also condemns treatments which are based on rigorous scientific research published in peer reviewed medical journals the world over. The appeal is going to be heard in the Divisional Court in December 2001.

Dr. F. ADAMS

Dr. Adams, formerly of Kingston, is a neuropsychiatrist and a diplomate of the American Academy of Experts in Traumatic Stress, American Academy of Pain Management, and the Royal College of Physicians and Surgeons of Canada. He has taught at Queen's University in Ontario, the University of Texas, and the University of Toronto. He established the pain service at the University of Texas at the world's largest cancer care center. His research was central to the recent major changes made by the US medical licensing boards and the guidelines for pain management formulated by the World Health Organization; Dr. Adams was involved with both during this process. He originally developed several of the standard tests used by neuro-psychiatrists worldwide also. He has directed many pain management centers for the US and in Canada. His CV of 19 pages provides information on his many publications in the world's peer reviewed medical journals on the editorial boards of many of which he also served.

Without a single complaint or known clinical misadventure he was brought into discipline by the CPSO in May 1998. No disclosure was ever given to Dr. Adams or his lawyer as to how this case commenced. Seven months later a report was provided by CPSO investigator Dr. A. McFarlane, who is not a neuropsychiatrist or even a pain specialist. The factual errors were so numerous, the CPSO withdrew the report. A new report was commissioned by the CPSO from Dr. D. Moulin. It was written without interviewing Dr. Adams or the patients whose charts were the basis of the report. The report was ready in July 1999. Before even commencing the hearings, the CPSO imposed restrictions on Dr. Adams' license.

None of the files taken for the investigations showed a single instance of harm done to a patient, not one instance of addiction having developed, lack of appropriate tests (such as liver function monitoring when potentially toxic drugs are used). Because of the exceptionally good results Dr. Adams had achieved in some of the most severe cases of chronic pain, and which the prosecution used as evidence for proving incompetence, the suggestion had been made by the editors of the Canadian pain journal, *Pain Research and Management*, that these cases should be prepared for publication.

Eight hearing days took place in September 1999. The defense introduced voluminous pain management literature, including Dr. Adams' own papers. One of his expert witnesses was the internationally renowned pain expert, Dr. Harold Merskey, professor emeritus of the University of Western Ontario and editor of the above-mentioned medical journal. The prosecution introduced as their primary evidence the Alberta Pain Management Guidelines. Since the CPSO's own were not completed until December 2000, they might have introduced the international guidelines adopted by the World Health Organization. That would have meant, however, judging Dr. Adams by guidelines he had helped to create. The authors of these Alberta Guidelines had some time previous to this disciplinary event submitted their document to Dr. Adams for review. Following his assessment, the authors of this review had declared their guidelines obsolete. This fact is not in evidence in the Decision rendered in April 2000; instead, the Decision states that by not following the Alberta Guidelines Dr. Adams was proven to be falling below the standard of medical practice. The transcripts of the hearings on September 9, 1999, provide the following interesting passage:

> "The idea of standards [of practice] is to avoid trouble," Mr. Donald Posluns, acting for the prosecution, stated. "The College doesn't have the burden to show you that patients are dead or disabled or actually toxic; the College is obliged to demonstrate that at the time the doctor did or didn't do something .... Not that there were some adverse consequences....certain patients showed improvement, that's true, but that's not the question."

The approach taken by the prosecuting CPSO here is once again one of the requiring a member to follow an arbitrarily imposed and selectively chosen standard of practice unrelated to recorded, empirical results and the needs and choices of the specific patient, in contravention of the spirit of the RHPA.

The CPSO's expert witness, Dr. Moulin, complicated the situation for the prosecution because he did not feel that Dr. Adams should lose his license. Even more astonishing was the following development:

A member of the CPSO Council who also sat on the Discipline Committee, Dr. Ellen Thompson of Ottawa, herself a pain specialist, submitted her protest against these proceedings in writing to the Executive Committee and then went public as well on the subsequent CBC television *Fifth Estate* program devoted to the Adams case. She declared the CPSO's attitude as being "in the pre-Cambrian era when it comes to pain management". This prompted censure from the then Registrar, Dr. J. Bonn, who faulted Dr. Thompson for not being a "team player". Indeed, the Adams case took place at the same time during which the US medical licensing boards declared pain the Fifth Vital Sign, which must be treated on par with the other four.

> Dr. Thompson, then a CPSO Council member, stated publicly that the discipline's process, in her experience as one of the Discipline Committee members, is "often fishing expeditions, which they [CPSO] abandon only if they can't find what they are looking for in the first place."

Because so many severely ill patients were affected by the Adams case, a storm of public protest arose. More than 8,000 (eight thousand) faxes and letters were sent to the Registrar by patients and family members of those patients. The media featured the case prominently (see items 13,14,15 in Appendix). Formal complaints were also lodged against the Registrar and the Deputy Registrar by both patients and doctors.

In support of the prosecution's desire to revoke Dr. Adams' license, CPSO lawyer Mr. Posluns produced during the summation phase of the proceedings a quotation from a *Medical Post* article. In it, some years ago, Dr. Adams passionately criticized pain management in dying cancer patients in Ontario's hospitals as being no different than Nazi medicine, i.e. merciless.

> Mr. Posluns declared that Dr. Adams "is incorrigible" and that nothing less than revocation of license was indicated because, in order "to change his ways he tells you he would have to become Nazi, which he will not do, so we have here a clear case of ego-centricity compounded by grandiosity". Mr. Posluns stated that "the CPSO cannot take responsibility for Dr. Adams like for a slightly retarded and unruly elementary school student who is lacking in prudent judgment." Only revocation of his license would ensure compliance, since Dr. Adams had made it amply clear that he did not intend to adopt the pain management ideas the CPSO wanted him to agree to. (July 21, 2000).

The context of Dr. Adams newspaper statement is important: Dr. Adams was commenting on the fact that Ontario palliative care wards were spending more and more money on physical restraints to keep thrashing and screaming patients under control, instead of providing full and readily available sedation. These circumstances, incidentally, led to the federal government's first Senate report on pain management in 1995. And indeed, at the same time that Dr. Adams' case was being heard at the CPSO, Senator Sharon Carstairs and her committee issued their second (July 2000) report severely criticizing the lack of pain management in Canada once again. One of the members of that committee, Dr. Helen Hayes, who was awarded the Order of Canada for her palliative pain work, made a point of writing to the CPSO expressing her criticism of the Adams prosecution and commending him for his outstanding contributions to pain research and management.

Presumably due to the escalating public protest covered throughout the mainstream media for months (e.g. *Macleans* magazine, *CBC Fifth Estate* and CBC radio's Michael Enright items 13, 14, 15) the Discipline Panel did not pursue revocation, but imposed a temporary suspension and ordered skills upgrading as well as long-term restrictions of such a nature that Dr. Adams found it was impossible to practice in Ontario.

At the same time, the then Registrar, Dr. J. Bonn, took the unprecedented step of devoting an editorial in the CPSO's *Members' Dialogue* (Appendix item 16) to the Adams case, assuring the membership that this had nothing to do with the use of opiates. However, his assertions did not reflect what happened at the hearings nor did it harmonize with the content of the Penalty. The contradictions are listed in item 16.

> **The Penalty states that its purpose is "to send a message as a general deterrent to all physicians". As the case centered specifically on the use of opiates, the "message" can only be about their use.**

Then Registrar, Dr. J. Bonn stated on CBC radio (Appendix item 14) that the CPSO had to prosecute Dr. Adams because he was not following any guidelines at all. In fact he was following the international guidelines already accepted in several provinces in Canada. The full story of the Adams case was well researched and presented by CBC's *Fifth Estate* (transcript in item 17 of the Appendix).

Significantly, the Federation of Medical Licensing boards of the USA and the federation of Canada's medical colleges have been formally affiliated with each other for many years. Part of that affiliation requires mutual recognition of each other's standards. Dr. Bonn's statement was, therefore, incorrect in many respects. In theory, Canada ought to recognize the US (and therefore also the international) standards on pain management and hence ought not to have prosecuted Dr. Adams at all.

Dr. Adams was ordered to take re-training and to be assessed by the CPSO-appointed preceptors at Queen's University. (They were surprised, as they felt that he should be **teaching** them pain medicine.) The report that was issued by Queen's University (see Appendix item 18) stated unequivocally that Dr. Adams' license should be restored and all restrictions lifted. However, then Registrar Dr. J. Bonn, without referring this matter back to the Discipline Panel or the Executive Committee for reconsideration, instructed Dr. Adams' lawyer that the license would be reinstated only if Dr. Adams guaranteed to abide by those very restrictions for the next three years (Appendix item 19).

Shocked by the rampant impropriety of this case, Dr. Merskey was joined by CPSO Council member Dr. E. Thompson, and they produced an analysis of the Adams case which actually does reflect the facts from the hearings and the Decision (Appendix item 20) and provided it to the media at a Queen's Park press conference on March 28th, 2001.

Unable to work in his field, Dr. Adams decided to leave Canada and return to the US where his license in Texas was renewed with that state licensing boards full knowledge of the actions taken against him in Ontario.

Prior to his departure, Dr. Adams spoke at that same press conference. (Transcript in Appendix item 21.) Dr. Adams made two significant points. Regarding the first he outlined that the CPSO had ordered him to see his most severe pain patients every 15 days for prescription renewals. Besides being medically not indicated and causing enormous inconvenience to these very sick people coming from all over the province, the financial implications were astounding for the province as well.

He said:

> "Every 15 days to see [these] patients would have been a financial windfall and I would have become quite wealthy over the next three years [the period for which this restriction was in place]. I calculated that I would have grossed better than $ 1.5 million billing the way the College wishes me to bill. Premier Harris is continuously upset by the burgeoning health care budget and has repeatedly asked physicians to bill responsibly...the College chooses to overlook that and has now not only mandated but actually commanded that, in essence, what I do is commit OHIP fraud for the next three years."

Because the Adams case is seen by the OMA Pain Section members as setting a precedent, the financial implications indicate a possible annual increase in OHIP spending of roughly $ 120 million, if the 300 pain doctors in the province have to accept the Adams Decision's deterrent. Lawyer Mr. Matthew Wilton, who specializes in medical cases, sees this as a very real possibility. (Appendix item 3.)

The second important point Dr. Adams made concerned the terrible human cost of his prosecution. **"I hold [Dr. Bonn and Dr. Carlisle] morally culpable for the incredible amount of physical pain that they have created in this province, when they suspended my license, and for the two hundred and some patients who then went without medication. I kept the office phone going for some time after my suspension... However, it was very difficult, no matter who you are... to tolerate hearing people on the other end of the phone screaming, crying, gagging, actively vomiting, describing a litany of symptoms and a litany of despair because they were out of medication."**

The main reason Dr. Adams, now 5 months without an income, left Canada was that the restrictions effectively stopped him from continuing to serve his patient population as he had done before. They were unable to receive from him, or any other doctor, the treatments that had worked for them and which are internationally accepted. Those patients who called the CPSO asking for help in finding a pain doctor were told that it was not the CPSO's job to find doctors for them. Other pain doctors either refused to take on former Adams patients, or told them outright that they feared being brought into discipline as well. In fact, the CPSO asked for reports on all Adams patients from those doctors who did take them on, without the knowledge of those patients.

To put pain medicine into perspective, Dr. Thompson told the media that the waiting list at most Ontario's pain clinics is about three years. At any time about 75,000 pain patients are without care. According to the *National Chronic Pain Association*, the suicide rate among chronic pain patients is 10 times higher than in the general population, and they tend to succeed on the first try. The cost to the public of **not** treating chronic pain is enormous: under his care the patients of Dr. Adams went off the public purse and returned to managing their work and families, which they were unable to do before. Some, who were suddenly cut off their pain medication following Dr. Adams' suspension, very quickly ceased to be able to function at work. (See the *Star* article on this specific issue of September 10, 2001.)

In June 2001 the medical licensing authorities of the State of New York commenced a formal hearing into Dr. Adams' case, as he is licensed there as well. The result of that board's deliberations, which oversees the largest medical jurisdiction in North America, was issued on July 10 (Appendix item 22). It states, that "findings of misconduct made other than in New York are binding in this hearing only if they constitute misconduct in New York." Following their review of all the documents and evidence which was the basis for the CPSO's decision, the New York authorities concluded:

> "The Hearing Committee is, to put it succinctly, dubious as to whether the standard utilized by the Ontario College [to assess Dr. Adams] are comparable to the applicable standards prevalent in New York."

They proceed to critique the CPSO's view that Dr. Adams was guilty of falling below the standard of practice because he did not do complete physical exams by agreeing with the Dr. Adams' defense experts. The defense had pointed out that psychiatrists do not do full physical exams when these have already been done several times over by the referring doctors.

> "Every 15 days to see [these] patients would have been a The New York medical licensing authorities noted the lack of pain management standards in Ontario at the time of the disciplinary proceedings and concluded: "This is not a case where it is appropriate to equate standards applied in a foreign country, especially in such a controversial and evolving area as pain management, with those prevalent here, without any proof as to what the latter standards are." Dr. Adams' New York license was renewed.

Since the Adams case, the CPSO has commenced with disciplinary hearings against yet another pain doctor discussed below.

Dr. S. S. KOONER

Dr. Kooner practices in Windsor specializing in asthma and allergies. He is exceptionally successful with children suffering from asthma; patients consult him from all over the province. Trained originally in India, he received his medical fellowship from the University of Saskatchewan. He is also trained as a clinical ecologist (environmental physician) and is a member of the *Pan American Allergy Society*, a medical organization with member physicians throughout the world many of whom teach at universities. The treatments developed by them are included in current medical textbook chapters, some of which were introduced by the defense in Dr. Kooner's discipline hearings in 2000. These treatment modalities are recognized by the Canadian federal government. The CPSO tacitly approves their use as "complementary" through their 1997 policy on complementary medicine (even though these asthma therapies were developed at mainstream universities as far back as the 1940s and are hardly complementary).

In 1996 a patient had an anaphylactic reaction (not anaphylactic shock! there is a significant difference) during testing, a very common occurrence. The full protocol published by the *Anaphylaxis Network of Canada* (distributed by the Ontario Ministry of Health) was immediately used and the patient was revived within a minute. Because of its frequency, allergists' offices are equipped with the instruments needed to deal with anaphylaxis. However, Dr. Kooner took the extra precaution to send the patient by ambulance to the hospital for observation and investigation. The boy was released within an hour and went back to school the next morning. As cases of anaphylaxis are registered with the *Anaphylaxis Network*, this case came to their attention.

For reasons unknown so far, one of the doctors associated with this registry contacted the mother of this boy about a year after the incident and suggested to her that she should lay a complaint against Dr. Kooner, so that "this does not happen again to anybody." The CPSO did not tell the mother that this is a common occurrence, which probably happens dozens of times daily in medical practices throughout Ontario. She was also not told that the standard protocol had been followed to the letter, and as there also was no demonstrable or lasting harm, there could be no substance to a complaint. Instead, a protracted cat-and-mouse game began during which Dr. Kooner was asked by the CPSO to make some adjustments to his letterhead, change his consent forms and the like. A Section 75 was at first not even mentioned.

Then, suddenly in January 1997 Dr. Kooner was informed of a Section 75 disciplinary proceeding, but instead of starting this accordingly, nothing happened for 3 and ? years, until August 2000 when hearing dates were suddenly announced **even though the negotiations with his lawyers were then ongoing, leading his lawyer to believe that the Section 75 investigation would be dropped.** Thus, the e defense lawyer, Ms Kirby Chown, was surprised, objecting that no time was allowed to get expert supportive opinion, that no full disclosure had been given, and that important evidence was still missing without the repeatedly requested explanation for their disappearance: the tapes done by the CPSO interviewing Dr. Kooner had been lost. She also questioned the very legitimacy of the invocation of Section 75 because every item the CPSO had asked for had already been complied with.

At this point, the CPSO offered Dr. Kooner a sort of last chance: he was asked to voluntarily stop all asthma work—or else go to discipline. He refused and the hearings began on October 2, 2000, with the CPSO seeking revocation of license. The defense's position was that every possible, universally agreed upon, standard protective measure had been observed in this simple case of an adverse reaction to allergy testing. However:

> Mr. Posluns, speaking for the prosecuting CPSO instructed the Discipline Panel as follows: "The outcome of treatment is not a useful concept. Even if he [Dr. K.] had killed somebody, it would be irrelevant...doctors can have bad outcomes. If we want to get into how many died and how many benefited, well this is not a murder trial and it is unfair to judge outcome. Only standard of practice is to be evaluated. You set the standards in Ontario, you have never heard of the *Pan American Allergy Society* and its treatment modalities, therefore you have to find the member guilty".

Dr. Kooner's patients organized a patient group and unleashed an intense public protest campaign with press conferences, town hall meetings and the like. Hundreds of letters of protest went to the CPSO also. One of his patients whose children had also been treated by Dr. Kooner was a character witness during the hearings. He stated flatly, "We are deeply offended by these proceedings against Dr. Kooner" and suggested the CPSO was conducting kangaroo courts. At the press conference held in Queen's Park the media was joined by many MPPs and MPP. Items 23 and 24 are letters from the Official Opposition to the CPSO asking for clarification in this case.

Two months after the hearings began, the Kwinter Bill was passed which specifically prohibits penalizing doctors for practicing unconventionally as long as patients are not hurt. In the Kooner case nobody was hurt and the defense provided plenty of judgements showing that even before the Kwinter Bill became law, the courts do not support preferential endorsement of one type of therapy over another, if both have published scientific support. The Discipline Panel did not take notice of the passage of the Kwinter Bill, but on July 11, 2001, gave their Decision, finding him "incompetent," "unfit to continue practicing", or "that his practice should be restricted" under s.52(1) of the Health Professions Procedural Code. The Decision is full of inaccuracies and irrelevancies, such that several people involved with this and other cases as well as with the preparation of this report, observed that the CPSO Decisions have the quality of "cookie-cutter" productions: the individual case's facts are simply kneaded into the dough and the same type of Decision is rendered regardless of the case.

Dr. Kooner's patients are terrified that the treatment they have received and which works for them (unlike the treatments they used to get) may suddenly be no longer available. As most of Dr. Kooner's asthma patients are children, the situation is serious. Dr. Kooner's Sentencing is to take place November 14 of this year.

How Health Canada Sells Us Out

Vitality Magazine March 2004

The blizzard that descended on central Ontario on the night of January 27th caused zero visibility, and so the course of the 401 was guesswork. With very few cars along that 500 km stretch on the road on the road to Ottawa, it was only the noise my tires made on the corrugated strip of pavement flanking the right shoulder that enabled me to know I was on the road. Thus, it took me over ten hours to make it to Ottawa, twice the usual time.

But my destination was worth risking life and limb for—a national symposium on Health Canada's proposed changes to our health protection legislation, hosted by the Canadian Health Coalition. This momentous event, attended by scientists, famous media personalities, and concerned citizens, created such a stir that it culminated in an "Open Letter to the Prime Minister" protesting the total sell-out of Canada's most precious natural resource—people—to the pharmaceutical and biochemical industry. It was signed by hundreds of Canada's most famous people—from Margaret Atwood to David Suzuki, thousands of ordinary people like you and me, and endorsed by 26 countries. Two days later, the roads were clear and the land resplendent in glittering winter garb as I drove home and tried to digest what I had learned. It occurred to me, that instead of "It is as bad as you think, and they are out to get you", we need a bumper sticker that reads: "They are much worse than you feared, and they have already got you."

Proposed Changes to the Food and Drugs Act

Our government has decided that the *Foods and Drugs Act* needs renovating and informs us in a 2003 "Report on Plans and Priorities" that the act has "too narrow a focus on safety…and does not allow for taking into account considerations other than safety and efficacy in managing health risks." The new act is supposed to "unleash business energies" and "reduce the regulatory burden on business", especially on the biotechnology and drug industries. Under the title "Health and Safety First", the government published its plans to give us all "a higher level of protection" through a new act:

- Instead of the current "duty to care" for Canadians, the act would be focused on risk management, a business concept that *includes* potential damage or death in its legal cost projections in the same way as a general calculates how many troops would get killed in a campaign. Even if a drug turns out to be carcinogenic (e.g. Paxil), not everybody gets cancer, so enough money can be made from people who don't complain to make the drug cost-effective. Risk management is literally the opposite of "duty to care", the latter does not permit conscious inclusion of dead bodies whose litigious costs can be financially managed from the drug's profits. Worst of all, according to German sociologist Ulrich Beck, the current environmental pollution caused by radiation and synthetic drugs with carcinogenic properties will be felt by people not even born yet.

- The precautionary principle, currently in the act, would disappear; proof of harm would be transferred from the drug company to the patient. Health Canada washes its hands of the problem because all safety issues would be dealt with by the producer; no independent evaluation or human trials would be required. The drug becomes the equivalent of a person and is assumed to be innocent until proven guilty. Like corporations, which are legal entities with the status of a person but without the liability and responsibility of a person, now the drug would have that status also, and not even the government could do anything about it.
- Health Canada would no longer be liable—for anything. Nice move, given the fact that they are currently facing $ 12 billion worth of liability suits for regulatory negligence, faulty medical devices, tainted blood, as well as civil suits for harassment of their own scientists for not bending to corporate demands for approval shortcuts.
- Direct to consumer advertising (DTCA) of drugs would also be permitted. According to Stephen Leacock, advertising "is the science of arresting human intelligence long enough to get money from it." The claims made in those ads would be based on nothing verifiable whatsoever. All scientific information concerning its efficacy and safety would be the "proprietary information" of that company. In the US, the sales from the 50 most advertised drugs account for 48% of the $ 20.8 billion *increase* in retail spending since advertising began big time in 1999—obviously an excellent business move. (From **www.yourlawyer.com**, Jan. 19, 2004)

The CHC's extensive critique (available on their website **www.medicare.ca**) asks, "Who exactly are Health Canada's 'clients'? The people of Canada? Or the industries that Health Canada is supposed to be regulating?"

The Human Cost of Big Pharma's Profits

So, what about the recommendations made by Justice Krever and the Romanow Report? They are gone with the wind that whistles around Parliament Hill, and thousands of Canadians died—not for nothing, oh no! They made some companies very rich before they died. Both Justice Krever and Roy Romanow made it clear that the government's role is to protect the health and safety of its citizens, not to further investment interests that carry risk to health and safety. Health Canada appears to treat us as if human sickness is an infinite resource and as if people, like the environment and natural resources, don't need the application of the concept of sustainability. Consider the fact that the cost of prescription drugs in Canada increased between

1985 and 2000 a whopping 344% and that drugs alone cost the state more than fees for doctors and hospital care combined. And why are chronic disease and antibiotic-resistant illness increasing constantly, even though the population is not?

FDA records show that drug mark-ups frequently are in the 800,000 % range, but unrelated to production costs. That is because "most drug companies have a pipeline problem" (J. Surowiecki, February 16th, *The New Yorker*). Thus, we read there that Merck devotes three billion dollars annually to research, but has produced zero new drugs for years now. The number of available chemical molecules is limited. That leaves price increases and mergers. The joke in this industry is that "you know you are in the pharmaceutical business when you have worked for five companies in the past two years and you are still sitting at the same old desk." They buy each other up in frantic haste to milk one more blockbuster drug. Surowiecki observes, "When the going gets tough, the tough go shopping."

As for their effectiveness, consider that the journal *Pharmacy Today* reported a couple of weeks ago that in their (super-conservative estimate) at least 200,000 American die annually from drug side effects. The prestigious Johns Hopkins Medical School pegged the number at 250,000 six years ago, and the estimate for Canada is at 100,000 annually—and all are avoidable. That's 959 people a day. Investigators agree that the cause is the wholesale sell-out of the regulatory system to the interests of the pharmaceutical industry.

Drug Deaths, Lawsuits, and Cover-Ups

This event was graced by stellar medical experts and internationally famous whistleblowers such as Dr. David Healy (antidepressant expert), Dr. Nancy Olivieri (blood disease expert), Terrence Young (former MPP whose daughter died from Prepulsid), Professor Barbara Mintzes (researcher in the effect of drug ads) of the University of British Columbia, Professor Joel Lexchin (specializes on the drug approval system) of York University, and Dr. Michelle Brill-Edwards, formerly of Health Canada who knows the system from the inside.

Terrence Young told the heart-breaking story of his daughter's death from Prepulsid, now the subject of an international class action suit involving the families of hundreds of victims. During the inquest the drug company's representative said "We see Health Canada as our best customer." In a meeting Young learned that Health Canada sees its job as "helping companies get their drugs to market faster." When he insisted that a report include the warning against "corrupt practices" at Health Canada, he later found those words changed to "management practices."

Dr. Olivieri told the story of her ongoing worldwide legal battle against a drug that causes liver damage or failure in many patients and irreversible arthritis in many more. Former Health Minister Allan Rock refused to meet with her because the manufacturer's headquarters are in his riding. The drug is of enormous financial importance because children suffering from malaria develop the blood disease it "treats" at exponential rates.

Dr. David Healy described the process by which drug experts like himself are systematically duped by the manufacturer, denied access to the actual data, and presented with reports containing mysterious language: thus a certain percentage of patients on antidepressants develop "emotional liability" which later turned out to mean suicide. Another percentage of patients become "hostile", which turned out to be plainly homicidal. The "scientific" reports come from authors "TBD", which means "to be determined"; they are written by anonymous industry writers. Indeed, all presenters discussed the fact that about half of all medical research publications are ghost written by the industry. SSRIs are also highly addictive in the biological sense. The manufacturers hide that fact by referring to patients suffering from withdrawal as having a "discontinuation syndrome".

Dr. Brill-Edwards related an event that sums it all up perfectly. When Dr. Olivieri tried to engage a Health Canada Deputy Minister in a discussion about drug safety, he said, "Well, tell us what's unsafe about it." Dr. Brill-Edwards interrupted and said, "No! You provide us the proof that it is safe. That is your duty under the act."

Take Action to Protect Your Health

We need to really understand the systemic ignorance in our health care system: *First,* our doctors are usually too busy to read the fine print in the CPS; that is the annually published *Compendium of Pharmaceuticals and Specialties.* Distributed free to every doctor's office, it contains what the drug industry must still admit to. Current legislation, does still require a minimum of safety information and it must list potential adverse reactions in small-print whispers. *Second,* our doctors tend to think, as we do, that Health Canada is checking the safety and efficacy of prescription drugs—so we are both duped. *Third,* hardly any doctor knows that the current approvals process is rigged because the evaluators have no access to the raw data. Everybody—from the Health Canada scientist down to the patient popping a carcinogenic antidepressant or Co-enzyme Q_{10}-depleting choles-terol-lowering drug—is kept in the dark and fed BS: "We are all mush-rooms," observed the representative of the Canadian Labour Congress.

All of us are exposed at some point to this Corporately Regulated Arse-nals of Pharmaceuticals (CRAP). Therefore, all of us must act. Here is a list of suggestions:

1. Support the Canadian Health Coalition (**www.medicare.ca**) because they are actually doing this job for us on a shoe-string and full-time. Your and my MPs have so far done nothing—but the Canadian Health Coalition made the CRAP hit the public fan. Supporting them is as important as eating organic and taking your vitamins.

2. Download the "Open Letter to the Prime Minister" from the CHC website or from mine: **www.kospublishing.com**, sign it, e-mail or mail it to the PM and send a copy to your MP and ask him or her what they are going to do about this criminal negligence being perpetrated on thirty million Canadians.

3. Take yourself to the documentary movie *The Corporation* and become politically enlightened.

Some helpful measures that came to my mind are: first, we need to raise the price of all prescription drugs (except the ones on the World Health Organi-zation's list of 350 necessary ones, which are 5% of what's currently pre-scribed) by at least 1,000% so people and even insurance companies can't afford them. That would reduce morbidity and increase our longevity to that of Spain and other poor western countries where the spending on drugs is less than one third of ours. (See TIME Feb.2, 2003)

Second, each drug should, like cigarettes, come with the appropriate warn-ings. Paxil boxes would read: "Taking this SSRI increases your chance of cancer by 750%." Or on a Lipitor box it would say, "Significantly reduces the enzyme your heart function depends on." Or good old aspirin would inform us: "Long-term use increases your chance of pancreatic cancer by 58%" (see proceedings of American Association for Cancer research, October 29, 2003).

Third, we must demand that our current legislation remains in force because its requirements for safety and precaution are excellent. "Safety and duty to care do not go out of date", the CHC report observes. Since it isn't actually enforced, as all the scandals from genetically engineered foods to drug after disastrous drug have shown, we need criminal accountability, as Terrence Young observed. In the spirit of the recently passed bill C-45, which makes corporations responsible for disasters such as the Westray Mine tragedy, and the recent Supreme Court decision making polluting companies responsible for clean-ups, we need court decisions that stop government collusion with industry and condemn this lucrative mass murder. Indeed, the choice for those responsible at Health Canada should be between Kingston and Penetang. Courts must establish if we are dealing with mere crooks or the criminally insane.

Fourth, we need the enunciation of a new human right. All international human rights treaties focus on life, liberty, fair trials, racism, labor laws and the like. The Helsinki Accord also mentions the right to informed consent in medicine. What we urgently need in this time of wholesale corporate criminality is the recognition that it is a *human right*, not to be lied to for profit, and that being told the truth, the whole truth and nothing but the truth, ought to be as fundamental a human right as life itself.

The CHC must have the last word: "If Health Canada's proposed evisceration of the Foods And Drugs Act is allowed, there will literally be no limit to what the corporations will put in our stomachs and our blood-streams"— and ignorance will not only cease to be bliss but will become death.

Sources and Resources

Dr. J.S. Cohen, *Overdose: The Case Against the Drug Companies—Prescription Drugs, Side Effects and Your Health,* Tarcher/Putnam, 2001 (A mainstream pharmacologist and university professor reveals the industry skullduggery and FDA collusion.)

H. Ferrie, *Hippocrates in the Land of Oz: A Survival Guide for Our Golden Age of Medicine,* Kos Publishing, in press for November 2004

Dr. D. Healy, *Let Them Eat Prozac,* Lorimer, 2003 (Everything you never believed possible about corruption in medical research.)

J. LeCarre, *The Constant Gardener,* Viking, 2001 (A novel by the greatest of spy story writers based on the Dr. Nancy Olivieri story.)

R.Pelton et al. *The Nutritional Cost of Prescription Drugs,* Morton, 2000 (This encyclopedia, available in two versions—for doctors and for patients—written by pharmacists informs about the known damage drugs can cause, all supported by mainstream medical journals. An absolute MUST-read before you fill a prescription or buy an over-the-counter drug. Take it to your doctors and blow their minds.)

Dr. F. Ravikovich, *The Plot Against Asthma and Allergy Patients,* Kos, 2003 (Everything you never thought possible about burying breath-giving cures for corporate benefit.)

J. Robinson, *Prescription Games: Money Ego and Power inside the Global Pharmaceutical Industry,* McLelland & Stewart, 2001 (now only available through **www.amazon.ca**) (The best one-stop overview of the nature of Big Pharma.)

J. Thompson et al. eds., *The Olivieri Report,* CAUT Series, Lorimer, 2001 (The full report by the Canadian Association of University Teachers on how Apotex, the University of Toronto, Sick Children's Hospital and Health Canada joined forces to protect a deadly drug from revenue losses.)

A comprehensive report on the financial cost of prescription drug harm is on **www.garynull.com**: *Death by Medicine* by Dr. C. Dean et al, December 2003

Many thanks to Dr. Carolyn Dean, Michael Downey, and Croft Woodruff for technical information and to Dr. Sherry Rogers for the acronym CRAP which for her means Cigarettes, Coffee, Refined sugars, Alcohol, Pop and Processed foods.

Update October 2004: *The FDA issued warnings against the use of SSRI antidepressants in children because of the increased risk of suicide, Health Canada followed soon after with a similar statement and also publicized the increased risk of cancer for all age groups taking antidepressants. The psychiatric community remains on auto-pilot and talks the predictable nonsense about ensuring the "benefits [which are they, pray tell?] outweighing the risk [suicide and cancer can be outweighed?]". Seeing medical education is predicated on the use of drugs, psychiatrists have little else to work with and can't, therefore, say anything new as yet. Prime Minister Paul Martin responded to this event in a letter dated April 26, 2004, in which he completely ignores the substance of this conference and reiterates that the changes to the Canadian health care legislation will be made, presumably as planned, which means to make Health Canada even more industry-friendly. He does not acknowledge any of the criticisms. Maybe he should hear from you?*

6

Perversion of Science

The Quackbusters—Busted!

Vitality Magazine May 2002

*"The great mass of people will more easily fall victim
to a big lie than a small one."*
Adolf Hitler, *Mein Kampf*, 1925

My first encounter with Quackbusters was on November 10,1998, when a public debate was sponsored by the American College of Toxicology in Orlando, Florida. The speakers on one side were Albert Donnay and Grace Ziem, both with Johns Hopkins medical school and experts on multiple chemical sensitivity. The Quackbuster representatives were its founder Stephen Barrett and Ronald Gots, the founder of the Quackbuster branch, Environmental Sensitivities Research Institute. Both men are also directors of the *American Council on Science and Health*, another branch of Quackbusters. Their presentations were later published in the prestigious *International Journal of Toxicology* (vol. 18, no.6, 1999) but had to be retracted.

The debate in Orlando focused on whether chemical sensitivity is a psychological or a biological condition. In front of an audience of several hundred people, and aware that the entire debate was being video- and audio-taped, Gots stated that prestigious university-affiliated authors of a (named) main-stream peer-reviewed journal had recently provided incontrovertible proof, on the basis of rigorous scientific study and experiment, that chemical sensitivity was a psychological condition.

Gots was followed by Johns Hopkins' speaker Albert Donnay who informed the audience that this prestigious study was fictitious. The authors were fictitious, too. Even the journal was fiction. A gasp went through the audience. Amazingly, Gots made no attempt to answer. Even more astounding was the body language of both Gots and Barrett. While the audience was audibly shocked and murmurs were going through the crowd, those two Quackbusters leaned back in their chairs, fiddled with their pens in the bored and relaxed manner of total self-assurance awaiting the next item on the agenda.

How is this possible? I asked myself. If this had happened to a university professor, his tenure would be in jeopardy and his chances of ever getting published again in a peer-reviewed journal would be zero. Sure, some university professors lie and cheat and fudge the data, and occasionally huge government investigations into science fraud are launched, such as recently in Germany—but never does this happen so outrageously, brazenly in full public view. If cooking the data to support a favorite theory is like the skilled production of counterfeit money in a secret basement operation, Gots' performance was like a bank robbery in full daylight.

A bona fide researcher, even if he is a crook, must at least appear to be honest. But if your work is supported by an infinite money source, nothing much matters. Gots' and Barrett's job seems to be to keep lies circulating so doubt remains strong and fuel is given to the self-defensive all-too-human tendency to dismiss unpleasant information as scare-mongering. Such propaganda provides a highly effective break for change and saves billions of dollars for those whose products and practices would otherwise be compelled to change radically. So, who funds Quackbusters?

The main Quackbusters are Ronald Gots, Victor Herbert (died of cancer in 2003 in his late 50s) and Stephen Barrett, retired non-practicing physicians all who appear in countless public venues, many high profile, to air their views on how untold millions are being poisoned by vitamin C, why we should fight for the right to have fluoride in our water, avoid unhealthy organic foods because they lack those protective pesticides we urgently need, and trust in the absolute safety of mercury amalgam fillings. Global warming is a silly scare perpetrated by individuals in need of psychiatric help, and vaccines cannot possibly cause health problems. On Barrett's web site one finds in-depth article on everything he believes is fraud (amounting to roughly one fifth of the US gross national product). The most personal and viscous attacks are reserved for the likes of Linus Pauling and many leading lights in current medical research.

For Barrett and friends nobody -absolutely anybody—has any authority. The alternative crowd is for them as bad as, the (alas!) progressively more and more deluded mainstream such as the World Health Organization, the NIH, the FDA, the White House task force on complementary medicine, Harvard and Johns Hopkins medical schools, and any other serious person or institution trying to make sense of the world's ills. As for good old-fashioned research, the only democratic tool humanity has got by which to establish what is real and what works—that's only permitted in Barrett's world as long as the results fit his opinion.

In the world of Gots and Barrett there are no surprises. They are trapped in a black-and-white movie from the early 1950s and they want us all to be trapped in it, too. In a detailed analysis of why doctors turn to complementary medicine, Barrett diagnoses them as suffering from paranoid mental states, fascination with the paranormal, profit and prophet motives, psychopathic tendencies, and boredom.

That last item is closer to the truth than even Barrett could stand: I have had literally hundreds of doctors tell me at international conferences on environmental and complementary medicine that they were bored to tears with prescribing drugs and have their patients return for more and more drugs, getting sicker and sicker. Then they switched to real medicine (the kind inspired by Hippocrates who 2,500 years ago taught about clean air, water and wholesome food) and being a doctor became exiting at last. "Life began when I stopped seeing drug reps," one said, and another sighed happily, "I haven't used my prescription pad in years. I am not sure where it is."

Barrett tells us that "Neither Quackwatch nor I have any financial ties to any commercial or industrial organization" and "Quackwatch has no salaried employees" and is funded by personal donations and profits from publications. "If its income falls below what is needed…the rest comes out of my pocket." His and Gots' pockets are interesting, to say the least. The funding sources of their organizations were readily available on the Internet until recently; in the early '90s he stopped disclosing such information. The last annual report to list donors was published 1991 where we find all our toxic friends: Monsanto and Archer Daniels Midland (both of genetic engineering fame), the Nutrasweet Company (neurotoxic aspartame etc.), Union Carbide (as in Bopal disaster), the producers of pesticides, fertilizers, and fluoride Dow Chemical, Dupont, Cargill etc., the biochemical warfare and pharmaceutical producers Eli Lilly, the Uniroyal Chemical Company, all the big petroleum and pharmaceutical companies, and various refined sugar producers and refined food producing giants. Two thirds of the world's economy is controlled by this list of North American Big Business. With friends like that, who needs to worry about telling the most fantastical lies in public?

To test Quackwatch's insistence that it is based on public support, I applied to become a member in 1999. First I was told that the annual membership fee was US $25,000. I said, "That's fine, send me the membership application form." Was I calling on behalf of a corporation? No, I informed the person, who then said, "We prefer corporate members."

Stephen Barrett, a retired psychiatrist, has written 49 books debunking what he identifies as health fraud. He also enjoys debunking UFO's and experiences of the paranormal. He operates six Web sites. In his CV he claims that he did peer reviewing for some of the top medical journals (e.g. *New England Journal of Medicine, Annals of Internal Medicine, Journal of the American Medical Association*). Since the peer review system is secret, there is no way of verifying this claim.

Of course, mainstream medicine has as much trouble discriminating between what's sound and what's dubious in medicine as the rest of us. So, it came as no surprise that in 1999 Quackwatch was able to convince the *New England Journal of Medicine* to co-host a conference on a critical appraisal of alternative medicine. The journal's justly famous then editor, Marcia Angell was the keynote speaker, but rubbing shoulders with Quackwatchers did not impair her find mind and sound judgment. All the hype and tongue clicking notwithstanding, the conference produced lots of sound stuff.

Angell's editorial integrity is now the stuff of legend, as she sounded the wake-up call for medical publication rules and standards of ethics with her June 22, 2000, editorial. She identified the rot by asking to whom the pharmaceutical industry is accountable and argued that it is time medical research does some serious soul searching. As of September 2002, the rules governing conflicts of interest in medical publication have been re-written worldwide. Barrett's friends are having a hard time, at last—as is his entire organization, because the law suits against Quackwatch are increasing in number and seriousness. Check out **jurimed@yahoo.com** for the details.

Quackwatch's Dr. Victor Herbert specialized in vitriolic smear campaigns. In one instance this backfired to the public's greatest benefit: Linus Pauling describes his many irritating meetings with Herbert in *Linus Pauling in His Own Words* (1995): "Here is this …. Victor Herbert, who to this day keeps writing papers and giving speeches saying that no one benefits from taking extra vitamins, and he won't even look at the evidence…. I finally became sufficiently irritated by this fellow that I decided I ought to do something about it. So I sat down one summer…and in two months wrote the book *Vitamin C and the Common Cold*." (1971)

Dr. Herbert was originally intended to be an "expert" witness in the CPSO's trial of Dr. Krop, but was refused by the defense lawyers as unacceptable. Dr. Abraham Hoffer, the father of orthomolecular psychiatry, met him in court and demolished Herbert's testimony against a psychiatrist accused of curing patients without drugs before a US regulatory tribunal.

Quackwatch's negative influence is formidable. The formula of their attacks on health freedom is fairly simple and easy to detect and its success depends on persistent repetition. The Quackwatch formula simply requires citing scientific literature that is outdated, irrelevant or non-existent. Only the specialist or nitpicking investigative journalist will ferret out the truth. In attacking the White House Commission on Complementary Medicine (annual budget of US $ 50 million at the National Institutes of Health) initiated by President Clinton in March 2000, Barrett devoted enormous amounts of cyberspace to its condemnation. Triumphantly, he (mis)informs the browser that even members of that task force have broken away in disgust and made their dissent known publicly.

What really happened can be found in the generally more reliable March 28, 2002, issue of the world's premier science journal *Nature*. Two members of that task force stated that more money should be allocated towards research into complementary medicine, and that the task force's final report would have been better if it had cited even more research to support its suggested program of action.

Quackwatch delights in using the medial regulatory systems to go after doctors who have strayed from the One True Barrett Path. The State of New York is currently holding hearings (the equivalent of a public inquiry) into the inappropriate way in which the disciplinary process has been used (with Quackwatch "expert" witnesses) to stop doctors from using complementary medicine. The popular radio show "The Touch of Health" was relentlessly attacked with viscous and insulting e-mails by Ontario Quackwatch member Dr. Polevoy until the show was closed down.

One of the worst examples of Quackwatch's power comes from Nova Scotia. In the early 1990s the faulty air filtration system at Halifax's Camphill Hospital caused 900 people to become seriously chemically injured and today more than 300 remain permanently disabled. When these cases began to come before Worker's Compensation tribunal in the late 1990s, it was Ronald Gots who appeared as the "expert". The expert opinion reports, accepted by the tribunal, weren't even signed by doctors and Gots explained that the secretaries could be trusted to know the physicians' intentions. Gots' expertise caused all claims to be denied and the claimants were encouraged to seek the help of a psychiatrist instead. So, to the rescue came Johns Hopkins researcher Albert Donnay who provided the whole truth and nothing but the truth, scientific and legal, to the appeals board. Since then case after case has been won on appeal.

(Added in 2004) The main focus of Quackwatch is environmental illness which it is their mission to discredit. How they do this is important to understand, because it elucidates the technique used not only by them, but also by pharmaceutical-industry-sponsored research: Ronald Gots and Stephen Barret wrote a book in 1998 published by their own company, Prometheus, and entitled *Chemical Sensitivity: The Truth About Environmental Illness.* They proceed, in chapter after chapter, to marshal the "evidence" that Multiple Chemical Sensitivity, Sick Building Syndrome, the relation ship between diet and hyperactivity, the toxicity of mercury amalgam, Gulf War Syndrome, fungal overgrowth (candidiasis) and more, all do not actually exist.

Each chapter is carefully organized to include references to existing medical literature. The problem is, however, that all their references, without a single exception, are totally outdated and are chosen from a time when the debate among scientists began in each instance. Naturally, they quote themselves, instead of primary research, most frequently. Most telling of all is the complete absence of any report from the World Health Organization which, with regard to most of these health conditions, was generally the first to recognize them and initiate research resulting in consensus statements supporting the existence of these health problems and the need for their treatment. The two instances in which the WHO is cited, the citations are incorrect (pages 78 and 97). Anyone who works for environmental illness patients ought to study this book carefully, as it is a virtual manual of all the dirty tricks used especially by the industry of environmental toxins to defend itself against liability.

Some time ago, a friend found me on the Canadian Quackwatch site described as "a doctor's wife who promotes quackery in public lectures." I am flattered. The information I provide must be dangerously accurate.

Update October 2004: *Stephen Barret, Ronald Gots and Quackwatch have suffered tremendous defeats in the courts since 2003, personally for fraud as well as with their organization, specifically in California, Oregon and Washington State where their testimony was thrown out by several judges, specifically with regard to the mercury amalgam issue and nutritional and homeopathic medicine cases. Quackwatch is currently defending itself against many legal actions launched against it by doctors and health agencies.*

Sources and Resources
The battle over access to safe medicine and knowledge of disease prevention is fought to a large extent over the Internet by which the news travels faster than through medical journals, government agencies and the courts. Therefore, the following sites and e-mail connections are recommended as most helpful:

If you are involved in work that requires knowing how the enemy thinks, surf the Quackbusters' web sites which are operated by Dr. Stephen Barrett: **www.quackwatch.com**; the Canadian counterpart is run by Kitchener pediatrician Dr. Terry Polevoy **www.healthwatcher.net**

To find out how Quackbusters really operates visit: **www.iahf.com/quackbusters.html; www.savedrclark.org;** and **www.internetwks.com/pauling/lie/index.html;** and **www.healthfreedomlaw.com** to find out what law suits are in progress against Quackbusters, and for what reasons, get on the e-mail list of Tim Bolen: **jurimed@yahoo.com**

For the science and current developments regarding mercury amalgam visit **www.iaomt.org**, the site of the *International Academy for Oral and Medical Toxicology* whose scientists have won many legal victories for non-toxic dentistry; many of these dental medicine scientists are associated with the World Health Organization and the National Institutes of Health and are advisors to the health authorities of the European Union.

For the scientific facts, international consensus, current research and personal help regarding Multiple Chemical Sensitivity, visit Johns Hopkins medical school associate Albert Donnay's site **www.mcsrr.org**

An excellent source of information on the current status of available clinical treatments and research in complementary medicine for cancer and many other environmentally mediated diseases is the National Institutes of Health site **www.CMBM.org**. You can download, free of charge, the entire text of all the presentations made by the world's top researchers at the NIH international conferences.

For facts on herbal medicine and a balanced interpretation of the ongoing debate battle between pharmaceuticals and natural remedies visit **www.herbalgram.com**

A first class source of information on the worldwide growing awareness about the effects of fluoride visit **www.fluoride.org.uk**

To learn about the dangers, science, and legal actions going on worldwide with regard to vaccines visit **www.909shot.com**; this is especially helpful with regard to the facts on the connection between autism and the MMR vaccine

If you want to be kept up-to-date on all of these politically loaded health issues (and many more besides!) request to be put on the e-mail list of one of the best sources of information: **croft@cwhealth.com**

An excellent source for information on health freedom issues, and especially newly developed treatments, is the news letter of the *International Council for Health Freedom* which operates in 17 countries; available through **ccichf@san.rr.com** tel.619-702-1282, Visit their site **www.ichf.net**

K. Ausubel, *When Healing Becomes A Crime*, Healing Arts Press,2000

J.P. Carter,MD, *Racketeering in Medicine*, Hampton Roads Publishing Co., 1993

M.L. Culbert, *Medical Armageddon*, C & C Communications, San Diego,1997

W. Duffy, *Sugar Blues*, Warner Books 1975(the first of this type, still a bestseller)

D. Haley (US Congressman), *Politics in Healing*, Potomac Valley Press, 2000

J. Lisa, *The Assault on Medical Freedom*, Hampton Roads Publishing Co., 1997

G. Lanctot, M.D., *The Medical Mafia*, Here's The Key Inc.,1995

What is Junk Science?

Vitality Magazine April 2002

The most frequently asked question put to me by my readers is: "How can one tell the difference between fact and lies in medicine?" Knowing how to identify reliable information about therapies is vital to your health. By not reading the fine print, today's health care consumers can get killed in the supermarket of modern medicine. Illness is a growth industry: bypass surgery costs US $ 10 billion annually. (**Note:** The New York Times *reported on September 27, 2004, that leading experts at the prestigious Cleveland Clinic working in bypass surgery, stents and angioplasty do not believe that these procedures do anything much to treat heart disease or prevent heart attacks, because it these interventions are at best of very short duration and their invasiveness is extremely dangerous. These procedures are done because, these surgeons said, "there is this embedded belief that fixing an artery is a good thing… it is ingrained in the American psyche that the worth of the medical care is directly related to how aggressive it is."*)The six largest pharmaceutical companies are worth US $ 500 billion. With advertising telling us how they all are determined to cure us, the fact is that annually illness increases: thyroid disease by 14%, depression 23%, hypertension 20%, gastric ulcers and pain each 10%. (The only good news is that antibiotic use has decreased in one year by 17%.) Impotence must be a really rampant (and fabulously lucrative) condition—how else to explain the astounding decision to let Viagra be advertised on television? Worst of all, many doctors fit the bumper sticker: "Don't follow me, I'm lost too." That is nothing new.

However, today we do have options. Being sick and faced with conflicting information from "experts" was always hell, not taking charge of one's life always potentially fatal. Anybody who still clutches the baby-blanket-thought, "But isn't my doctor supposed to know?" better grab a soother, too. This article is not for the faint-hearted.

On April 9, 1998 the world's premier science journal, *Nature*, reported that Vitamin C might promote improper cell mutations—i.e. may cause cancer. This was front-page news worldwide only because Vitamin C's importance in prevention and treatment, from cancer to the common cold, is so well established. In order for this "news" to be true, patients and scientists worldwide would have to find a new explanation for their thousands of main-stream reported positive clinical results with Vitamin C (the count is currently around 26,000 articles). It's rather like somebody suggesting that the earth may be flat after all; continuously verified experience to the contrary is universal. Anthropologists tell us that hunter-gatherers get on average 20,000 mg of Vitamin C daily. They have none of our chronic diseases, nor cancer, which the World Health Organization warns, every second person is now expected to get. Yet, those Vitamin C-stuffed bushmen replicate their DNA without cancer-causing mistakes. Interestingly, experimental and zoo-kept monkeys and apes are given 50,000 mg of the stuff daily to ensure their optimal health. Fortunately, medical scientists from universities all over the world demolished this report in a joint response published in *Nature* on September 17 that same year. So what's wrong?

Simple: the experiment was conducted in a test-tube, not in a living organism. Vitamins function as catalysts in complex living systems. At any moment some 100,000 chemical events take place in a cell, all inter-related. Vitamin C speeds up anti-oxidation, affecting the whole system. Removing the entire living context of a bio-chemical event leads to irrelevant results. Some 80 years of real-life, real-time experience with Vitamin C is not affected by a test-tube abstraction. Later, it was reported (not on the front page, of course) that the graduate student who handled the DNA samples made some mistakes his boss didn't notice. Oops. (Another report suggested that it clogs arteries—later shown to be an interpretation mistake: Vitamin C causes the walls of blood vessels to become thicker and stronger, thereby preventing nutrient loss into surrounding tissue.)

The Medical Post reported on November 20, 2001, the results of a study involving 3,654 diabetics randomized to be given 400 IU of Vitamin E or a sugar pill (placebo). Not surprisingly, the first group did no better than the second. Since the blood vessels of diabetics slowly turn to stone through calcification, Vitamin E is essential prevention. Where is the mistake? Simple: the daily recommended allowance (RDA) of this vitamin for *healthy* people until 2001 was 400 IU (now it is 1,000 IU). Diabetes is characterized by an inability to maintain adequate levels of nutrients. Giving such patients the previous RDA (measured to be just enough to keep *healthy* people ticking), is like putting out a house fire with a garden watering can. Did the researchers who designed this study not know Vitamin E's known mode of action? Why didn't they bother to check those diabetics' blood levels of this vitamin and compare them with the norms for healthy people? Why did they not check the current medical literature on Vitamin E in diabetes and give them amounts known to make a dramatic difference? Were they persuaded/paid to mis-design the study? Well, the study was paid for by pharmaceutical companies.

The (in-)famous arthritis drug Celebrex provides a good example for industry's corrupting influence. The *Journal of the American Medical Association* warned in 2001 that taking this drug **in**creases a person's chance to get a heart attack by 55%. While reducing arthritic inflammation, it increases blood pressure and frequently causes "rhabdomyolysis", i.e. rotting away of the heart muscle causing death. In the US this drug is now under FDA review—the body count made it necessary. In Canada it is still celebrated in full-page color ads in most major national magazines. (For an excellent overview of Big Pharma's deadly effect, read the transcript of CBC Ideas of March 13, 2001.) What Third World countries achieve in death tolls with civil wars, we do just as effectively with drugs. While the former ruin their economies, we make deadly medicine central to our economy.

Chelation therapy is a non-surgical intravenous procedure that removes arterial plaques; it is cheap and has never had a fatality. By-pass surgery is expensive and has a mortality rate of ca. 20% and doesn't last. A report tabled before the US Congress in 1993 by chelation doctors revealed that many heart surgeons, when they or their families become sick with heart disease, prefer chelation.

On January 23, 2002 the *Journal of the American Medical Association* published a study showing chelation doesn't work. Yet, what about the many studies showing the opposite published ·in equally reputable journals and involving much larger cohorts? Chelation therapy was developed by US military medical researchers in World War II and is now taught by the American Academy for Advancement in Medicine. It isn't a skill a doctor acquires by reading a manual. The protocol is some 50 years old and, through experience with close to 2 million patients has been much refined. Reading the details of the treatment protocol used in the above study reveals that it wasn't even approximated. Especially serious is the omission of vitamin E supplementation, central to chelation therapy. Of course, the study was sponsored by Pfizer, the world's largest manufacturer of cholesterol-lowering drugs—a huge market threatened very seriously by chelation therapy. Since mainstream doctors rarely know about chelation, they sadly tend to believe this nonsense.

Happily, the best and most thorough research exposing stupidity and corruption currently comes from the mainstream. There are at least as many truth-seekers as there are paid liars. (See, for example the August 2004 book by Marcia Angell, *The Truth About the Drug Companies*; she was the editor of the prestigious *New England Journal of Medicine* for twenty years.) Last year a large international study was published by one of the world's top journals, *The Lancet* (vol. 358, 2001), re-evaluating the usefulness of mammography for breast cancer screening. The Canadian Medical Association (CMAJ March 5, 2001) did the same for prostate-specific antigen (PSA) testing used for early detection of prostate cancer. Both concluded that these testing methods have done nothing to reduce mortality, but a lot for increasing unnecessary surgery and radiation because of the frequent false positive results. The evidence also has considered undeniable that radiation exposure from repeated mammography *causes* breast cancer. These studies are challenging a multi-billion dollar industry. (For radiation-free breast screening call Cycle of Life Technologies in Toronto)

The November 2000 issue of *Geriatrics and Aging* reported that movement disorders in elderly patients are generally caused by the cocktail of drugs they get without anybody bothering to check how these chemicals interact. They impair the central nervous system seriously, which then causes broken hips and loss of independence. This tragic situation is primarily the result of carelessness. Most elderly are on drug plans. Giving them yet another prescription (without checking the readily available information on adverse effects and interactions) is the fast way out. In January of this year, The *Annals of Emergency Medicine* reported that adverse effects due to drug interactions in the elderly is the primary reason for their hospitalization.

If we ask ourselves: "What do the great detectives of literature—Sherlock Holmes, Hercule Poirot, Miss Marple, Judge Dee, Father Brown, and Chief Inspector Morse—have in common?" we get three answers that apply equally to medicine and murder. Their seemingly extraordinary powers are founded on one mental quality: doubt in what appears obvious. Secondly, their success comes from one carefully considered question: "Who benefits?" Third, and most important, they never shrink from the truth, however awful it may turn out to be, when they find it at last.

The days are gone where medical knowledge was inaccessible to lay persons. We have the Internet and there are many excellent newsletters and books written by doctors who find curing patients more exciting than pharmaceutical company perks. Fortunately, corruption is neither absolute nor uniform, and as its activities, in the long run, inevitably must self-destruct. In 1998 the American Medical Association reported that over the last 30 years the side-effects from properly prescribed and correctly taken drugs cause annually more deaths than from AIDS, suicide and homicide combined: the equivalent of a jumbo jet going down daily. That statistic caused the tide to turn.

Mainstream medical research is as fed-up as patients with the spin-doctoring, the Big Pharma bullying, and the shoddy science designed to deceive. (On February 6 this year the *Globe & Mail* reported that 87% of doctors have ties to the industry and that CMA ethical guidelines are being drastically revised.) In September last year all the medical journals of the world joined forces and announced new guidelines for research submissions. Big Pharma is reeling. The Canadian Association of University Teachers published the Olivieri Report providing hard-hitting recommendations which show how deep the rot has become. The editorials in the Canadian Medical Association's journal often sound like the outraged articles in the alternative medical press. The CMAJ of Sept. 18, 2001: "The duty of universities is to seek truth. The duty of pharmaceutical companies is to make money for their shareholders... universities that subordinate the disinterested search for truth to other ends, lose credibility ...research can either serve or subvert the public interest." The war has begun.

In North America, according to the FDA and the *Journal of the American Pharmaceutical Association*, the cost of serious drug side effects is now annually US $ 177 billion. For every US $ 1.11 spent on a prescription drug another US $ 1.77 is needed to treat the harm it does. Here is what you can do to protect yourself during times when you must use a prescription drug or need to wean yourself off one.

Adverse side effects are caused by their toxicity and because they cause depletion of vital nutrients. When supplemented during periods when some of those drugs might be unavoidable, you can prevent getting even sicker while the drug does its work. No known adverse interactions are known with these. If you want to know more about interactions between drugs and neutraceuticals: **www.NaturalDatabase.com** . To see for yourself what the drug industry must admit to regarding serious side- and long-term effects, consult the *Compendium of Pharmaceuticals and Specialties*, updated annually and available for you to see at any pharmacy; take a photostat copy of the info on the prescription drug home to consider carefully. Never take a drug merely on the basis of the short blurb handed to you with your prescription: that and the 30-second explanation (if any) your doctor gave you is NOT "informed consent", as federal law requires.

Antibiotics are vitally important emergency drugs, but they deplete good bacterial gut flora and knock out your Vitamin C and Magnesium reserves very fast. Always take these at the same time as well as acidophilus and other probiotics. None of these interfere with the antibiotics' desired activity.

Antidepressants, also sometimes a necessary emergency drug, deplete B vitamins, Selenium, Zinc, L-Gluthathione, Calcium, Magnesium, Vitamin C, and essential fatty acids. Take all of these at the same time.

Drugs for ADHD reduce brain blood flow patterns and need to be supplemented with Vitamins B complex, C, Selenium, Magnesium, essential fatty acids and Ginko Biloba. These are especially important when weaning a person of these drugs.

Diabetic medications deplete Chromium, Vitamin C, Magnesium, Vitamins B6 and B12, Folic Acid and essential fatty acids must be supplemented.

All hormones (synthetic only!) such as estrogens, progesterone, the Pill deplete B-complex vitamins, Calcium, Magnesium, Vitamins C, E, Beta-Carotene and essential fatty acids. Why take the synthetic stuff when the natural stuff is available in compounding pharmacies everywhere and without depleting any of the above? Indeed, the natural stuff *increases* absorption of all of the above as well as Melatonin production, so you sleep well again.

Arthritis medications deplete Calcium, Magnesium, Vitamin C and B-Complex, Folic Acid, Glocosamine sulfate and essential fatty acids and need to be supplemented.

Corticosteroids should be used as an emergency drug only; long-term use frequently causes osteoporosis, growth problems in children, and depression. It depletes and needs supplementation with the following even short-term: Vitamin C, B Complex, Potassium, Zinc, Selenium, Calcium, Magnesium, Co-Enzyme Q_{10} and essential fatty acids.

Diuretics and all the "statin" drugs used for cardiovascular disease drastically reduce: potassium, Calcium, Magnesium, the B- complex, E and C vitamins, zinc, Co-Enzyme Q_{10} and essential fatty acids.

Any drug that reduces the B-complex vitamins has the potential for serious mood-alterations ranging from depression to suicide and homicide (see David Healy's book). Hence so many suicides and homicides are associated with drugs like Prozac, a classic B Vitamin enemy; it has had more adverse reactions recorded by the FDA than any other drug in pharmaceutical history. Similarly, any drug that lowers Vitamin C levels has the potential to be carcinogenic.

Sources and Resources

J.Thompson et al., *The Olivieri Report*, Canadian Association of University Teachers, Lorimer Ltd., 2001

D. Haley, *Politics in Healing*, Potomac Valley Press, Washington DC, 2000

D. Healy, *The Anti-Depressant Era*, Harvard, 1997

A.Hoffer, *Vitamin C and Cancer: Discovery, Recovery, Controversy*, Quarry, 2000

A. Hoffer, *Factoids: Or Lies Some People Tell You About Vitamins*, $10, e-mail: **hoffer@Islan Net.com**

T. Moore, *Deadly Medicine*, Simon & Schuster, 1995

T. Moore, *Prescription Disaster*, Simon & Schuster, 1999

J. Robinson, *Prescription Games*, McClelland & Stewart, 2001

croft@cwhealth.com join his e-mail list for information on drugs, therapies, medical politics

Center for Health and Policy Studies, University of Calgary, **sj.lewis@home.com** and ask for information

National Network on Environments and Women's Health for safety issues on drugs **nnewh@yorku.ca**

International information on medical safety **hai@hai.antenna.nl**

A website devoted entirely to Vitamin C : **www.orthomed.com/#point** as is **www.abic.net** .

6. For the monthly goldmine of information on medicine, medical politics, and therapies that work, nothing beats the *Total Wellness* newsletter by Dr. Sherry Rogers: 1-800-846-6687 or **www.prestigepublishing.com**

For the best (guaranteed bull-shit-free!) medical journal accessible to the general reader, written by doctors and researchers subscribe to *The Townsend Letter for Doctors and Patients*, 360-385-6021 or **www.tldp.com**, e-mail: **tldp@olympus.net**

Canadian Schizophrenia Foundation, 16 Florence Ave., Toronto, M2N 1E9 for booklets containing mainstream studies showing the beneficial effect of vitamins and minerals for mental health problems.

This article is dedicated to my friend Lynne Burke of Orangeville, Ontario.

Stoned by Prescription

Vitality Magazine October 2003

Imagine the media informing you that a jumbo has gone down, killing all on board. Imagine being informed of such an event every single day of the year—year after year for four decades. That's about 140,000 people a year. And that's what's happening: the victims are people treated with properly prescribed legal drugs for properly diagnosed illnesses. They die from prescription drugs—not from their diseases. Some deaths are caused by the 187,000 known drug interactions nobody thought to check for, but most are from the drugs themselves. Add to these *reported* adverse reactions another 10 to 50% for the unreported cases. (April 1998, *Journal of the American Medical Association.*)

Millions don't die, of course, and for them these drugs work—for a while. They live (sort of) with the so-called side effects: *Aspirin* seriously depletes vitamin C making you vulnerable to infection. *Diuretics* deplete potassium vital for heart and muscle function. The Pill depletes folic acid and vitamin C and vastly increases your risk of cancer, as do other synthetic sex hormones. *Antibiotics*, taken frequently, kill favorable intestinal bacteria and cause systemic candidiasis, which can trigger both cancer and autoimmune disease. The SSRI *antidepressants* (selective serotonin re-uptake inhibitors like Prozac, Paxil, Zoloft etc.) deplete the B vitamins, the detoxicant Selenium, the brain food zinc, the nerve and enzyme food magnesium, the bone builder calcium, the cancer preventives L-gluthathione and vitamin C (some diabetic medications do all of this also), and they are associated with cancer more than tobacco and an increased risk of suicide. Many SSRIs are addictive, tend to ruin your sex life, most are toxic to the liver, and they can reduce blood flow to the brain as well. All *statin drugs*, meant to lower bad cholesterol to prevent heart attacks, deplete Co-enzyme Q_{10}, the very stuff your heart needs most to function, and they greatly increase your chance of developing one of the worst autoimmune diseases: Lupus. *Arthritis medications*, steroidal or non-steroidal, deplete all of these vital nutrients, some are suspected carcinogens, all deplete essential fatty acids making one vulnerable to depression, psychosis, skin diseases and more. The non-steroidal ones called NSAIDs (non-steroidal anti-inflammatory drugs) are even worse than Aspirin (*see the news on the September 2004 world-wide withdrawal of Vioxx*). Steroids after prolonged use are no longer absorbed by the stripped cell receptors. They seriously depress the immune system.

Among the "oops!" variety we find drugs like Thalidomide in the 1960s which caused tens of thousands of terrible birth defects before it was pulled off the market. In the 1980s the heart drug Tamocor killed literally thousands of people before it was pulled. CBC's *Ideas* (March 13, 2001) aired the research into deadly drugs by Thomas Moore, a health policy analyst and author of *Deadly Medicine*. Moore observed, "So deeply embedded is the human desire to a have a pill…. [we] have suspended our normal critical faculties when it comes to drugs. We have something that every consumer should know is their right, and they never get it, and that is the right to informed consent."

Consent is messy when big bucks are at stake. The main players in Big Pharma, as these companies call themselves, are Merck (market value in 1998 at US $ 140 billion), Bristol-Myers-Squibb ($100 billion), Johnson & Johnson ($ 93 billion), DuPont ($ 87 billion), Dow Chemical ($21 billion), Monsanto ($33 billion). Four-fifth of Big Pharma's total budget serves only one fifth of the world's population. As Robinson observes, "The drugs that are needed are not necessarily the drugs that sell" because drugs that work have expired patents and are needed by four fifth of the world without money.

I was stunned and fascinated (and absolutely sickened) by the fabulously researched and heart-poundingly well-written new bestseller by Jeffrey Simpson: *Prescription Games* and Eichenwald's *The Informant*. Reading these requires a strong stomach and a serious case of lust for truth. For four decades these companies have consistently been first in return of revenues, assets, and equity, fifth in profit growth and fourth in total return for investors. Drug profits surpass all other Fortune 500 companies, and they have for forty years outperformed Standard & Poor's 500 Index by 10% every year. All this mind-boggling wealth is made on drugs for cancer, cholesterol, smoking, hair loss, impotence, ulcers, menopause and depression. "Blockbuster drugs are harvested out of chronic diseases," Simpson reports.

These astronomical profits (1,000% mark-up over production cost is the norm) became supported by taxpayers money, which pays for most of the actual drug development costs, ever since former Prime Minister Mulroney's 1993 Bill C-91. In 1997 the US allowed pharmaceuticals to advertise to the consumer directly, exponentially increasing profits. Harvard University's Jerry Avorn proved that prescription habits by doctors are overwhelmingly influenced by drug reps. Research has further shown, that what the drug reps tell the doctors is mostly hot air.

For example, to ensure that sales for Prozac, whose patent expires this year, don't drop too painfully fast for the manufacturer Eli Lilly (also the world's premier manufacturer of biological warfare materials), it is now recommended for Premenstrual Syndrome. (PMS is well known to be mediated by magnesium, progesterone and essential fatty acid deficiencies.) Pharmaceutical reps wine and dine doctors, send them on vacations, offer up to $ US 40,000 per patient recruited for studies, or as Dr. T. Rohland of Nova Scotia reported in *The Medical Post* (Feb.9, 1999): "If [the drug companies] can no longer appeal to our greed by giving us gifts, then a new tactic is needed. How about our raging uncontrollable hormones? Enter the gorgeous, young, model-type drug reps." One doctor kept track of drug rep visits and mailings (*Medical Post* May 22, 2001) which came to 452 promotional encounters in one year.

In Canada, only Quebec and British Columbia have legislation prohibiting pharmacies from selling information on doctors' prescription patterns to Big Pharma. In all other provinces this information is available and also used to influence the licensing bodies, the Colleges of Physicians and Surgeons, to conduct witch hunts against doctors who treat diseases instead of being accessories to making patients into cash cows.

The World Health Organization has recognized this "inherent conflict of interest between legitimate business goals and social needs" for a long time—

to no effect. Former Health Canada scientists, Dr. Michelle Brill-Edwards, provides the reason for this. She told Robinson: "The dilemma of those in power is not 'Do you serve citizens versus do you serve corporations?' That's a no-brainer. People in power serve the corporations because they have the money." But sometimes the human conflict can happen right within a pharmaceutical company: Merck's CEO was appalled to learn that millions of Africans go blind every year from river blindness, a disease easily prevented with a derivative of the cheap heart-worm medication we give our dogs. He ended up defying his own board of directors and angry investors and donating millions to stop this illness—successfully.

Interestingly, these same companies also make the pesticides which cause all of the diseases in the first place, either directly by ingestion, skin contact or inhalation, or indirectly by dangerously depleting the nutrients in the foods. What an amazingly effective business strategy! Part of this strategy—logically—is to control research. This is a typical North American problem. In Europe most research is government funded and out of the reach of direct business interests. That's why we get all that exciting research on nutritional and environmental medicine from Europe.

In Canada and the US research is primarily funded by drug companies whose contracts always contain gag clauses preventing researchers from reporting negative findings, should these occur. Controlling research and clinical practice starts in the medical schools with the drug reps' pizza parties. When MacMaster University, frustrated, declared their interns off limits to pharmaceutical reps, instructing these doctors of the future to read their research journals instead, the Pharmaceutical Manufacturers Association threatened to withdraw all funding (*The Toronto Star*, Dec. 3, 1999).

Internationally famous blood researcher, Dr. Nancy Olivieri, found a drug to be toxic to the liver and wanted to change patient consent forms accordingly. Sick Children's Hospital and the University of Toronto fired her to please the manufacturer Apotex. That backfired. Nobel laureates, Oxford and Harvard universities demanded an end to gag clauses. She was reinstated and this month and the US based Civil Justice Foundation awarded her the prestigious Community Champion Award. The last recipient was Erin Brockovich.

Canada seems to figure prominently in this resistance movement. Internationally renowned researcher Dr. David Healy, hired by U of T was fired following a speech about the dangers of Prozac (suicide, violence, and brain damage). This one backfired even worse. The editors of the world's most prestigious medical journals issued joint editorials on September 12th condemning Big Pharma's attempt to control research and clinical practice. They will henceforth refuse publication of Big Pharma-funded research unless all the data are made available and gag clauses vanish. At the same time, 27 internationally famous medical scientists, among them 2 Nobel laureates, published a condemnation of U of T's treatment of Dr. Healy, declaring its reputation "poisoned".

It is gratifying that all of this information you have read here is published by first-rate researchers and produced by mainstream publishers. The tide is turning against biotechnology and drugs. Perhaps war and drugs will not drive world economy forever. We are not as stupid as they think we are.

What You Need to Know

1. Always assume the drug prescribed is toxic—unless proven otherwise. Browsing the internet sites of the US Federal Drug Administration (FDA) and Health Canada will tell you which drugs are currently under review because of serious problems.
2. There is no such thing as a "side effect"; it is exactly what you can expect to experience, at least in part, along with whatever primary effect the drug is intended to have. Air pollution is simply part of car design.
3. Assume that any drug is at best a necessary emergency measure, rarely a long-term requirement, and almost never a cure. There are situations, in which they are imperative and life saving, but on most of those the patent has expired. They are the tried and true pharmaceutical arsenal, and not aggressively marketed nor advertised because they have no stock value.
4. Always ask your doctor for a full explanation of the prescribed drugs: what is the active ingredient? What so-called "side-effects" can you expect and how high is the percentage of those? Is there any record of addictive properties? How did it fare in human trials? Did it ever have human trials? If it didn't—ask yourself if you are ready to be that human trial.
5. Always ask your doctor for the source of his/her information: did it come from personal reading of a medical journal or a drug rep? If the source is a drug rep, treat the information with a ton of salt, turn to the internet to find out more also about the entire family of drugs it belongs to, what side effects they consistently have, and what safer and cheaper alternatives exist. Did your doctor have good results with this drug with his/her own patients, or are you a guinea pig?
6. If you don't have access to the internet, and before taking the newly pre-scribed drug, go to your library and get out the latest copy of the CPS: *Compendium of Pharmaceuticals and Specialties.* Look up the drug and

learn all about the side effects and clinical trials, which by law the manu-facturer must publish annually. While much is not fully reported, this information is generally scary enough to make you think. Photocopy those pages and ask your doctor for explanations. If he/she doesn't have the time or doesn't want to make the time—change doctors. Your busi-ness is to become healthy, not accommodate your doctor.

7. Treat Over-The-Counter (OTC) drugs with exactly the same caution as you would prescription drugs.

8. If you have been prescribed an anti-depressant, a so-called psychotropic drug (for mental health problems ranging from schizophrenia to severe depression or eating disorders), a drug that influences the heart, your cholesterol levels, your endocrine system (i.e. anything at all hormonal), or a cancer drug—buy or borrow the books listed at the end and find out its commercial and biological history first. Again: your business is to become healthy, not make the undertakers wealthy.

9. Always, always discuss nutritional, herbal and vitamin /mineral supple-mentation as an alternative to whatever pharmaceutical treatment your doctor suggests. If he/she knows nothing about it—back to the library and internet. This is equally true for any surgical procedure whatsoever.

10. Beware of experimental drugs—especially for chronic illness (cancer, autoimmune and cardiovascular disease, anything expected to influence cell division). Well-researched, scientifically proven treatments and out-right cures have been around for whatever ails you for a long time. Resist being the playground/victim for the human fascination with new, high-tech toys.

11. If you are asked to enter a clinical trial designed to be "double blind and placebo controlled", think twice. A huge body of scientific literature ques-tions the medical ethics of giving sugar pills to people in control group patients who are just as sick as those getting the active drug. Inquire about toxicity. The chemistry of the experimental drug will be known. Ask who is paying for the drug trial: if it is a pharmaceutical company, they want to bring this drug to market and expect a healthy return for their invest-ment. Negative results will be discouraged.

12. The more authoritarian and rushed the doctor behaves, the less he/she really knows. The more collaborative, encouraging of exploration the doctor is, the more likely you will improve. If you "can't talk to that guy"—don't. Change doctors (there are many other excellent ones) or go

to a herbalist, homeopath, or naturopath. (The word "doctor" originally meant "teacher", and medicine must return to teaching.) True, they are not covered by OHIP, but the toxic sludge you might be prescribed, is expensive and may ruin your life.

13. Corruption and ignorance are part of the fabric of life, therefore, research the alternatives as carefully as the mainstream solution. Not all supplements are created equal, and money is an object. Toronto has excellent compounding pharmacies that specialize in supplements. They will tell you which products are best, have the least artificial ingredients, and how they interact with conventional medication or each other.

Update October 2004: *If you enjoyed the revelations in the books discussed above, you are in for an enormous treat if you read 2004 book published by University of California Press,* The $ 800 Million Pill *by M. Goozner, a financial expert and investigative journalist now with the prestigious organization* Science in the Public Interest. *This book has been on the New York Times bestseller list for months. Already mentioned and recommended again here is the August 2004 book by Marcia Angell, the former editor of* The New England Journal of Medicine, *entitled* The Truth About The Drug Companies, *Random House.*

Sources and Resources

K. Eichenwald, *The Informant: A True Story*, Broadway Books, 2000

J. Glenmullen, *Prozac Backlash: Overcoming the Dangers of Prozac, Zoloft, Paxil, and Other Antidepressants with Safe, Effective Alternatives*, Simon & Schuster, 2000

D. Healy, *The Antidepressant Era*, Harvard, 1997

D. Healy, *Let Them Eat Prozac*, Lorimer, 2003

J. Robinson, *Prescription Games: Money, Ego and Power Inside the Global Pharmaceutical Industry*, MacClelland & Steward, 2001

Dr. Sherry Rogers' newsletter is still the best for scientifically reliable information on the truth about drugs and effective treatments: for subscriptions to "Total Wellness" call 315-454-8119, **www.prestigepublishing.com**, $ 40 per year.

International Society for Orthomolecular Medicine, 16 Florence Ave., Toronto, M2N 1E9, tel. 416-733-2117

OMA Section on Complementary Medicine, Chair: Dr. L. Rapson, 416-968-1366

Canadian Environmental Medicine Association, Chair: Dr. J. Molot, 613-521-2391

The following article by my husband was written for psychotherapists in Ontario in order to inform them about the suppressed information in mainstream science on the lack of safety and efficacy of antidepressants, specifically the SSRIs such as Prozac. What this article doesn't mention is something we found out later: the alleged 10,000 patients who were enrolled in the definitive trial that was the basis of Prozac's FDA approval some twenty years ago, were in fact only about 200 in number. Harvard Medical School Psychiatrist Peter Breggin decided to contact every single person who was enrolled in this trial. See his book, *Toxic Psychiatry*, 1994.

SSRI's—How Effective and How Safe?

By Robert Ferrie

(General Practitioners' Psychotherapy Association's Newsletter January 2004)

In my practice, I have seen a fairly large number of people who are already medicated with various SSRIs when they come to me for the first time. I have found, that not only are they *not* improved, as a result of the medication, but are actually worse off. They have usually gained a lot of weight, their sex drive is gone which affects their relationships, they have difficulty concentrating, and often they have tics or experience numbness and tingling in various parts of their bodies. They are still depressed and, therefore, seek out psychotherapy. They also report feeling emotionally numb generally which makes it very difficult for them to respond to psychotherapy and to get at the cause of their original symptoms which is often a trauma. These traumatic antecedents are such that they could be fairly easily resolved, were they not medicated.

I became seriously interested in the problems SSRI's seem to cause when a 17-year old patient of mine became so violent 30 minutes after restarting Celexa, that a SWAT team had to be called. So, how true is the claim that SSRI's are safe and effective?

There are two important books dealing with these issues: *Prozac Backlash*, by Harvard's John Glenmullen (2000), which came to my attention because it was reviewed in *Nature* (a vote of confidence from the leading scientific community), and *Let Them Eat Prozac*, by David Healy, published this year by the Canadian Association of University Teachers (CAUT). We all know Dr. Healy, the keynote speaker at our 2003 conference. These are must-read books for anybody working in psychotherapy. Not to know what these researchers have unearthed could be literally fatal for our patients.

Effectiveness

M. Zimmerman, a professor at Rhode Island Hospital, found that, "as few as 15% of 346 depressed patients [in his own clinic] would have met the eligibility requirements of a standard drug trial" as conducted by drug companies to meet FDA approval. Astonishingly, among the *exclusion* criteria for the manufacturer's studies was suicidal ideation. (See *The Medical Post*, Feb. 28, 2002, and **www.brown.edu/Administration/News**). Yet, these drugs are used specifically to treat suicidal patients. So, on what basis is this use justified?

Kahn, Warner and Brown, writing in the *Archives of General Psychiatry* (2000; 57:311-17) had obtained the FDA's data base, through freedom of information legislation, on the approval process for Prozac, Zoloft, Paxil, Wellbutrin, Remeron and Effexor. In contrast to what we have been led to believe about the "new and improved" effectiveness of SSRI's, it turned out that there was virtually no difference between these new drugs and the older tricyclic drug used as the comparator: 40.7% symptom reduction for the new drugs versus 41.7% for the comparator. Even worse, placebos were 30.9 % effective, which means that there is a negligible statistical difference between these new drugs and a sugar pill. Does a 10 % difference justify the advertising hoopla ?

Wolfgang Fleischhacker et al. (*Arch Gen Psychiatry*, 2003;60:458-64) carried out a meta-analysis reviewing *placebo*–controlled trials and found that *active*-controlled studies were superior ethically and scientifically. (An active controlled study compares substances of known effectiveness with the new drug being tested.) They concluded, that it is neither scientific nor ethical to compare the efficacy of a new drug to an inactive placebo. Yet, the majority of studies used to gain approval and used by the industry to promote their products, are placebo controlled trials. The placebo-controlled study is not necessarily the appropriate measure of scientific rigor.

The *Romanow Report* recommended that the Canada Health Plan should not pay for a new drug unless it is shown to be substantially superior to established comparators and demonstrated that such a policy would result in huge savings because the various provincial drug plans spend more on drugs than on physicians services. At the very least, we ought to avail ourselves of the Canadian Medical Association's information booklet on how to save on drugs by using older, equally or more effective and safer drugs.

Safety

Two facts stand out in the critical research. The first deals with the *lack of selectivity* of the "SSRIs". The second deals with raised prolactin levels these drugs cause. Apparently, SSRI's do *not* selectively raise serotonin *in vivo*. But they do have other effects. Significantly, Y. Sheline found a *drop* in metabolic products of serotonin in humans. In other words, the SSRIs studied actually lowered serotonin *in vivo* (*Journal of Clinical Psychopharmacology* 1997, vol. 17 (1): 11-14).

J. Ichikawa and Stephen Dewey separately found that Prozac and Celexa, respectively lowered dopamine approximately 50% in animals. (*European Journal of Pharmacology* 281 (1995) 225-61 and Glenmullen p.49). The decreased dopamine levels are cause for serious concern because the antipsychotics are known to have caused tardive dyskinesia by lowering dopamine. Guy Chouinard of Montreal researched extra-pyramidal affects induced by antipsychotics. He found that exposure to them of 15 years or more leads to almost certainly to tardive dyskinesia (Glenmullen p. 53). Tics and symptoms of tardive dyskinesia are showing up in patients on SSRIs for varying lengths of time. Astonishingly, even though it is known that drugs like Prozac, potentially lower dopamine, no long-term studies have been done on this problem. The regulatory system does not require long-term studies. To prevent harm, doctor must re-assert their position as gate-keepers of the system. FDA or Health Canada approval does not absolve doctors from critical thought.

Perhaps, the most serious side effect associated with SSRI's is akithesia, a sense of intense agitation, also thought to be due to lowered dopamine levels. It is according to Healy's research the probable cause of the many suicides, incidents of violence, and murders that have been the focus of successful lawsuits against Eli Lilly, the manufacturer of Prozac. I say "successful" meaning that settlements were made with the plaintiff—huge settlements, all with gag orders attached. (See Healy's and Glenmullen's books for the details). However, in one case the gag order ceased to have legal effect when a divorce court ordered disclosure of a husband's assets. This resulted in the public learning about these enormous settlements.

Prolactin, the pituitary hormone which induces lactation and suppresses sexual drive, is of central significance to the issue of safety. It causes breast luboalveolar epithelium to proliferate (*Harrison's Principles of Internal Medicine*, 2001). Meltzer (Glenmullen p.122) found, that within a week of taking Prozac, patients showed a seven-fold increase in prolactin. Does this explain the 50 –75% rate of sexual dysfunction and weight gain on SSRIs? And what about the documented seven 7-fold increase in breast cancer amongst patients taking Paxil found by M. Cotterchio in a study of the Ontario Cancer Registry (*American Journal of Epidemiology* 2000, vol. 151 (10):951-7)?

David Healy considers the danger of suicide associated specifically with Prozac nothing less than an ongoing "public health disaster". As psychotherapists we rightly worry about suicide, but the rates of suicide, upon careful analysis, as Healy shows, are *higher* on these drugs than on placebo (this also applies to the newer ones like Remeron and the antipsychotics, e.g. Risperdal).

We read in a recent *Toronto Star* that Freudian analysis is dead and has been replaced by SSRIs, implying that psychotherapy is not scientific, but that the "selective" drugs to correct your "chemical imbalance" are based on real science. Perhaps the Freudian form of psychotherapy, which was never examined in a controlled manner, is indeed dead, but what about other forms of psychotherapy that have been rigorously studied such as EMDR and CBT. What does science show about psychotherapy vs. drugs?

The evidence is startling: relapse rates at 2 years for Major Depressive Disorder with psychotherapy are 20% compared to 78% with drugs. (Blackburn, I.M. *Journal of Affective Disorders* 10, 1986: 67-75). In a similar study at three months there wasn't much difference between drugs and CBT, but at the end of four years, 70% on drugs had relapsed compared to 35% with CBT. (Fava G.A. *American Journal of Psychiatry* 153, 1996: 945-47). Bessel van der Kolk recently presented a study at the International Society for Traumatic Stress Studies in Chicago. He compared treatment of PTSD with EMDR to Prozac. After termination, *all* Prozac responders had relapsed, but there was *no* relapse in those who responded to EMDR. (verbal communication; in press).

Depression is often a traumatic syndrome. Drugs, in my view, seem to prolong the misery and in some cases make it almost impossible for the patient to ever be cured. On high doses they are emotionally so flat and lacking in affect they cannot engage in any effective therapy. If they try to reduce the dose, the distressing withdrawal symptoms trigger the original traumatic memories, and that makes it very difficult for them to do without the drug. They are then often told: "it is your original disease", when in fact it is serious withdrawal which the manufacturers euphemistically refer to as "anti-depressant discontinuation syndrome" (see Glenmullen p. 76). We don't have any extensive studies on adverse effects by *independent* researchers. I am still searching for them.

A note of caution, going off these drugs must be gradual and carefully monitored for withdrawal reactions. Some have no difficulties, but the degree of reaction seems to be directly related to the total dose over time, the type of drug, and the number of drugs used. How many patients are properly informed before going on these drugs? And how many doctors, the only real gatekeeper in the prescription system, are informed?

(A complete bibliography and the overheads from my presentation at the EMDR Association of Canada Conference November 2003 is available upon request by e-mail from: **dilmun@inetsonic.com**)

A Visit with Big Pharma's Marketing Managers

Vitality Magazine April 2004 and Canadian Center for Policy Alternatives' *Monitor* September 2004

On March 4 and 5, a conference at Sunnybrook Estates allowed me to peek into the world of Big Pharma. My media pass to the **Canadian Forum on Pharmaceutical Marketing** stated: "*Hear how the world's leading pharmaceutical companies are modernizing their global branding, internet marketing and competitive intelligence techniques to improve shareholder value.*" Speakers came from Big· Pharma giants Pfizer, AstraZeneca, Merck Frosst, Bayer, Wyeth, leading medical biotech firms, the Canadian Medical Association, and government. Presentations covered "strategies for the evolving global market", trends in "biopharmaceuticals", "competitive intelligence... for long-term gains", "maximizing loyalty in patients", and Direct To Customer Advertising (DTCA). Even a panel discussion was included on "marketing and ethics." Participants had to fork out $ 1,500. For me it was a freeby, lunch and all.

Being used to the high energy of medical conferences and political activism events, I wondered what people would be like who work for the world's second largest industry (after armaments). Strangely, only 35 people attended, including the speakers, technicians and me (the only reporter). Almost everybody was dressed in precisely tailored black, white, and grey suits with perfect hairdos and make-up, males and females equally represented, everybody focused and cool. But the mood was subdued to the point where I thought to myself, "They are either on Prozac or would like to be." It quickly emerged from the power-point presentations' pie-charts, graphs and statistics that the fever chart of world drug sales suggests ill health. Paul Getty, possibly the richest man ever, supposedly said, "A billion just doesn't go as far as it used to"—exactly Big Pharma's own diagnosis, as presented at this forum.

Martine Richard of Canada's Patent Medicine's Pricing Review Board, stated that in 2002 sales in the "major world markets" rang in at US $ 638.8 billion, obtained from sales in the US (53.4%), Canada (2.6%), and Europe (19.1%) totaling 75.1% and representing about 600 *million* people (that is US$ 1,060 for every individual!). The rest of the world, being a few *billion poor* people with malaria, TB, regular infections, and AIDS are not part of the "major" market. They can't pay for patented drugs.

This drug habit is driven by shareholders' interests, and this conference was devoted to them. So, presenters focused on obstacles to growth and how to generate more consumption (more sick people). The key-note speaker, Pierre Gaudrault, represented Pfizer which, incidentally, was rated 17th among the world's top 100 corporate criminals (**www.MotherJones.com**). He identified the problem as: the limits of chemistry, governments frantic to reduce health costs, cheaper generic drugs, and popular pressure to change patent laws. As of 2004, only 3 new active substances have been submitted for patenting, as opposed to 10 in 1999 and 29 a couple of years earlier. Big Pharma calls that the "pipe-line problem"—no new potential blockbuster drugs in the works: synthetic chemistry is finite. The cost of research and development has simultaneously gone through the roof: in 1988 it cost US $ 150 million to bring a new drug to market, and now it's about US $ 1 billion, and evidently, a few more billion are unlikely to produce a new blockbuster. His solution was to exhort everybody to "capture customer loyalty, enthusiasm, and commitment around the world". He ended with an inspirational quote, known to all environmental activists, from the great Rene Dubois: "Act locally—think globally!"

In 2002 in North America alone more than 100,000 drug reps were working the doctors' offices, a three-fold increase from 1993, or 1 rep per every 5 doctors. The return on investment for every US dollar spent in 1996 was US $3.34, but by 1999 it had decreased to US $ 1.94. Marketing in 1996 cost US $ 6.1 billion, but only three years later Big Pharma was throwing US $ 9.4 billion at marketing and advertising (from Sawaya, 2002).

So, dirty tricks increased: financing phony patient support groups (*Toronto Star* Feb.7, 2004); inventing new diseases (Pfizer's "social anxiety disorder", supposedly treatable by Zoloft, was invented by a Fred Nadjarian of Roche in Australia for which he faced a public disgracing); attempting to use Children's Aid Society wards without their knowledge as human research subjects for antidepressants (*Hamilton Spectator* Dec. 11,2002); the widespread sale of doctors' prescription patterns by pharmacies to Big Pharma in contravention of current privacy laws (see outraged editorial in the March 2,

2004, *Canadian Medical Association Journal*); and many more are told in *Prescription Games*. Almost every major drug is under legal challenge annually costing hundreds of millions of dollars in out-of-court settlements or fines (see the documentary *The Corporation*).

Much of the discussions focused on that magical solution to a troubled market: DTCA! Various speakers described how it had increased sales by close to 70% annually in the US, and reading from a February 4th FDA memo, they noted that DTCA especially increases customer *compliance*! It lasts a little longer after the adverse effects emerge, especially on lucrative antidepressants and cholesterol-lowering drugs, but the speakers cautioned, Canadian activists are astonishingly successful in blocking DTCA. Most depressingly, even though Canada has the ultimate "industry-friendly" Health Minister, Monsieur Pettigrew, he told Big Pharma that there was no reason to introduce DTCA because there was "just no evidence to show that this enormous increase in drug consumption in the US had improved health overall." Amazingly, nobody laughed! This was black humor of the finest vintage and nobody noticed. When the question of ads for vaccines was raised, audible sighs of relief were heard and everyone was reminded to take heart as, thankfully, those are exempt from Canadian DTCA rules. Vaccines are the new frontier of corporate medicine.

Of course, there is a statistic, mentioning which in this meeting would have been equivalent to farting at a royal reception: The world's most prestigious medical school, Johns Hopkins in Baltimore, published last year numbers indicating that drugs and doctors' mistakes may be the primary leading cause of death in the US, costing the economy US$ 80 billion annually. (Full details and sources at **www.mercola.com**; view all research on **www.garynull.com**).

Dr. Andre de Villiers was different. He reported on his medical biotech company which markets the technology and chemicals used to treat certain cancers and surgical transplants. This technology identifies cancer cells for targeted destruction while leaving healthy cells intact. Similarly, donor rejection can frequently be solved without killing the patient's entire immune system with immuno-suppressant drugs by zeroing in on only those immune factors that are causing the rejection: high tech medicine that works for life. Having lost a daughter in 1986 to a disease this technology now routinely cures, I was deeply impressed. He pointed out, understandably smugly, that his was "good marketing because it's a good product and good science." Good point.

Considering that the *American Journal of Cardiology* last August published findings indicating that heart disease and cholesterol may have no link at all, a finding supported by European research, the blockbuster drug Lipidor may soon prove that even blockbusters aren't what they used to be as their supportive science winds up to be neither.

The ethics panel revealed just how mad the medical profession has become. McGill University's ethics expert Dr. Eugene Bereza and University of Toronto's Dr. Michael Gordon were vocal, charming, eloquent, satirical, blunt and devastatingly truthful. Supporting the recent editorial in the CMAJ (Feb. 17, March 2) they agreed that current wholesale bullying of researchers (allowed to publish only drug-supporting results) and doctors (bribed and coerced into prescribing new drugs) is unacceptable. Citing the Nancy Olivieri case (see my March article), Dr. Gordon observed, "Just how bad does this have to become!"

While conceding that many drugs are indispensable, they observed, (like a battered wife without a job might to her SOB husband), that research dollars today come virtually only from Big Pharma, and that this abusive relationship does not promote excellence. Shareholders need more and more sick people, while scientists want to *cure* sick people. Some serious efforts are being made to stop this abuse: McMaster Medical School teaches its students Ten Commandments for handling drug reps. The first being: "Physicians should maintain control" of the encounter. The rest focus on demanding scientific proof for every claim made, and the last insists the doctor may not "commit to the use of the product", but merely indicate that "it will be given further consideration." The ethicists also suggested that Big Pharma should consider self-restraint with all its coercive dirty tricks. What a concept!

When the discussion was opened for questions from the floor, not even one was posed. Nobody appear to wonder *why* everybody is so ticked off, what might possibly be wrong with the products, prices or (God forbid) drug effectiveness, and what alternate marketing strategy should be considered. Imagine Mercedes, BMW, or Volvo being told their cars are dangerous to drive and that people are mad about their engineers lying and cheating about the physics involved in their manufacture resulting in many people driving crippled or killed. Since those cars are synonymous with excellence, this is unthinkable. With Big Pharma's products and its Dark-Lord-business-practices this is what most people associate with this industry, yet not a single question was raised.

At a book table Dr. Lou Sawaya of Ottawa sold his publications on drug rep education. His 2003 *The Reader is not an Idiot—He is your Doctor*, includes a joke (here abbreviated): the US president and the CEO of a pharmaceutical company consulted God. The US president asked, "Lord, when will our unemployment problem be solved?" God replies, "In the year 2020." The president walked away, crying bitterly. Then the pharmaceutical CEO asked, "Lord, when will the public image of our industry become favorable again?" God thought for a long time, and then God walked away, crying bitterly.

A Short Survival Guide for Dealing In Drugs

As the ethics panel pointed out, US judges ruling on Big Pharma cases agree that this industry is the cause for the corruption of medical science, education and practice. So, whom do you trust and what can you believe? The simple rule of thumb is: look who paid for the study. But if sleuthing through journals is impossible when you have to make a quick decision, having just been handed a prescription, here are some suggestions on how to navigate the minefield of pharmacology:

1. **Always consult the** *Compendium of Pharmaceuticals and Specialties.* The **CPS** is the annually updated compendium of all Health Canada-approved drugs sent to every pharmacy and doctor; it contains the chemistry, cautions, and dosages the manufacturer must by law provide—**always** ask your doctor or pharmacist to explain these in ordinary language. Refusal is a contravention of the *Canada Health Act* which requires informed consent.

2. Avoid taking a drug that is listed as potentially **"hepatoxic"** (toxic to the liver) and requires regular liver function tests. Remember, the majority of liver transplants are done because the liver was killed by a drug—not a disease.

3. Avoid drugs that interfere with any **"cytochrome"** (portion of a cancer-protective gene), even if just "in combination with ..." some other drug. Messing with genes is a shot in the dark and neither the doctor nor manufacturer understands: whatever happens is usually irreversible.

4. Anything that reduces **"dopamine"**, or any other neurotransmitter's function, generally causes *irreversible* neurological harm, such a tardive dyskinesia.

5. A drug that lowers **immune function** (T-cell or B-cell production or activity), such as cortisone-based substances, chemotherapy drugs, and antibiotics have serious lasting effects. Research this on the Internet or in the library and look for alternatives. If unavoidable, you can limit negative effects and enhance the drug's intended effectiveness by taking supportive nutrients in high, therapeutic doses. Negative interactions are mostly myths. <u>**Example**</u>: you supposedly can't take pro-biotics, such as

acidophilus, with antibiotics; in fact, taking them prevents candida over-growth. For known interaction consult the annually updated *Natural Medicines: Comprehensive Database*, also on **www.NaturalDatabase.com**.

6. If **"long-term effects are unknown"**—check the Internet and find out more. This is a vitally important warning. Sometimes, such a drug may be helpful and unavoidable for a short period, but taken for more than a month may be bad news. Read the books below to find out how and why.

7. Anything that cautions use in **lactating or pregnant women** indicates a *systemic* effect (crossing the placenta and blood-brain barrier). Such drugs are potentially *teratogenic* (causing birth defects): they can cause irreversible damage before birth, or organ damage later.

8. Drug manufacturers are *not obliged to inform about* **nutrient depletions** caused by all (!) synthetic drugs, so the CPS is no help. Check the com-pendium by pharmacists Pelten and LaValle listed below; if the drug is a must, protect your body by taking those nutrients it depletes. **Example**: all synthetic "blood thinners" and lipid-lowering drugs require simulta-neously potassium, magnesium and Co-enzyme Q_{10} to avoid *increasing* the risk of heart failure.

9. **Information must come from somebody** *other* **than the manufacturer, Health Canada, or patient groups funded by drug companies.** Send the group (especially those working for lucrative illnesses such as asthma, cancer, diabetes, Multiple sclerosis etc.) an e-mail and ask who funds them. If they identify themselves as *"Survivors of ..."* antidepressants etc. etc, their information is likely trustworthy.

10. Three areas that require your total attention are **hormones** (e.g. menopause therapy for women, cortisone for asthma etc.), **cardiovascu-lar disease,** and **depression**. Cholesterol (or lipid)-lowering drugs, anti-depressants, and *synthetic* (as opposed to natural!) hormones are harmful—in the highly informed opinion of *mainstream* medical researchers (see PharmaWatch 604-687-6613, **www.drugintel.com/ drugs/statins** and list below).

11. Always look for the *generic* brand (cheaper) or for *older* versions of the same drug (which are less toxic). The best source for alternatives to drugs is *The Textbook of Nutritional Medicine* (look for most recent edition from Third Line Press) and "orthomolecular medicine" (**www.orthomed.org**).

12. The World Health Organization lists only some 350 drugs as "essential". *None are still patent-protected*, and they constitute only 5% of Big Pharma's offerings; the remaining 95% is therefore suspect and demands your most

careful critical scrutiny (visit the international leader in exposing Big Pharma's product misinformation, Dr. Peter Mansfield, at **www.mja. com.au**).

Sources and Resources

www.cbc.ca/news for Health Canada's 162,000 plus adverse reactions from 4,621 frequently used drugs; obtained by the CBC through legal action under Freedom of Information legislation

www.canadiancoalitionforhealthfreedom.ca

Dr. James Lunney, MP—Ottawa office: 613-992-5243 or **lunney0@parl.gc.ca** (support his bill to stop nutritional supplements from becoming prescription-only; the bill is back in parliament as of October 2004 and needs your support even more than before, as we now have a minority government and one has a chance at getting something done)

www.medicare.ca (Canadian Health Coalition)

J. Bakan, *The Corporation: The Pathological Pursuit of Profit and Power*, Viking, 2004 (the book on which the documentary is based)

J. Robinson, *Prescription Games*, McClelland & Stewart, 2001 (available through **www.amazon.ca**

For full information on psychiatric drugs, get the consent form *International Journal of Risk & Safety in Medicine*, Jan. 1998 available from its author **David.Cohen@umontreal.ca**

www.garynull.com most comprehensive source on *mainstream science* on vitamins, minerals, etc; alphabetically organized. Next time your doctor states: "There is no scientific evidence on vitamin C …." download that section. On this site also: "*Death By Medicine*" by Dr. Caroline Dean who assembled the scientific evidence on the death toll caused by drugs and unnecessary surgery

Dr. J.S. Cohen, *Overdose: The Case Against the Drug Companies: Prescription Drugs, Side Effects and Your Health*, Tarcher/Putnam, 2001

Dr. D. Haely, *Let Them Eat Prozac*, Lorimer, 2003

R. Pelton & J. VaValle, *The Nutritional Cost of Prescription Drugs*, Morton, 2000

Dr. F. Ravikovich, *The Plot Against Asthma and Allergy Patients*, Kos, 2003

Dr. A. Saul, *Doctor Yourself: Natural Healing That Works*, Basic Health Publications, 2003

7

The Big Shop of Horrors

Dr. Sherry Rogers on
Multiple Chemical Sensitivity

Vitality Magazine November 2002

"When I had chemical sensitivity, I felt as though I had joined the disease-of-the-month club. I was actually afraid to answer people when they asked me how I was, because I couldn't recall which symptoms they might be referring to. I had so many symptoms, it was embarrassing; for when medicine is stumped, hypochondriasis is a cop-out diagnosis to save face."

These are the words of a frustrated patient who happens to be a doctor also—a doctor who came to the end of her tether and realized that nothing medical school had taught was providing solutions. A strikingly beautiful woman, US-based Dr. Rogers was suffering from such horrible eczema that people would ask her, "What on earth happened to you?" when meeting her.

She was plagued by years of insomnia, brain-fag so bad she totaled 5 cars in less than so many years. Her body was a Candida factory from all the antibiotics she had taken. Increasingly frequent headaches were virtually paralyzing. A range of bizarre neurological symptoms came and went, but mostly came, due to mercury amalgams, formaldehyde outgassing furniture, and vinyl wallpapers. Pesticides assaulted her endocrine system; her ovaries were dead at age 44. In addition, her love of horses caused her to break her spine six times in riding accidents resulting in total dependence on heavy pain killers adding to the toxic environmental load about which she knew nothing then.

"I had been through 13 years of medical school and had no clue about what was wrong with me," she observed. Indeed, this is what is so scary about MCS: the current medical paradigm, which looks for bacteria and viruses, is unprepared conceptually as well as by virtue of doctors lacking basic training in toxicology, for the systemic responses to toxic chemicals and pesticides. Medicine needs to start thinking of people the way pesticide manufacturers do about bugs and pests, and the way toxicologist *know* all of these substances work. Dr. Rogers is trained in this manner and has the added advantage of knowing what MCS is like from the patient's point of view.

Dr. Sherry Rogers has all the right stuff: an M.D. and membership with the prestigious American Board of Family Practice and a Fellowship with the even more prestigious American College of Allergy and Immunology. However, as it turned out, the finest and most useful part of her education commenced when she found herself to be a fellow E.I. (Environmental Illness) patient entering a fellowship with the vast majority of all patients, everywhere.

The overwhelming research evidence is rapidly forcing standard medicine to understand that the epidemic diseases of our time (cancer, asthma, the autoimmune diseases, neurological and psychiatric illness) are the price we pay for a civilization built without forethought about its consequences for human health.

A deeply religious person, she says that "God sent me all those illnesses and gave me the task to find a cure for them. Now, at 58, I am healthier than I ever was in my entire life." That positive attitude which affirms, as part of the wholeness of life, even the greatest afflictions combined in Dr. Rogers with the spirit of a medical detective. The result was embarking upon medicine's "road less traveled " which provides an education in modern environmental toxicology and nutritional science.

Her greatest support has come from her husband, she says. Dr. Rogers dedicated almost every one of her many books to her husband, nicknamed Luscious. In love with him for the past three decades, he is a frequent presence in her books by way of anecdotes showing how his keen observation and intuitive understanding helped to find ways to heal. Learning of the neurotoxicity of carpet backing and glues, he ripped them out one day. Dr. Rogers walked into the devastated office and "felt like walking on air. I could breathe and my mind was clear at last!" Together, Sherry and Luscious found Dr. Jo Miller in Alabama who taught her all about food allergies (deadly nightshades in her case, i.e. potatoes, tomatoes, peppers etc.) and cleared up her eczema for good. They learned that the paints, glues, varnishes, insulation materials, and pesticides they had exposed themselves to, during the renovation of their 200 year old farm, were the source of everything else she was suffering from. Patients need to be as grateful to Luscious as to Sherry.

The ancient Greeks believed that Asclepios, the god of medicine, was "the wounded healer" because he limped due to an injury inflicted upon him by Zeus, the CEO of the Greek pantheon. He is depicted accompanied by a dog who represents his instinctual guide and a small child carrying a lantern signifying the child's open mind which illuminates the doctor-patient relationship. Thus good doctoring has been gained through suffering. In Dr. Rogers' case this included deliberately becoming a guinea pig. In the 1980s she smoked heavily "in order to get hooked so I could teach my patients how to get un–hooked". She observed with amazement that it took until 1990 before smoking was outright forbidden at medical conferences.

Dr. Rogers, the eldest child of a large and very poor family, says: "I should not have succeeded. "Nobody in my family for generations had finished even high school. In my area, in the 60s, coming from such poverty, being a woman, I could expect little. But I put myself through university and became a doctor." Her training was traditional: "During medical rounds, we went to see the gall bladder in #326," she recalls, "not a human being." Standard medicine labels, she says, and misses the reality that "among 100 arthritis patients, the cause of arthritis in each may be a different one." Illness as a bio-individual event, shared humanity, and the need to follow Hippocrates' advice on clean air, clean water and "Let food by thy medicine", are the eternal biological truths that doctors like Sherry Rogers are reviving.

A Fellow of the American Academy of Environmental Medicine, she has written many excellent books, lectures internationally, teaches courses at universities, publishes original research with the US National Institutes of Health and leading mainstream medical journals, and runs a practice that serves patients who seek her out from all over the world. She edited the environmental health section of the *International Medicine World Report.* Like her great teachers, Dr. Thereon Randolph (the father of environmental medicine) and Dr. William Rae of the famous Dallas, Texas, environmental health clinic, she too had that amazing experience of a medical Alice in Wonderland: she fell into that rabbit hole and learned that nothing in health and disease is as she had thought it was.

Her illness made her see with the eyes of the activist who recognizes the arrogance and Big Lie of the dark side of medicine. She is an outspoken critic of the automatic-pilot drug-pushing medicine which not only does not inquire into causes, but has forgotten that finding causes is what medicine is all about. "A headache is not a Darvon deficiency," she insists. "Time to test your cardiologist?" or "Time to fire your doctor?" she challenges the readers of her marvelous monthly newsletter, *Total Wellness.* She never seems to miss an opportunity to tell the truth about the latest blockbuster drug touted by Big Pharma as the answer to whatever ails us, though it almost always does more harm than good.

Introduced by her oft-repeated saying, "How the sick get sicker quicker" Dr. Rogers provides the full scientific information on these drugs and tells how the side-effects are carefully concealed, the statistics falsified, and what the financial implications are for patient and industry. In 1993 industry managed to get the *American Journal of Clinical Nutrition* to publish a tobacco-science type study designed to protect their patent-dependent lucrative products against the increasing preference by patients for more effective natural substances. Diabetics, who benefit dramatically from high doses of this neuropathy preventing vitamin, were given less E than the daily recommended allowance (RDA) for healthy people—in order to make it appear that natural substances such as Vitamin E are useless.

For Dr. Rogers we are all under a huge MACC Attack (multinational agricultural and chemical corporations) from the disease-producing industry (pharmaceutical companies and genetic engineered food and pesticide producers). She teaches how to survive and thrive in this toxic world, what foods confer health, what strategies protect against pollution ("The solution to pollution is dilution"—read her books to find out how). That begins with cutting "out the CRAP" (cigarettes, coffee, refined sugars, alcohol, aspirin, processed foods). Central to health is the abandonment of SAD, the Standard American Diet with its nutrient-depleted and toxin-laden refined foods.

Dr. Rogers' parable of the Twelve Boxes explains the central concept of this new medicine, the notion of the "Total Load". The body can handle lots of toxins and emotional stress, but as the chemical flood tide increases beyond our evolved capacity to cope, we become sick. Unlike the mechanistic model of standard medicine, which masks the symptom or attacks a specific organ, environmental medicine teaches that the road to health begins by reducing the total load: identify food allergies, and/or identify and desensitize chemical sensitivities, and/or increase good nutrients, and/or heal absorption problems such as a leaky gut, and/or correct the imbalance of intestinal flora such as in Candidiasis, and/or reduce emotional stress etc.

"I like to think of the total load as being analogous to a boat filled with twelve marked boxes. All of us are set adrift in the sea in the same type of boat with the same twelve boxes", and we all develop leaks. "Some of us have a leak near the gunwales so we only need to throw overboard a couple of boxes to stop taking on water. Others have their leak toward the keel and need to throw over many boxes." And what is in those boxes? "The total environmental overload." Box 1 through 11 contain inhalants, pollens, dust mites, molds, animal danders, food allergies, specific environmental sensitivities, hormone deficiencies, the infamous Leaky Gut, deficient nutrition, heavy metal poisons, emotional stress, electromagnetic field sensitivities etc. The 12th is the "mystery box" which could be the worst killer because it contains "the patient's unwillingness to take responsibility for his own health." Understanding requires action, so one must chuck that gas cook stove, stop eating processed foods, and remove mercury amalgams. Tragically, this box may contain the "worst of all: a spouse who is unwilling to learn and become a partner in healing."

Dr. Roger's Treasure Chest As a devoted reader, I will give you an overview of her work, which has become absolutely indispensable to my family and me personally as well as to my own medical writing. All are available through Prestige Publishing in Syracuse, N.Y., at 1-800-846-6687, as is her invaluable monthly newsletter, *Total Wellness* (about Can. $ 45 per year). Excellent videos showing how Dr. Rogers works with patients, and the specific test kits she developed (not available through standard doctors) can also be obtained. Phone consultations with her can be arranged by calling 315-488-2856.

The E.I. Syndrome took over 3 years to write. Its first edition appeared in 1986 when being an environmental physician was far more dangerous to one's professional health than today. Dr. Rogers did the research and writing while battling environmental illness herself. She was treating patients like herself, lecturing on environmental medicine, and writing this book while slowly healing herself. This is the real thing suffered through chemical by chemical, researched, and applied to herself and others. All her subsequent books are expanded forays into specific illnesses providing new and up-to-date medical insights into each.

To gain an appreciation for Dr. Rogers' achievement, consider her description of life during the writing of this book: "In 1986, even though I was infinitely better than I had been in the previous one and a half decades with E.I., I was still so profoundly affected that when I lectured in Chicago that year, I had to rent 3 tanks of oxygen on wheels and use them delivered through a ceramic mask just so I would know my name!"

You Are What You Ate gives an outline for the treatment of "resistant diseases of the 21st century". It is a first-rate how-to book for both diagnosis and treatment options to be explored. It is also a most valuable crash course in the principles of environmental medicine explained through lots of patient case stories and personal experiences as a patient and as a doctor. This book is especially valuable for people suffering from Candida-related problems.

The Cure is in the Kitchen provides you with the long and the short of macrobiotics, its principles, history, medical and biochemical bases, recipes and shopping guides. This book took years to put together as Dr. Rogers studied with the world's foremost expert on this diet, Michio Kushi. The case histories make this a dramatic cookbook which is an indispensable tool especially for cancer patients. Humor is its most welcome and notable feature, as the intrepid Dr. Rogers describes how she managed to experiment with this strange diet. It is important to mention that Dr. Rogers explains the applicability of various diets, as the strict macro diet is not appropriate for all situations.

Macro Mellow is for people with chronic illnesses who need not go as far as the totally strict macrobiotic diet and who want to keep their families from running away from them at dinner. It is strong on issues such as cholesterol and specific nutrients required in the various chronic illnesses.

Chemical Sensitivity is a 48-page booklet that deals with the basics of environmental illness, its scientific basis, its identification, and answers the most common questions asked. *The Scientific Basis for Selected Environmental Techniques* provides patients suffering from environmental illness with the tools they may need to educate their doctors with incontrovertible scientific and epidemiological evidence, bring some relevant new information to PTA meetings, help their lawyers working to establish the validity of workplace-related chemical and other environmental injury, and handle insurance companies. Written for Americans, the facts are equally useful to Canadians in our parallel battles.

Tired or Toxic? Guides the reader through the world of environmental illness: causes, diagnosis, treatments, their underlying biochemistry is explained for the lay person; every conceivable question is answered. Most importantly, the politics of modern medicine is explained with excellent references, showing why standard medicine is often so abysmally ignorant and kept in the dark by economic forces (see the chapter, entitled "When medical evolution becomes revolution"). This book is like an extensive consultation with Dr. Rogers' herself.

Wellness Against All Odds addresses the needs of the patient with serious and potentially fatal illnesses. In it she provides the nuts and bolts of environmental medicine: how to get rid of accumulated toxins and correct nutrient deficiencies in serious illness conditions through the use of up-to-date therapies.

Depression Cured At Last, a book of some 700 pages focuses on all the ways by which our brains get attacked by environmental toxins and nutritional deficiencies and how to regain control over your mind and soul. (This one is my favorite, I must admit.) It is a marvel of research meticulously referenced and shows how seamlessly mind and body, biochemistry and spirit, interact to make a meaningful life possible.

No More Heartburn focuses on the diseases of the bowel giving practical solutions to all those who have been through years of toxic drugs and debilitating surgery. Finally, in *Pain Free in Six Weeks*, Dr. Rogers' latest book, she deals with the causes, biochemistry, and range of successful treatments of all forms of pain—about which she knows more personally than anybody would care to know—in arthritis, fibromyalgia, fractured discs, cancer, Gulf War Syndrome.

Far from being exclusively focused on environmental illness, her books (and especially her newsletter) provide a wealth of information on prevention. You learn how to heal, eat, live and raise your family in the spirit of Hippocrates.

"Detox or Die"

Vitality Magazine October 2002

Dr. Sherry Rogers is coming to town. Rise out of your heavy metal-induced depression, take your pesticide-mediated anxiety seriously, and declare war on whatever ails you by attending the November Health Expo. She and other Environmental Medicine leaders (such as Dr. Jozef Krop and Dr. Zoltan Rona) will tell us how to fix what our environment did to you and me and how to clean up this home planet of ours for ourselves and our descendants. Dr. Rogers scared the hell out of us at last year's Health Expo with her immense knowledge of environmental medical science and also gave us real hope and usable tools for even the most awful illnesses. Author of many excellent books, she has now published a zinger of a book that makes one shout Hallelujah! Its title, in true Sherry Rogers fashion, pulls no punches: *Detoxify or Die!* The health information she gives adds a whole world of meaning to the great New Testament saying, "The Truth shall make you free." Have courage and read what is below, there is light at the end of the tunnel.

"Those scary media reports of hidden toxins in our environments are a spit in the ocean compared with what really occurs," Dr. Rogers writes. So, here I am to tell you that it is worse than you thought: the world's garbage crisis—usually confined to political hot-potato-fights over where to open a municipal dump—has become a profoundly personal crisis within the bodies of every living thing, especially in ours. The line between the personal and the political, which feminist Gloria Steinem once declared to be blurred for women's issues, has totally disappeared when it comes to the universal human issue of health. For the truth is that it is our bodies that have become the world's toxic dumpsites. The billions of dollars worth of pesticides, plastics, petroleum products, and heavy-metal containing technology have made the industrial world rich beyond belief and threatens human survival as it conquers the earth. As in the story of King Midas, whose touch turned everything to gold—even his wife and children—our economy is killing us.`

"We have conquered the world with pollution. There are no more pristine areas left without a trace of man's manufacturing might" writes Dr. Rogers. Indeed, every living thing now has DDT in its tissues and its toxic effects are increasing over time. The World Health Organization informs us that for purposes of scientific research, there are no control groups (organisms uncontaminated by toxic synthetic chemicals) to be found on planet Earth. Every aspect of life and all political policy are directly or indirectly affected by the sociological importance of environmental illness (see the excellent survey by S. Kroll-Smith in the sources below).

No environment is untouched. Pollution is found in smoggy and in clean-looking air, murky and clear water, and especially in our food—from the Arctic to the rain forest, from downtown Toronto to the Himalayan village. Smog alerts have increase by 500% in the last 25 years (World Watch Institute). Nothing is too private not to be affected—from our brain cells to our hormones. Every bodily system and organ has its distinctive spectrum of outraged response to this arsenal of artificial stuff against which our organism has no defence, it wasn't evolved to deal with these chemicals. Without employing detoxification strategies for their elimination, one organ or another succumbs—and so we have epidemics of cancer, chronic disease and immune system failures no amount of fancy genetics will explain away.

We are so used to blaming suffering on God or the Devil, that the genetic "program" seemed the perfect new candidate for taking on the responsibility we try so hard not to accept. But neither God nor the Devil, and certainly not our genetic program, will take the blame for what is our responsibility. On June 13th 1999 the *New England Journal of Medicine* published the results of an international study which examined the lives of more than 90,000 twins to see whether the incidence of cancer was indeed familial—or genetic. It turned out that genetics has absolutely nothing to do with who gets cancer; the environment and unhealthy lifestyles were the only indicators.

Human breast milk is so contaminated with Dioxin (the active ingredient in Agent Orange—another one of Monsanto's gifts to humanity, along with neurotoxic aspartame and genetically engineered foods) that its disposal would have to be done according to toxic waste regulations. Within the first year of life a baby raised on it may ingest eighteen times a life-time's quantity of its "safe" limit. The EPA announced that 100% of the North American population carry the carcinogen styrene in their bodies, thanks to styrofoam cups; styrene is the main culprit in the last decade's 200% increase in childhood cancers.

Semen, human eggs, and our entire endocrine system are so contaminated with the toxic residues from plastic products, heavy metals and pesticides that even conservative scientists agree that detoxification of *both* parents' bodies *before* getting pregnant would be a good idea. Our bodies took some 7 million years to evolve, but not until 50 years ago did our enzymes and detoxification organs encounter the half million different synthetic chemicals never smelled, felt or ingested on this earth before. We are unable to metabolize any of this synthetic garbage. It passes right on to our offspring and damages parent and child in the process. It sabotages the cell replication process in DNA of mother and fetus, causing cancers or chronic diseases; or it blocks the work of hormones which control developmental timing, and then our kids are further damaged during pregnancy.

The carcinogenic phthalates found in plastic products also at the very least, target the brain—"and we sure have enough ADHD to prove that to be true" observes Dr. Rogers. The thyroid is the target organ of pesticides. Dr. Rogers mentions in passing that ex-US president George Bush, his wife and their dog Millie all developed thyroid disease. Since they are three unrelated creatures of two different genera, one can only conclude that their thyroids were unable to cope with whatever chemicals the White House lawns and roach-fighting brigades exposed them to.

The EPA confirms that 100% of all people in the world have traces of heavy metals like mercury, lead and cadmium in their blood which target the immune system, the memory areas of the brain, and the nervous system. These come to us through dental amalgam, paints and the like to give us Alzheimer's, Parkinson's, Multiple Sclerosis, Myasthenia gravis, Chronic Fatigue Syndrome and Multiple Chemical Sensitivity. These connections are proven, and published in the mainstream literature. This year, the *Journal of the Canadian Medical Association* published an excellent series of articles (see citation below) reviewing the methods and research of environmental medicine. As anybody knows who has ever read a book by Dr. Rogers, the worldwide scientific proof of both diagnosis and treatment methods are all painstakingly recorded in a bibliography that could scare a seasoned medical researcher.

And so, where are we now? Well, we now live in a time on this precious planet, when a gallon of clean water (the very stuff of life from which all life evolved some 5 billion years ago) costs more than a gallon of gasoline. Dr. Rogers writes that "to get clean ice [for climate research purposes] scientists have to drill a core down to a level that was formed before the 20th century." We live in a time in which the rapidity of species extinction is greater than in any other previous, natural, geological era before us.

And our homes are the most contaminated and dangerous places of all where we encounter, routinely, about 500 of the worst disease-causing chemicals of all. An average carpet outgases about 200 volatile organic chemicals which include carcinogens and neurotoxins like formaldehyde, chloroform, phenol, xylene, toluene and many more. Carpets and perfumes (my personal pet peeve) in aftershave lotion (guys, take it from me—you smell great without that toxic crap, just wash your pits), women's perfume, hair spray and shampoos share the carcinogen benzene. Our drinking water contains some 500 toxic substances last time the EPA looked, and many of those substances are toxic medication prescribed to somebody other than yourself.

Our techniques for understanding the damage we are doing to our environment and our bodies have become so sophisticated, we could begin to use these tricks for crime detection; each compound has its specific speed of entry into the blood stream and its individual time of residence there. Therefore, Dr. Rogers explains: "...if a crackerjack detective wanted to know where you had been all day and what you had done, all he has to do is draw a blood level of your chemicals. Trichloroethylene would tell him that you picked up the dry cleaning...benzene would tell him you probably stopped to gas up the car; and toluene could betray that you might have picked up the your kids at the gymnasium with a polyurethaned floor."

The good news is that the evidence has become undeniable—current US president G.W. Bush proving the exception that proves the rule—and the research basis is all mainstream. The mainstream media and even the movies cover the stories of our toxic world. Close to home, on October 17th David Suzuki's CBC TV show "The Nature of Things" aired a fabulous program on the toxins found in one's home and what can be done about it (get a video or text copy of "Up Close and Toxic" from CBC's customer service).

The creative minds of thousands of medical researchers are at work to understand the causes of environmentally-mediated illness, trace the biological pathways, find ways to help living organisms rid themselves of these toxins and develop ways to begin the repair. Nothing in life and death is ever uniform and monolithic, so the inevitable variation gives rise to new ways of understanding. That is why hope is not silly but the only realistic and viable attitude.

Dr. Rogers gives her readers the unvarnished truth, but this is not a tale of doom. She offers a marvelous range of solutions for cleanup, healing, and prevention. This book, she tells us, is not only based on several decades of medical practice as an expert in environmental medicine, but on the research results of more than 300 pounds of toxicology textbooks and EPA reports. Best of all, her advice is based on the firm and unshakable ground of personal experience with pesticide and urea formaldehyde poisoning which nearly killed her.

The successful treatments of environmentally mediated disease include specialized diets, Far infrared sauna treatment (probably one of the very best detox and healing treatments!), specific detoxification protocols for various substances, and essential clean-up protocols (e.g. removal of mercury amalgam) all clearly explained and backed by sound, verifiable science and personal medical experience. Among the most powerful remedies is food—good food, pesticide-free, non-GMO-contaminated food. Seriously ill people, of course, require far more powerful intervention through nutrient supplementation and other regimes. For example, consider the following deceptively simple study of otherwise generally healthy people, aimed at seeing how far just a tiny little bit of quality food would actually go to guarantee health in the long run.

"To show how powerful food is, in one study they just had folks eat good wholesome foods and eliminate the junk. The diet contained 2 tbs. of sesame butter, 2 slices of whole wheat toast, raisins (3 small boxes) and 2 tbs. almonds or pecans for snacks, ginger tea and (2 cups) green tea, 1 tbs. wheat germ oil, 6 servings of fruits and vegetables, beans, whole grains (1/2 cup each) and optionally 3 oz. Meat, fish, poultry (for the week), nonfat dairy and eggs. Disallowed were white flour, junk processed foods, and whole milk products. The result? Dietary fiber, vitamin E, vitamin C and carotene levels in the blood increased 160, 145, 160 and 500% respectively! Cholesterol dropped 13% and the bad cholesterol, LDL, dropped 16%." Furthermore, blood tests showed that those substances our bodies use to fight disease, oxidation stress (aging), and to repair DNA damage all increased dramatically as well to optimum levels. "Thus, with a mere whole food diet and getting off the junk, you can dramatically slow down aging and disease, as this study proved. This translates into a small miracle, nothing that any medicine or gene therapy is capable of even coming close to duplicating. Wow! A 500% increase in beta carotene is what Harvard researchers used to turn cancer genes back into normal genes—the chemistry necessary to reverse cancer."

The implications of this one research example are staggering. By individually controlling our most immediate environment through simple, sound decisions about food (and homes and gardens free of toxic chemicals) we gain control over our health and transform—systematically and most assuredly—the way the world lives and eats. No more need to blame any God or Devil or the faulty genome for the "slings and arrows of outrageous fortune". Health is knowable and achievable. The journey to healing ourselves is also the journey to healing our polluted world. All problems have hidden within them solutions—often elegant, simple and obvious. In the midst of our dismal personal and planetary mess, Dr. Rogers has provided us with a first rate map showing the way back to health and the celebration of Nature. To hear and learn more, see you at the Expo!

Sources and Resources

Ashford, N. & Miller, C. *Chemical Exposure: Low Levels—High Stakes*, 2nd ed. Van Norstrand Reinhold, 1998

Kroll-Smith, S. et al eds. *Illness and the Environment: A Reader in Contested Medicine*, New York University Press, 2002

Walker, M. et al. *The Chelation Answer*, Second Opinion Publishing, 1994

Journal of the Canadian Medical Association series by L. Marshall et al., Vol. 166 nos 8-13, April 30th—June 25, 2002

CBC's October 17th, 2002 program on D. Suzuki's *The Nature of Things*: "Close Up and Toxic"

Healthy Home Services Inc. 416-410-4247

DG Medical Corporation, London, Ontario, provides a full line of detoxification products for heavy metals which are excellent. I recommend these unhesitatingly because my family and I take them. Call *Institute for Integrated Medicine* 519-659-7971 (NOTE: I derive no financial benefit from endorsing this or any other products.)

The best combo source for truths about toxins and what you can do to prevent illness and heal yourself and your family is found in these two doctors' books:

Dr. Sherry Rogers, *Detox or Die*, Sandkey Co., 2002

Dr. Jozef Krop, *Healing the Planet—One Patient At A Time: A Primer in Environmental Medicine*, Kos Publishing Inc., 2002 (call 519-927-1049)

Recognizing Multiple Chemical Sensitivity

Vitality Magazine October 2003

It is said, that when you come to the end of your rope, tie a knot and hang on. For those whose lives have been devastated by Multiple Chemical Sensitivity and who have been hanging on to that knot for quite some time now, this determination is finally paying off. It appears, that with regard to MCS, Canada is beginning to live up to its reputation of striving for a just society. I am reporting on developments which I have been part of since April.

Canada's most senior Senator, Herb Sparrow, had personally observed a CPP appeal hearing of one of his MCS-afflicted constituents from Battleford, Saskatchewan. This person had become disabled from a massive exposure to pesticides. Events at that appeal convinced him that the federal pension and disability program is indeed influenced by some serious bias against people diagnosed with chemical injuries. He reported the procedural abuse he had witnessed to the Minister of Human Resources, the Hon. Jane Stewart, requesting her help –which she provided with grace and speed and charm.

On April 10th the Minister gathered in her office Senator Sparrow, representatives of RAINET (the advocacy organization working for this CPP applicant), and me at RAINET's request. The files of this and several other MCS cases, similarly tainted with procedural bias, often for many years and with heart-breaking effects, were formally given to the Minister. A lively discussion about health and environment unfolded. Believing that nobody can ever have too much education, I presented the Minister with a copy of the book my publishing company had recently brought out: Dr. Jozef Krop's *Healing The Planet One Patient At A Time.* To my delight she not only leafed through it with spontaneous interest and asked many pertinent questions, but began to tell us about people in her own Brantford constituency who had become ill from environmental toxins. She requested detailed reports from RAINET and from me for the senior administrative staff of her department to assist with the process of drawing up new guidelines for MCS-afflicted applicants.

RAINET (Research Advocacy and Information Network) was founded by Hilary Balmer, a nurse who became disabled due to chemical injury. Her organization wants to have "chemically/environmentally induced injury and/or illness an officially recognized disability". In partnership with workers' advocacy groups and medical organizations, Hilary has helped many people. With the unexpected help from the Senator, Hilary's efforts have matured into truly meaningful discussions with the federal government. In her report to the Minister, Hilary observed (supported by ample documentation) that "pervasive prejudice against persons with disabilities such as...MCS...permeates the agencies charged with the responsibility of adjudicating applications for disability benefits. The incapacitated person is perceived as merely a psychological misfit and thus undeserving of disability benefits."

The subsequent meeting with senior Human Resources administrative staff was friendly and collegial. New guidelines are being created and some messed-up cases have already been fixed. Existing legislation is excellent because it focuses on how disabled a person is, regardless of the diagnosis which may change or be difficult to make. Between 1998 and 2003 three Supreme Court and one federal appeals' court decisions have spelled out how the government must interpret the law governing disability benefits and what characteristics a reliable expert opinion has. In 1998 the court stated that the law must be understood "in broad and generous terms so that any doubt arising from the language of such legislation ought to be resolved in favour of the claimant" (*Rizzo*). In 2000 it ruled that applicants must be "accommodated" according to their level of disability (*Granowsky*), and in 2001 clear "tests for disability" were defined (*Villani*) to protect the "benevolent purposes of the legislation". In May (*C.U.P.E. 2003*) the Supreme Court defined experts as requiring the qualities of "neutrality, independence and proven expertise".

Nevertheless, the reality is that when a person carries an MCS diagnosis, the competing interests of insurance companies, employers, and government programs often erect seemingly insurmountable barriers for the applicant. Furthermore, not only is MCS a new disease, but it is caused by substances upon which industrialized economies depend. This situation began some 200 years ago when coal-fired industries caused asthma, allergies and cancer to appear in unprecedented numbers. Since then tens of thousands of even more toxic substances have become part of everybody's environment—with a predictable increase in corporate and public attempts to avoid responsibility.

Lawyer Matthew Wilton of Toronto has defended many doctors who diagnose environmental illness, such as the internationally renowned environmental medicine expert Dr. Jozef Krop and the asthma expert Dr. Sukhdev Kooner who works in Canada's asthma capital, Windsor. These physicians often run into trouble with regulatory agencies and industry because they stand up for their patients against insurance companies and government agencies which deny the reality of MCS and even traditional environmentally mediated illnesses, such as mold toxicity.

A large part of Matthew's practice is devoted to clients with insurance claims. The typical case is that of a disabled person whose private insurance is running out and whose employer wants to fire him or her. Insurance companies turn to their own doctors who are trained by their organization, the Canadian Association of Independent Assessors, in the fine art of discrediting a patient's application. A few years ago, a formal complaint was lodged by Ontario doctors with their licensing authority, the College of Physicians and Surgeons, objecting to this obvious lack of medical ethics when a doctor actively works against a trusting patient's interests. The College replied that this wasn't unethical because the patient was merely referred and not actually the doctor's own patient—a twisted logic arising from the fact that representatives of the insurance industry sit on the College's council and sometimes are even members of the disciplinary committees prosecuting doctors who stand up to the industry.

These "independent assessors" assert that MCS is just another form of panic attacks. "Experts" are produced who insist that nothing else is the matter with this person. Their "proof" is in each case boringly the same: outdated medical literature is cited, current medical research results are ignored, meaningless tests are demanded, and the physician who treated this disabled patient on a regular basis, and is thus qualified to defend her case, is dismissed as being ignorant. Often this medical garbage becomes part of applicant's file with Canada Pension and Disability—and so both the private and public insurance processes become fatally flawed.

Matthew insists, however, that this systemic injustice can be overcome successfully. "Don't ever think it's useless to fight!" Generally, judges fully understand the difference between an "expert" from the insurance industry and the informed opinion of the regular, treating physician. "Judges understand that the GP has nothing to gain by stating the truth about a person's disability, while the insurance doctor certainly does stand to gain by denying that disability." As long as your own doctor stands by you, the applicable legislation, especially the Ontario Human Rights Code and current employment laws, will generally support your claim. Of course, most people in this situation are close to destitute as well as browbeaten, so Matthew often handles them on a contingency basis, an approach that is almost always successful for all concerned.

What is it about MCS that brings out the best and the worst in people? Simply put, MCS challenges the way we run our world. It challenges the chemical industry the way cancer did the tobacco industry. Both brought their products to market before their safety was established and both have to face the fact that these products are not and never will be safe.

In the early 1950s allergist Dr. Theron Randolph had a patient who had severe allergic symptoms unrelated to the usual suspect triggers. Careful observation showed that her symptoms were present only when certain wind patterns brought high concentrations of petrochemical particles into the Chicago area. This was the first recorded case of environmental hypersensitivity, as Dr. Randolph called her untypical allergy. In 1965 he founded the American Academy for Environmental Medicine which, to this day, teaches doctors from all over the world how to diagnose and treat illness caused by many environmental toxins, fossil fuel products, pesticides, organic industrial solvents and carbon monoxide poisoning being chief among them.

Today, the illness is called Multiple Chemical Sensitivity (MCS); it consist of a whole family of diseases of which the best-known ones are Fibromyalgia, Chronic Fatigue Syndrome, Gulf War Syndrome and Cacosmia (the MCS variant in which people lose all tolerance for scents, toxic or otherwise). The international consensus statement on MCS syndromes was published in June 1999 (*Archives of Environmental Health* vol. 54/3). The definition states that symptoms are reproducible with repeated exposure, that the condition can be chronic, low levels of exposure cause symptoms which improve when the offending chemical is removed, many substances can cause reactions, and many organ systems are involved in the MCS patient.

The most common complaints include acute intolerance to light, noise, and chemical smells of all kinds, extreme fatigue, muscle pain, swollen joints, muscle weakness, shortness of breath evolving frequently into asthma, anemia, chronic urinary tract infections, nausea, diarrhea, migraines lasting days, tingling in hands and feet, irregular heart beat, watery and itchy eyes, generalized itching and more. Harvard University's environmental medicine publication, *Environmental Health Perspectives,* published a survey in September of this year showing that about one third of MCS patients became ill from pesticides, another third from solvent exposure. Similar results were obtained in a study done by the University of Toronto and submitted to the Hon. Jane Stewart by Dr. Lynn Marshall, the director of the Environmental Health Clinic at Sunnybrook & Women's College Hospital.

Rachel Carson's research in the 1960s into the health effects of the pesticide DDT, a declassified biological warfare chemical from World War II, showed that small, frequent exposures to a toxic chemical can cause permanently disabling illness or cancer. This finding turned upside down the traditional notion that the amount of a poison determined how sick one became. In 1960 approximately 10 billion pounds of toxic chemicals were released into soil, air and water. Currently, about 35 billion pounds of pesticides, organic solvents and other products containing heavy metals are released annually. Most have never been tested for their health effects. However, as more and more people are affected, scientific investigation has increased rapidly: in the 1950s the world medical literature had 5 articles on the subject; in 1997 only 120 research studies existed; today more than 10,000 are listed.

In 2001 the Ottawa based Environmental Illness Society of Canada (now no longer in existence) commissioned the first socio-economic study of MCS. This showed that about 4 million Canadians are chemically sensitive, about 500,000 severely so, some 5,000 are relatively disabled as a result, and roughly 50 to 60 people are forced to seek assistance, such as federal pension benefits. Among the most severe cases about 60% attempt suicide. This illness costs $ 10 billion in lost productivity, about $ 1 billion in lost taxes and another $ 1 billion in avoidable health costs.

The subject of medical research worldwide, MCS now has many clearly defined biomarkers and sophisticated as well as very simple and inexpensive tests are available to establish a clear diagnosis for each of the different MCS syndromes. In 2000 the Canadian government published a report urging reform of the pesticide legislation (which was been done), and recommending that MCS be officially recognized and its treatment covered by Medicare (not yet done). But now that the *Canadian Medical Association Journal* published a whole series of research papers (April through June 2002) on the health effects of the environment and the Ontario College of Family Physicians is hosting its first conference on the subject this October, maybe MCS will become fully recognized at last. The Ontario Human Rights Commission already instructed the Ministry of Health on April 9th, that people sensitive to pesticides must be protected from any spraying for west Nile virus.

While justice for the severely disabled MCS patient is now within their reach and the recognition of this condition fully recognized by medical science, the battle is not over. Consider the fact that the same month when the international consensus on MCS was published (June 1999) the College of Physicians and Surgeons of Ontario found environmental medicine expert Dr. Jozef Krop "guilty" of diagnosing MCS and reprimanded him for it in September of this year—when simultaneously the federal government began to remove the systemic bias against MCS disability pension applicants. So who else is still opposing the fact of MCS? One powerful group is the Environmental Sensitivities Research Institute established in 1995; it accepts only corporate members (I tried to join and was refused!) and its board of directors consists of the major pesticide producers of North America such as

DowElanco, Monsanto, Proctor & Gamble, and the Cosmetics, Toiletry and Fragrance Association. The chairman is the CEO of the pesticide industry association called RISE.

Indeed, the chemical industry's worries about its future are justified— and encouraging. However, we may take comfort in the fact that humanity has been through such ethical crises before and society always emerged much improved by the experience. The last and most brutal example being the end of slavery which was an equally unavoidable economic earthquake for society. Facing the truth of MCS has started the process making the world cleaner and healthier, and it is nice to have one's government lend a hand.

Sources and Resources

American Academy of Environmental Medicine, tel 316-684-5500 helps you find a doctor trained to diagnose MCS in Canada

RAINET P.O. Box 943, Uxbridge, ON, L9P 1N3, tel. 905-852-2676

Matthew Wilton Law Office, specializes in disability issues; 127 John Street, Toronto, M5V 2E2, tel. 416-860-9889

Environmental Hypersensitivity Association of Ontario, Box 1250, Station K, Toronto, M4P 3E4

Environmental Health Clinic, Women's College Hospital, 76 Grenville Street, Toronto, M5S 1B2

Ontario Medical Association's Section on Complementary Medicine, call 613-432-3240

www.mcsrr.org is the most comprehensive and helpful web site with information on everything you want to know about MCS

Alternative Medicine Guide, *Chronic Fatigue, Fibromyalgia & Environmental Illness*, Future Medicine Publications, 1998

P.R. Gibson, *Multiple Chemical Sensitivity: A Survival Guide*, New Harbinger, 2000

K. Glenn, *I'm Sorry But Your Perfume Makes Me Sick: And So Does Almost Everything Else That Smells*, Bluebird Books, 1997

T. Kerns, *Environmentally Induced Illness: Ethics, Risk Assessment and Human Rights*, McFarland, 2001

J. Krop, MD, *Healing The Planet One Patient at A Time: A Primer in Environmental Medicine*, Kos Publishing, 2002 (call 519-927-1049 to order)

T.G. Randolph MD, *An Alternative Approach to Allergies*, rev. ed. Harper Collins, 1990

Recognizing Multiple Chemical Sensitivity (MCS)

A Report Prepared for the Ministry of Human Resources of the Government of Canada October 2003

By Helke Ferrie

INTRODUCTION

The following is the written version of my oral presentation made on June 27, 2003, at the offices of Human Resources and Development Canada. I did so at the request of RAINET (*Research Advocacy and Information Network*) in support of that organization's efforts to have citizens with an MCS diagnosis treated equitably when applying for CPP or similar benefits. On April 10, 2003, RAINET had presented the Minister for Human Resources, the Hon. Jane Stewart, with files on applications for CPP which appeared to have met with bias because of the applicants' MCS diagnosis.

Senator Herb Sparrow was also present at the April 10th meeting with the Minister because he had been a witness to one such RAINET case at a Canada Pensions and Disability Review Tribunal hearing. Important technical aspects of this case also were (1) the fact that the applicant, who was too sick to attend in person, was not accommodated as required by the recent Supreme Court decision (May 2000) known as *Granovsky v. Canada*, and (2) the manner in which her MCS diagnosis was dealt with may not have followed the direction given in August 2001 by the Federal Court of Appeal's *Villani* decision, which defines the test for a disability's severity.

Following our meeting with the Minister, another meeting took place on June 27 with the Department of Human Resources' senior administrative and management staff. Our delegation was told at the outset that the fundamental legislative criterion guiding the Human Resources Department in assessing a disability application is a person's *observable, measurable and verifiable disability—rather than a generally accepted diagnosis.* This is so because diagnoses may change over time, different disease states with various diagnostic names can lead to one or more disabilities, a particular diagnosis can lead to serious disability in one person but not necessarily in another, a person can be clearly disabled but the diagnosis may take time to established (e.g. Multiple sclerosis), or an illness may not yet be understood but clearly leads to serious disabilities, such in the case of AIDS. Therefore, we were told, *objective disability is what matters and diagnosis is secondary.* As an example, we were given the case of AIDS. When AIDS patients first began to apply for CPP, they were *routinely accepted* until a better understanding of the disease led to treatments that reduced disabilities in many people, and an individualized approach to each applicant became more appropriate. The parallels between MCS and AIDS are, in my view, significant and will be dealt with at the end of this report.

Every application for CPP must, however, be based on some medical assessment which necessarily includes a diagnosis focusing on a disability's cause. Therefore, recognition of a disability is always somewhat dependent upon a diagnosis. A person would not even come to the attention of the Department unless a doctor identified some disabling condition, whatever the diagnosis. Not surprisingly, problems are to be expected, even if the granting or denial of a CPP application is primarily focused on whether this person is able to function. Therefore, our delegation was told, we could be helpful to the Department by *providing our analysis of how medical science views MCS at the present time; this information might assist the Department in the creation of guidelines appropriate for the assessment of MCS cases.*

ABOUT THE AUTHOR OF THIS PRESENTATION

I became ill with MCS myself, hence I am speaking with the authority of a patient. I studied environmental illness when I started to recover, and began to write about health and environment issues and especially medical politics. Eventually I became a publisher. Copies of my first publication, *Healing The Planet One Patient At A Time: A Primer In Environmental Medicine* by Dr. Jozef Krop were given to all who attended these two meetings. Currently, several books by environmental physicians specializing in asthma, infertility, endocrinology, holistic dentistry, and by a medical law attorney are in preparation for publication. My work enabled me to interview and meet at many medical conferences leading researchers in MCS and public health. It was through my articles that RAINET became aware of me and we began to work together on MCS issues.

In addition to my own illness, one of my sons (now 30 years old) developed MCS as seriously as I had, following two farm accidents in 1995 and 1996 while working on a summer job; both events involved being completely drenched in pesticides for a few hours. His T-cell count went down to the level of an AIDS patient. His immune, gastrointestinal, and nervous systems were all seriously affected and the struggle for his recovery began in 1996 when we finally understood what was wrong with him and we found a doctor trained in environmental medicine, namely Dr. Jozef Krop in Mississauga. By spring of this year, my son's T-cell count reached low normal and most of his symptoms are gone. He has returned to university and his doing his PhD in the philosophy of physics at McMaster University.

Like many MCS patients, we did not know that this condition had a name and that specialized treatments were available. Over time, I developed a full-blown "traditional" neurological disease generally thought of as "idiopathic", namely Myasthenia gravis, a neuro-muscular disorder. Other people with MCS may develop "traditional" illnesses such as asthma, Multiple sclerosis, chronic dermatitis, porphyria, Parkinson's or Alzheimer's disease, severe anemia, Lupus, or cancer—depending on the nature and duration of the chemical exposure they experienced and the vulnerability of the target systems. I was at the time in my PhD program (physical anthropology) at the University of Toronto, where I was also teaching. The underlying causes, as objective tests soon indicated, were decades of exposure to DDT while living in India, years of antibiotic treatment for various tropical infections, and systematic poisoning of my immune system from mercury through dental amalgam (as later established through standard laboratory tests; for the mercury levels the World Health Organization's toxicity scale was used).

As can be readily surmised, the fact that MCS victims can and do often develop "traditional" chronic diseases has far-reaching implications for medical theory as a whole and challenges the concept of "idiopathic". It also sheds light on the epidemic rise of chronic idiopathic diseases. As for government policy, such as Medicare, Human Resources and Labor, MCS may prove to be as significant for medical history as the discovery of bacteria which launched public health and hygiene measures. Indeed, the discovery of bacteria changed the understanding of disease throughout the world; environmental toxins will do so, too. Researchers N. Ashford and C. Miller state in their classic book on MCS:

> *"We may be dealing with an emerging new mechanism or theory of disease. According to this theory, a two-step process occurs; (1) an initial salient exposure event(s) interacts with a susceptible individual, leading to loss of that person's natural prior tolerance for everyday, low-level chemical inhalants, as well as for specific foods, drugs, alcohol, and caffeine; (2) thereafter such common, formerly well-tolerated substances trigger symptoms, thus perpetuating illness."* [1]

The technical name Ashford and Miller coined for this condition is **Toxicant-induced loss of tolerance** (TILT)—a symptom that is observed in MCS, its related illnesses such as Fibromyalgia, Chronic fatigue and Gulf War Syndrome as well as in conventional illnesses when various agents (toxic or otherwise) can also produce this response. Hence, a new theory of disease is a justified prediction.

However, the basic principle of scientific medicine, as first enunciated by Hippocrates 2,500 years ago, remains unchallenged, namely that an exterior agent, hostile to an organism's ability to function, may cause disease or systemic malfunction. Bacteria, organophosphates, viruses, solvents, radiation, transfatty acids in processed foods—they are all very similar, when seen in the light of this fundamental concept.

The subsequent treatment (for my son and me) consisted of detoxification treatments developed by nutritional and orthomolecular medicine following the removal of all "silver" dental fillings; my son had none, but the necessary removal of lipophilic pesticides in his body required installation and long-term use of a far infra-red sauna. Drastic environmental interventions were necessary also, such the replacement of gas cooking and water-heating appliances with electrical ones, a shift to a 100% organic diet, air-purifying equipment throughout the house, substitution of clothing requiring dry-cleaning with cotton garments, and removal of all cleaning materials of synthetic chemical nature as well as avoidance of all scented products etc.). I was unable to work or even manage my household unassisted from 1994 until approximately 1997; most of 1995 I could not drive a car and was unable for many months to handle a telephone or read due to seriously blurred vision. Fortunately, I did not need the help of my government, as my husband, a physician, was able to take care of me and our son, and we could afford the treatments not covered by Medicare. The total, estimated cost of my recovery is about $ 20,000 and for my son about $ 26,000.

Today, I work fulltime out of my environmentally-safe home meeting monthly deadlines for articles published in Canada and the US and working with my prospective authors. I agree with the great Canadian psychiatrist and nutritional medicine physician, Dr. Abraham Hoffer's definition of health: according to him, people are healthy when they are *1. usually free of symptoms, 2. get along reasonably well with their families, 3. get along in their communities, and 4. pay taxes* [2]. I pay taxes and employ people, especially those who need accommodation, and make sure that my books are printed on fully recycled paper using vegetable inks free of scents and synthetic chemicals such as glues; that increases production costs, but chemically sensitive readers can safely read them.

I am even able to attend—on a short term basis and not too frequently—

events such as conferences and meetings held in environments that are commonly unsafe for MCS sufferers, such as the windowless Human Resources building which has wall-to-wall carpeting; but thankfully all participants were free of aftershave lotion and perfumes. It takes a day or two to recover after such an event, thereby reducing my work pace due to extreme fatigue and headaches, but so far I always recovered.

My son and I were fortunate. Many such severe MCS cases do not recover. Looking over the past 5 years, it is clear that medical science is advancing in this area—both with regard to diagnosis as well as effective treatment and the recognition that prevention is key. Public and political appreciation of this condition is also progressing, especially in Canada, which pioneered much of the political and social integration of MCS.

HISTORY AND OVERVIEW OF MCS

MCS is a condition medical science began to recognize in the 1950s[3], when it was exceedingly rare and initially had no agreed-upon name. Its name implies the presence of synthetic chemicals. Today approximately 80,000 synthetic chemicals exist which had not yet been invented in 1950 when DDT, a biological warfare agent declassified for agricultural and garden pesticide use, was the most widely used toxic chemical. Since 1960, synthetic chemical production rose from approximately 10 *billion* pounds per year to the current estimated annual release of about 35 *billion* pounds into soil, air and water in the US alone. Of these only about 600 are *known* to be carcinogenic, neurotoxic and/or teratogenic **because the rest have never been tested for safety** [4]. By 1999 MCS was integrated into mainstream medical research and supported by animal and human experimental investigations, theoretical explanation, therapeutic interventions, and some statistical and epidemiological data. That same year the international consensus statement on MCS was published by the US National Institutes of Health [5]. It is based on observations going back to the 1950s and essentially systematizes those observations published by Dr. Theron Randolph. It states:

1. The symptoms are reproducible with repeated chemical exposure.
2. The condition is chronic.
3. Low levels of exposure (lower than previously or commonly tolerated) result in manifestations of the syndrome.
4. The symptoms improve or are resolved when the incitants are removed.
5. Responses occur to multiple chemically unrelated substances.
5. Symptoms involve multiple organ systems.

A list of the signs symptoms commonly observed with MCS

The main source for the list given below is the research done by the University of Toronto published in the *Archives of Environmental Health*, September 2001.

Central Nervous System

Increased sense of smell, problems with concentration, fatigue, confusion, headache, temporary memory loss, dizziness, sleep disorders (some people can't sleep, others sleep 14 hours every night), anxiety, hyperactivity, and generalized sense of disorientation and confusion (following exposure) known as "brainfog" (sometimes also called "brain fog"), a term coined by a famous MCS patient, the Chief Librarian of the United States Library of Congress (he was a patient of Dr. Randolph's), intolerance to bright light and to heat and cold.

Musculoskeletal Symptoms

Joint pain, backaches, muscle spasms, swollen joints or limbs, muscle twitching, and severe muscle weakness.

Respiratory System Symptoms

Frequent colds or bronchitis, asthma, heavy chest, shortness of breath.

Hematological System

High or low platelets (depending on status of immune function), easily bruised, anemia or leukemia.

Genitourinary Symptoms

Water retention, frequent urination and urgency, inability to void, chronic infections of urinary tract, enuresis, infertility.

Gastrointestinal Tract Symptoms

Nausea, diarrhea, bloating, constipation or all of these in rapid succession, often followed by vomiting.

Cardiovascular Symptoms

Rapid heart beat, irregular beat, hypertension, severe flushing of the face (sometimes involving the whole upper body) when exposed to an offending chemical or reduced oxygen supply), tingling in hands and feet.

Ear, Nose and Throat Symptoms

Chronic stuffiness and runny nose, earaches, frequent ear infections, watery and itchy eyes, frequent sinus infections, intolerance to noise.

Dermatological Symptoms

Rough skin, sores, generalized itching, intolerance to certain fabrics.

It is important to note that MCS patients may have many of these symptoms at the same time, not necessarily in the same order or combination, or progressing to the same severity level. This makes them such a challenge for doctors not trained in environmental medicine who attempt to treat all these many symptoms traditionally: one at a time, or refer the patient to a psychiatrist—the doctor of last resort. Of course, each of these symptoms could also, when presented in *isolation and without a history of chemical exposure* at home or at work, be responsive to standard medical intervention. In the final analysis, the **history** and the **multiplicity of symptoms** should alert the doctor to the possibility of environmental illness. [6]

A person severely ill MCS will virtually never be free of symptoms; only the severity will fluctuate. And consequently impaired functioning will vary also. Such a person *will have difficulty keeping appointments for a future* date because he or she may be totally unable to function (e.g. unable to predict if they may be able to drive a car, speak without a slur, as was the case with me, have breathing problems such that climbing a set of stairs would be out of the question, muscle spasms and joint pain making movement difficult etc.). Many *MCS patients become socially progressively more isolated*; their families often cannot understand what is happening, and making them understand is at first difficult: in my case, visiting family members may need to take a shower and wash their hair immediately upon arrival at our home and use borrowed fresh clothes free of scented detergent; the scents that cling to them from subway and bus rides can ruin the family gathering for my son and me, so my other sons and daughters readily comply.

On a fairly "good" day, when such a person is managing basic chores satisfactorily, a *single exposure* to aftershave lotion (often one of the worst incitants) on the mailman delivering a parcel, or driving behind a diesel-fueled truck in slow traffic may cause within minutes a migraine size "12 on the Richter scale" (the measurements used for earthquakes), as I used to describe the experience. Eating a dish of fresh strawberries (there are more pesticides on strawberries and peaches than any other fruit) can cause stomach cramps, convulsions, and muscle spasms within a few minutes. A Human Resources worker wearing hairspray or perfume who visits such a person and sees her doing dishes and vacuuming would perhaps find it hard to believe how totally disabled this person may be half an hour later due to exposure to the worker's perfumed products.

Because of the unpredictability of a severe attack, MCS patients are often embarrassed by their condition. MCS can make you feel like a complete idiot and be frightening at the same time. One example: one day in 1993 I was teaching a class in an Anthropology 200 course at U of T (introduction to world prehistory), when in mid-sentence, while discussing a prehistoric human skull (of all things) my lower jaw and my tongue would not move. My arms felt heavy, and it required tremendous effort to breathe. My class looked at me in astonishment, waiting for me to continue speaking. I turned my back to the class and struggled through several slow, deep breaths and simply waited. Slowly, my tongue began to move and so did my jaw and I completed the class without further incident.

These are, of course, classic Myasthenia gravis symptoms—as I know now. The neurotransmitter responsible for muscle contraction was briefly blocked at the neuro-muscular junction. Today, I also know that neuro-transmitters, hormones, as all known types of messenger molecules, are reduced in their numbers and ability to function because the organs that produce them (especially the thyroid, the thymus, the hypothalamus, the adrenal glands etc.) are primary targets of pesticides, solvents, and heavy metals—the chief chemicals involved in MCS.

Today, thankfully, such events happen very rarely and always to a much milder degree, but just as suddenly if, for example, I am exposed to dry-cleaning fumes, a room full of heavily scented people, confined places like elevators in sky-scrapers, and lawyers' conference rooms which usually are full of books, documents, plastic plants, photocopiers, computers and print-ers, wall-to-wall carpeting, and those real knock-out air-fresheners often found in the bathrooms of public buildings and offices—all releasing neuro-toxic benzene, limonene, and many other chemicals hostile to organisms (most of which are, incidentally, also on the official EPA list of known car-cinogens). I do my best to avoid such situations and request meetings in places I know to be safe for me.

While the wide range of symptoms in MCS are nothing new—they cover the spectrum of reactions an organism can have to an exterior stimulation—the fact that such a *range* of symptoms and *all major bodily systems* can be involved has presented a major challenge to medicine: *MCS does not fit the classic model of diagnosis because it appeared in a post-classical period.* As an anthropologist I would add, that since science knows, for example, when and how conditions favorable to infectious diseases evolved (over the past 20,000 years) and what environmental and social conditions are required before a chronic disease can arise, the appearance of a new diseases should not be totally surprising, indeed it should be expected. The anthropological community would fully support my prediction that we will have many more events in the future, such as we have recently had with AIDS, MCS, SARS.

MCS is unique because of the following characteristics:
1. The *"one cause—one disease"* model which guided medicine since the Roman physician Galen (130-200 AD) *cannot apply to MCS* because chemicals do not come in isolation; we live in a veritable chemical soup the interactive effects of its huge number of component parts being virtually unknown to science. Different chemicals may effect different bodily systems and the interaction between these substances increases their power to effect body system. Classic medical theory, as guides most doctors today, is ill-equipped to understand such dynamic complexity. However, *MCS yields to pattern analysis*, as has Fibromyalgia (one of the forms of MCS) and enables formulation of diagnostic criteria. Doctors are trained to think in a Newtonian, linear fashion, which results in patients being sent from one specialist to another, a different specialist for each bodily system's complaints, with the result that the underlying cause is not even looked for, and Medicare costs go through the roof.
2. *MCS does not follow traditional models with respect to its expected course and prognosis.* The patient might remain "stable" by remaining sensitive to a lot of chemicals in the environment, from pesticides to perfume, or develop a traditional, well known illness, such as asthma, cancer, MS, chronic infections etc. Size and duration of the exposure, pre-existing health condition, and unknown factors, such as chemical interaction and DNA response all play a part.
3. Unlike traditional illnesses, such as infectious diseases, *pharmaceuticals usually do not help, but tend to make the patient sicker.* Most drugs used for chronic illnesses contain certain synthetic chemicals also found in those very chemicals that made the person sick in the first place (e.g. antibiotics are also hormone disruptors and carcinogens, other standard drugs further slow or inactivate the detoxification pathways of the liver or deplete detoxification substances such as glutathione, serum vitamin C levels etc.). Standard drugs cannot control the symptoms of MCS because standard treatments were not designed to deal with a dynamic multi-systemic disease.

4. *Avoidance of the offending chemicals is the first line of defense, remains the main defense, and is one of the most important preventive measures,* even after the patient has become free of symptoms: in an MCS patient the immune system appears to remain on hyper-alert for life. Such people can function well and may need no medical care as long as they work in an environment free of those chemicals and gases that made them sick. Furthermore, traditional approaches like immunization are not likely to be possible: immunization is based on the assumption that the vaccine interacts with a potential *biological* invader which the human immune system is expected to recognize. In MCS the immune system is depleted or in a state of perpetual alarm because it is confronted with a synthetic invader which it does not know how to handle. This can result in the worst-case scenario in which an MCS victim's available defense mechanisms are altered forever and can never again be exposed to those chemicals that caused the illness. Furthermore, as is discussed in more detail later in the section presenting Albert Donnay's material, some of the most toxic substances act *as neurotransmitters* (e.g. carbon monoxide) and effectively disable the body's defence protocols.

5. *MCS has turned upside down the classic notions of toxicology* first formulated in the Middle Ages by Paracelsus who taught, "the dose makes the poison". Modern toxicology teaches that *small, frequent exposures* to a toxic chemical substance may cause MCS, certain cancers, birth defects, and infertility. (See the appended "ABCs of Modern Toxicology".)

However, *classical methods of investigation have proven so effective,* that the 1999 consensus statement was possible. The following can today be asserted with confidence (the sources for these items are provided and discussed in more detail later on):

   a. MCS is reproducible in animals.
   b. MCS yields clear results with *in vivo* tests such as PET scans and MRI, liver enzyme tests and many others.
   c. The statistical number of occurrences of MCS is predictable across populations in relation to specific chemical agents.
   d. Classic epidemiological and statistical analyses have proven very useful.
   e. Now we even have hints that genetic markers for MCS susceptibility are identifiable, thereby helping to explain why some people become MCS victims and others, equally exposed, do not.
   f. We have extensive data on what treatments work, and why they work when they do work, with entire medical organizations dedicated to

this field (e.g. American Academy of Environmental Medicine, Pan American Allergy Society, several Canadian organizations, and organizations of the same kind in the UK, Australia, Japan, and Germany).

g. Most importantly, we know MCS is not a psychiatric illness, even though MCS patients may understandably also be depressed and some may also be suicidal.

A MEDLINE search showed that by 2001 there were 10,741 entries on MCS, all from mainstream medical journals. Of those approximately 20% related to solvent sensitivity, 14% to perfume sensitivity, and 50% to multiple chemical sensitivity. As recently as 1997 only 120 entries existed. In the late 1950s only 5 entries existed. (For details visit **www.asehaqld.org.au/chemical-injury-issues-paper.htm**.) The current edition of *Harrison's Principles of Internal Medicine* includes discussion on environmental causes of many illnesses and mentions the 1999 consensus statement on MCS as does the 2003 edition of the MERCK Manual.

As is the case with all new diseases, there is inevitably a political component to the recognition of the illness, but the task is to take care of the needs of such patients now. A new disease implies the identification of new causes, and these imply the need for prevention and treatment—all carrying an economic impact for those who will inevitably be "blamed" and those who will work to prevent or treat its victims. MCS presents a serious problem for the chemical industry, just as cancer proved to be a problem to the tobacco industry. Both brought their products to market before safety was established, and they both battle against recognition of evidence proving that these products are not safe. Similarly, the discovery of bacteria forced 19th century governments to undertake immense public-works programs to provide clean water and sanitation to stop the great epidemics. Coal-fired industry brought us classic IgE mediated allergies, unknown until the early 19th century, as well as the recognition of the existence of carcinogens. The effort to make this industry responsible for causing asthma and other diseases is ongoing, as are the current battles between scientists and the public and toxin-producing industries[7].

The world's economy is, in the words of Cornell University's Sandra Steingraber, a Senior Advisor to the World Health Organization, "chemically addicted", and if our economy is not cured of it, experts on environment and health issues agree, the extinction of the human race is a real possibility. [8] While cancer is the recognized outcome of our chemically polluted environment (now the second leading cause of death—up from 5th in 1960[9]), MCS is an illness affecting far less people, but with the potential to affect many more over time—especially children in whom MCS often progresses to asthma or even leukemia.

Unlike cancer, MCS carries with it the possibility of a cure for many victims, if given time and proper treatment. Even in serious cases, accommodating MCS patients in various ways allows them to continue being meaningful and effective members of society and keeping their families in tact and paying taxes, as Dr. Hoffer would say. MCS victims can achieve that status, even if the remain sensitive to the chemicals that once made them sick and must continue to observe strict measures of avoidance to remain functional.

The financial impact of MCS is backed by interesting research done in Canada. The Ottawa-based *Environmental Illness Society of Canada* commissioned the first study on the socio-economic impact of MCS on Canadians and published it in 2001. The results showed the following:

> Approximately 4 million Canadians are affected by chemical sensitivity, half a million of whom are severe cases, with 5,000 being disabled by this condition; of those **annually 50-60 persons apply for CPP**. About 60% of the most severe cases also involve suicide attempts and about the same figure applies to family breakups (suicide attempts and family breakups overlap for obvious reasons.)

The impact of MCS victims on Canada's economy is estimated to be as follows:

> $ 10 billion are lost in productivity, roughly $ 1 billion is lost in taxes, another $ 1 billion is used in avoidable health care costs, and about $ 1 billion in (avoidable disabilities) are paid.

These statistics are very similar to those obtained by the University of Toronto and in various areas of the USA through similar studies conducted by State governments and the EPA (see appendix to this report; April 9, 2003, letter by Dr. L. Marshall of the Environmental Health Clinic of Sunnybrook & Women's College Hospitals, Toronto.) A recent study by Philip Landrigan of the Department of Community and Preventive Medicine at Mount Sinai School of Medicine in New York, estimated the cost of environmentally mediated pediatric cancer to be as high as US $ 600 million a year; for neu-

rological and behavioral illnesses of known environmental origin the cost
was estimated as high as US $ 18 billion per year[10].

THE RECOGNITION OF MCS

MCS is today recognized to include a family of diseases. Recognition began
with *Sick Building Syndrome* which followed the energy crisis in the 1970s and
the efforts to conserve energy through improved insulation [11]. The other
members of the MCS family are *Chronic Fatigue Syndrome, Fibromyalgia, Gulf
War Syndrome,* and *Cacosmia* (MCS involving primarily smell: inability to tolerate petrochemical products, perfumes, tobacco smoke etc. which may
produce severe symptoms). Collectively, the whole family is also known as
Environmental Illness (EI); and they share certain biomarkers and the hallmark
EI characteristic of many organs and systems being involved simultaneously.

MCS was first recognized and described by Dr. Theron Randolph in 1951
who called the condition "environmental hypersensitivity". One of his
patients with multi-system complaints became sick in a seasonal pattern
which did not agree with classic allergy—Dr. Randolph's specialty. Through
a painstakingly careful history extending over a few years, Dr. Randolph
established that the cause was exposure to petrochemical products brought
into the patient's area through seasonal wind-patterns. Avoidance caused the
symptoms to disappear, and experimental exposure reproduced them. This
was, at the time, a total revelation, even to him. To a specialist in allergy and
immunology it was astounding that the body would produce allergic symptoms and even anaphylactic reactions in response to low-dose exposures to
petrochemicals. Randolph devoted the rest of his life to the study and treatment of environmentally induced illness and called this new area of medicine "clinical ecology". The *American Academy for Environmental Medicine*
was founded in the 1965. Later, through his collaboration with Linus Pauling
and Dr. Abraham Hoffer, Dr. Randolph went beyond mere avoidance measures and the AAEM developed the treatment methods used today.

The AAEM trains environmental doctors to this day; some graduates
work in Canada.[12] It works cooperatively with the *Pan American Allergy
Society* and some international medical organizations as well as some departments of occupational medicine that are university-based. The AAEM's
annual courses and training seminars are recognized for continuing education by the Canadian, British, Australian, American, Japanese and German
Medical Associations, and some of their members are professors at medical
schools throughout the world, including Canada. Their research is published
in standard peer-reviewed medical journals and textbooks. Some of the

treatments and tests were originally developed at Johns Hopkins Medical School and the Harvard School of Public Health, the two medical schools of primary importance to MCS research. The World Health Organization now endorses some of those treatments as the treatment of choice [13] In the USA, research in MCS is supported by the Departments of Defence and Veterans Affairs, the CDC's Agency for Toxic Substances and Disease Registry, the EPA, the National Institutes of health, the National Academy of Sciences, and many universities.

The 1960s brought the research of Rachel Carson to international attention and introduced a new concept into toxicology, namely that low and frequent exposures carry the high risk of often irreversible damage. (However, both high and low exposures can cause MCS.) The phenomenon of "sick buildings" brought about major changes in architectural protocols in which Canada led the way in 1984 by establishing building guidelines for chemically sensitive people under the auspices of the *Canada Mortgage and Housing Corporation*. Indeed, the recognition of MCS in both Canada (first) and the USA (later) was facilitated through the housing departments of both countries. In 1985 the Ontario Government sponsored the *Thomson Report* on environmental hypersensitivity disorders, making 30 recommendations covering research, clinical practice, and Medicare issues. Thus, Canada was the first country to examine MCS for purposes of medical research, development of therapies, and recommended its inclusion in the public support system.

In the USA, recognition of MCS was forced upon the government and the medical community through an event that occurred in 1987 in the headquarters of the Environmental Protection Agency (EPA). When 27,000 square feet of new carpeting was installed, hundreds of employees became seriously ill from the (now known to be neuro-toxic) glue fumes. Of these 75 individuals never recovered fully and are, to this day, working out of their homes [14]. This event led to the first serious medical investigation in the USA by Cullen (Cullen 1987) [15], and the criteria he developed for the recognition of MCS were eventually accepted internationally in 1999. A similar disaster took place from 1988 to 1993 in the Camp Hill Medical Centre in Nova Scotia where hundreds of people became disabled due to an error in the installation of the air ducts resulting in formaldehyde and other toxic substances being pumped into the building at low, steady levels. [16] One of the doctors there, Dr. Roy Fox, became ill with MCS himself. Eventually, in 1994, he became the director of Canada's first environmental health clinic (funded federally and provincially) in Nova Scotia. He also taught environmental medicine at Dalhousie University.

Subsequent workshops and research projects sponsored by the US National Academy of Sciences (1987) and the 1989 EPA report to the US Congress on MCS led to a full investigation of chemical neuro-toxicity by the Office of Technology Assessment in 1990. The Dallas, Texas, Environmental Health Clinic, founded, in the 1960s, to this day trains doctors from all over the world. In 1990 Health Canada was the sponsor of the first government-initiated international medical conference on MCS in Ottawa, and that same year the US department of Housing and Urban Development (HUD) recognized MCS as a condition requiring special accommodation. That year also the landmark book on the subject was published: *Chemical Exposures: Low Levels and High Stakes* by Nicholas Ashford and Claudia Miller of the Massachusetts Institute of Technology and the National Institutes of Health respectively. It was based on a report commissioned by the New Jersey State Department of Public Health; for that effort the World Health Organization awarded New Jersey a prize.

In 1991 the EPA and the National Academy of Sciences recommended that MCS be integrated into medical research and clinical practice. The US Justice Department included MCS sufferers in their Disabilities Act Guidelines, and by 1992 the US Social Security Administration included MCS for coverage. That same year environmental health clinics were started in Australia, Germany, China and the UK. In 1994 the Ontario government started the environmental health clinic at Women's College Hospital which is affiliated with the University of Toronto (see letter by the clinic's director, Dr. L. Marshall of April 9 to the Hon. J. Stewart). In 1996 the Ontario Human Rights Commission made several rulings in favor of MCS victims.[17]

The 1999 consensus statement discussed above was based on research by several renowned experts in occupational medicine and toxicology, the most important being K. Kilburn, one of the world's most famous toxicologists and neurologists (current editor of the National Institutes of Health journal *Archives of Environmental Health*).[18] Kilburn's research into the neurotoxicity of substances relevant to MCS and the changes observable in the brain are key in MCS research[19].

Two carefully designed research projects set out to prove that MCS was a psychological or psychiatric condition—one by Ryan in 1988 and the other by Davidoff in the early 1990s[20]. Both failed to prove the psychological basis of the illness and, instead, reached the inescapable conclusion that MCS is biological in nature and mediated by toxins in the environment. Subsequent investigations involving positron emission tomography or PET scans showed that MCS sufferers have *temporal lobe* impairment, while schizophrenics and other psychiatric patients have frontal lobe damage. [21] With single photon emission computed tomography (SPECT) central nervous system function has been investigated in MCS victims and shown clear deficits consistent with known neuro-toxic chemical damage.

In May 2000 the Canadian government issued a report entitled, *Pesticides: Making the Right Choice for the Protection of Health and the Environment*. Its primary aim was to reform the antiquated national pesticide legislation, which was done. Its recommendations included specifically the recognition of MCS and that its treatment be funded by Medicare (p. 55f), which has not yet been addressed.

In 2002 the *Canadian Medical Association* published a series of six articles (see appendix to this report) designed to teach doctors how to diagnose and treat patients presenting with symptoms of environmental illness. In October of this year the *Ontario College of Family Physicians* is holding its first medical conference on environmental illness in Toronto. The conference is supported by the *Ontario Medical Association* which granted the appropriate study credits. Earlier this year the *Ontario Human Rights Commission* specifically directed the Ontario Ministry of Health to protect and accommodate citizens with chemical sensitivity in case of pesticide spraying for West Nile Virus. (See appendix to this report).

A full list (up to the year 2000) of government agencies and medical organizations which have recognized MCS, and a representative list of legal cases won in favor of MCS sufferers, are found in the appendix to this report.

THE DENIAL OF MCS

An overview, even as brief as this one, of MCS in modern medicine would be seriously flawed if it didn't mention the fact that doctors practicing environmental medicine have been seriously persecuted, especially in the US, Canada and the UK, by the pesticide, pharmaceutical, and insurance industries, primarily through the industries' involvement with medical licensing authorities. This observation is supported by the findings published in the *Journal of the American Medical Association* (vol. 287, p. 612-17, 2002) showing that 87% of all physicians responsible for creating practice guidelines have financial ties to the pharmaceutical industry; 59% of these doctors recommend the products of those companies in the guidelines they authored. All of those relationships were in place when those physicians were selected for the committees charged with drawing up practice guidelines. The pharmaceutical industry also produces all of the pesticides and most of the chemicals implicated in MCS. [22] In Canada, for example, until last year most of the 30 council members of the *College of Physicians and Surgeons of Ontario* (CPSO), the provincial medical licensing authority, were directly or indirectly connected with the chemical industry (e.g. pesticides, pharmaceuticals and insurance industries), as evidenced on their publicly available CV information.

For purposes of this report, it is important to point out that there are blatantly biased physicians whose "expert" opinions are sometimes part of files submitted to the Department of Human Resources; these physicians are not only directly connected to the insurance industry in most cases, but are openly hostile to anything involving MCS or chemical injury. RAINET has ample documentation to prove this statement with respect to specific doctors. The most prominent of them all is Dr. Arthur. Leznoff in Toronto whose reports assisted materially in the rejection of applications by seriously disabled Canadians. The appendix to this report includes a transcript from a disciplinary trial in which a sworn statement was submitted by Dr. Gerald Ross, the first director of the Nova Scotia Environmental Health Clinic and co-director of the training clinic in Dallas, Texas. This statement speaks for itself and deserves the serious attention of the Department of Human Resources. Of special interest is the fact that Dr. Leznoff is **not** trained in occupational medicine, nor is he trained in environmental medicine, but describes himself on his letterhead as an expert in environmental sensitivities. In a report written by him *this year* (available from RAINET) he claims, in clear contradiction to his official CV, to be an expert in those fields and makes the following astounding assertion:

> "The major medical societies in the United States and Britain have published position papers on the disorder called Environmental Sensitivity or Multiple Chemical Sensitivity. These position papers all declare that there is no acceptable published evidence that, in these cases, it is the chemical, scent or food that is the direct cause of the patient's symptoms... this symptomatology can all be explained as manifestations of anxiety, panic or other psychological reactions."

This statement is unsupported by any references and, of course, ignores the international consensus on MCS. In the 1980s such position papers did exist, but all are superceded by subsequent research as well as new position papers—a fact conveniently ignored by Dr. Leznoff. He merely appended, in support of this assertion, to this 2003 opinion on a serious MCS case, two articles: one by him from 1997 (pre-consensus) and the other from 2000 co-authored with others, which curiously gives no references past the mid-1990s—when the explosion in MCS research began (see above p. 10). It is as if the whole of international research on MCS simply does not exist for Dr. Leznoff—yet, his blatantly bias opinion has ruined many perfectly legitimate applications.

Today, after the May 2003 Supreme Court decision which defines experts and expert testimony, the Department will need to re-examine the qualifications of doctors offering opinions on MCS cases. In *C.U.P.E. v. Ontario (Minister of Labour) 2003*, the Supreme Court defines an expert as somebody who is seen to be an expert by people in that same field of work, has a track record in that specific area, and has the qualities of independence, neutrality and proven expertise.

In this connection it is interesting to note that the organizations currently known to oppose the recognition of MCS are the *American Academy of Allergy* and immunology (of which Dr. Leznoff is a member) and the *Environmental Sensitivities Research Institute* (ESRI) established in 1995; it accepts *only* corporate members and its board of directors includes representatives from DowElanco, Monsanto, Proctor & Gamble, and the Cosmetics, Toiletry and Fragrance Association; its chairman is the CEO of the pesticide industry association RISE. [23]

In 1990 the *Chemical Manufacturing Association*, a US-based lobby group, submitted to various government agencies in the US and Canada a "position paper" which has since been made public by the *Environmental Illness Society of Canada*. To get a feeling for the importance of the timing of this publication, compare the list of events for that year given above. At that time, MCS was becoming part of mainstream scientific research and was being recognized in law and by government policy; research supporting MCS was coming especially from *publicly* funded medical schools. This position paper objected to MCS being recognized and states as follows:

"The primary impact on society would be the huge cost associated with the legitimization of environmental illness. Should the environmental illness advocates succeed in their efforts it would also impact on society and on many industries. Potentially affected industries include textiles, clothing, lawn care products, household cleaners, dry cleaners, paints and solvents [manufacturers], perfumes, hair treatment products, plastics, paper and many other consumer goods industries."

This position paper concludes with the following strategic advice: "*Should environmental illness arise as an issue, a coalition with the state [and provincial] medical associations is absolutely necessary.*" And from that "coalition" the persecutions of environmental medicine practitioners arose in large numbers, as documented in the Glasnost Report (see my web site: **www.collegeofphysicianswatchdog.com**) and my forthcoming book.

While the politics of medicine can indeed be astounding in its maliciousness against patients and the doctors who want to and can help them, this sort of struggle isn't exactly new to the history of medicine or any other human enterprise. The chemical industry—including gasoline, perfume, pesticides, various toxic synthetic drugs and endocrine disruptors—is for very good reason fighting hard for its survival. Indeed, the industry's anxiety about the economic impact of the eventual and certain end of the use of toxic substances is perfectly rational. However, one can take comfort from the fact that humanity has been through this sort of crisis many times before and society emerged much improved. The last and most brutal example being the end of slavery, which was an equally unavoidable economic earthquake for society.

THE CURRENT DIRECTION OF MEDICAL RESEARCH IN MCS
The appearance of MCS has effectively set medicine on a new course. Just how important the MCS issue has become is illustrated by the editorial of the 2003 "Grand Rounds" issue of the National Institutes of Health journal *Environmental Health Perspectives*. Its editor, Dr. H. Wu of the Harvard School of Public Health and Medicine summarizes in the introduction to this issue how central environmental medicine has become to all medical research. It is a masterly analysis of the issues; a copy is attached in the appendix to this report.

Canadians who apply for CPP, because they have become disabled, are faced with having to prove that they are indeed disabled, and the investigation process requires some kind of biological support or verification of the person's disability. That brings up the question of *biomarkers and objective tests.*

The view is often expressed that there are no real biomarkers or definitive tests to establish MCS (discussed in next section below). Even if that were true—which it most certainly is not—one should remember that many well-established and fully recognized diseases face the same problem, such as Multiple Sclerosis, Alzheimer's, clinical depression, schizophrenia, to name just a few. All *eventually* provide clear-cut biological evidence permitting a correct classification, but generally by that time the disease has already progressed very far. Unlike these traditional diseases, MCS provides powerful clues about its identity at an early stage (see especially the material by Albert Donnay in the appendix). In short: the reality of MCS should not be subject to a double-standard when it comes to scientific proof; what is considered an acceptable work-in-progress approach with other illnesses, should also apply to the evolution of MCS research.

In common with traditionally hard-to-diagnose illnesses, experts in environmental illness agree, MCS is most effectively diagnosed on the basis of an *exhaustive history,* and its characteristic feature, the large number of *"symptoms which involve multiple organ systems",* as the 1999 Consensus Statement asserts. However, definitive biomarkers do exist. The appendix to this report includes information on biomarkers and the appropriate tests from the medical literature.

THE LATEST INFORMATION ON MCS

It might be helpful to present the latest research on MCS. This is important because it points to what public policy will soon have to deal with. Four items are presented below which show the direction this research is taking. Each has relevance to your Department's concerns.

The **first** of these is the work of Martin L. Pall of Washington State University. This university issued a press release on January 4 this year announcing the publication of an article entitled "NMDA Sensitization and Stimulation by Peroxynitrite, Nitric Acid, and Organic Solvents as the Mechanism of Chemical Sensitivity in Multiple Chemical Sensitivity" in the prestigious journal FASEB (Federation of American Societies for Experimental Biology, 2002, vol. 16, pp. 1407-1417).

Pall suggests that MCS (including Fibromyalgia, Chronic Fatigue Syndrome, Gulf War Syndrome), as well as the psychological condition known as Post Traumatic Stress Disorder (PTSD), have a common biological mechanism which he describes as *"a vicious chemical cycle".* In this case, "chemical" is interpreted as being stress-induced through toxic chemicals within the body (such as stress hormones) as well as foreign toxic substances. PTSD is accompanied by an overproduction of stress hormones during an emotionally highly traumatic experience, but the subsequent chronic condition is not understood. Similarly, MCS is usually precipitated by an exterior chemical injury, but the subsequent chronic condition is also in need of explanation. The common area of investigation for Pall became the way in which the organism processes the internal or external chemical influx so as to wind up with a chronic condition.

The press release stated, "In the United States about 10 million people are afflicted with multiple chemical sensitivity...the onset of the condition can usually be traced back to an exposure to certain chemicals, but why the initial exposure results in an often life-long, incurable condition has been a mystery." Describing Pall's work, the press release summarizes, "Pall's new theory is [based on the observation that MCS involves] excessive levels of two chemicals in the body—nitric oxide and its oxidant product peroxynitrite. He suggests certain mechanisms act to keep levels of the two compounds elevated, thus producing chronic [organic] changes." Pall also suggests that this explanation complements an earlier theory proposed by environmental physician and researcher Dr. Iris Bell of the University of Arizona, namely that "neural sensitization in the brain" produces the chronic effect after initial exposure.[24]

Pall said, "What my article reports is that if you assume both theories are correct, you come up with a fusion that explains all the most puzzling features of MCS. It explains why MCS is induced by a previous chemical exposure and why MCS sufferers show such a high level of sensitivity to a wide range of chemicals." Pall discusses the research which shows how hypersensitivity in the brain is created following initial exposure, the subsequent production of these two chemicals, and how they increase hypersensitivity even further.

"Ordinarily these activities are highly regulated," Pall observed. "acting only on specific synapses in the brain where they are involved with learning and memory. The MCS response is produced when chemical exposure produces excessive responses over large regions of the brain. In this way normal and important mechanisms may act to generate this chronic illness. Thus, not only is the brain constantly inundated by chemicals to which it is normally somewhat sensitive, but the brain of a person suffering from MCS becomes abnormally sensitive to the chemicals—from 100 to 1,000 times more sensitive than in an unaffected person." Pall discusses two other known mechanisms which facilitate the accumulation of these toxic chemicals to much higher levels in the brains of MCS victims.

In PTSD virtually identical chemical activity has been observed following severe emotional trauma, and Pall suggests, "The notion that a biochemical vicious cycle may underlie [both]…suggests that this is a major new paradigm of human disease."[25]

Further research will expand on these observations, but it is clear that public policy will be powerfully influenced by this finding, if proven. The effect could be as powerful as the science that finally explained what smoking and exposure to second-hand smoke does to people's health. The parallel to smoking is helpful, as in both populations (MCS and smokers) there is a percentage of individuals who do not get cancer or other tobacco-induced illnesses. Even so, protecting the public interest demands that the consequences for the people who do get sick take precedence when formulating legislation. As far as the mandate of this department is concerned, the fact that this research is happening will hopefully help in evaluating MCS victims' applications; no matter how things turn out in detail, the science behind MCS has embarked on a road that will lead to further proof, not disproof of the condition's reality.

The **second** item of current research concerns genetic predisposition. On April 16 this year, the National Institutes of Health in Bethesda, Maryland, held a press conference during which it was announced that their Environmental Genome Project has sequenced "200 environmentally responsive genes [which] included links to vascular disease and leukemia." [26]

The implication of this research is that with MCS we are again dealing with a phenomenon like tobacco-induced diseases for which the genetic basis of the causes are well understood. It is known which cancer-protective genetic mechanisms are disabled by the toxicity of tobacco products, thereby allowing faulty cell reproduction to take off unchecked.[27]. Furthermore, the research into oncogenes has shown that predispositions for cancer exist in everybody, as apparently may also be the case with MCS. However, neither predisposition need be expressed, unless a chemical assault takes place. For both MCS and cancer the observation of oncologist Dr. Susan Love applies who famously said, "We start out with a perfectly good body until some chemical comes along and screws it up."[28]

An interesting parallel for this genetic basis of predisposition exists in the field of chronic pain research. In a recent interview with pain expert Dr. Ellen Thompson of Ottawa I learned that research has shown that about 17% of people have genetic markers which are known to predispose a person to developing chronic pain if injured seriously. Of course, not all 17% of the potential chronic pain population does get injured. Her remarks were in connection with the ongoing battles pain experts have with insurance companies and with other agencies that fill disability claims. Dr. Thompson pointed out that only a certain number of people would ever come into this system and that the fear of a stampede of chronic pain victims depleting the coffers of such agencies (or the government's) is totally unfounded. However, unfortunately, with MCS the potential for disability is much larger and, additionally, there is the danger of new epidemics evolving for which we appear not to be prepared at all.

The **third** and final research item worth mentioning concerns the research by Dr. G. Nicholson at the Institute of Molecular Medicine in California. Dr. Nicholson is probably the world's foremost expert on Gulf War Syndrome. He addressed the Canadian Defense Department at a 2001 conference initiated by that Department. His research investigated the *infectious potential* of Gulf War Syndrome and other forms of environmental illness.

One of the most characteristics of MCS which is especially alarming is the fact that it *can sometimes become an infectious disease*, primarily due to an impaired immune system which provides the opportunity for infectious organism to develop about which medical science knew nothing until about a decade ago. Dr. Nicholson studied 60 families where one member developed MCS and the rest of the family, not exposed to toxic chemicals, also became ill with the same characteristic set of symptoms and subsequent hypersensitivities to chemicals they had never been exposed to. The result of the last 10 years of his research has been the discovery of *mycoplasma* which, like other less frequently encountered bacteria (e.g. clamidia etc.) in an MCS victim become unusually virulent and develop opportunistically due to the chemically-induced impaired immune function of the host. Further research showed the presence of these mycoplasma in other chronic diseases, generally known as auto-immune diseases such as arthritis, Multiple Sclerosis, Lou Gehrig's disease (ALS), and Lupus, generally in about 40% of cases. When treated with certain antibiotic cocktails in combination with therapeutic doses of certain vitamins, enzymes and minerals, most of the victims of MCS and the other traditional illnesses recovered fully so as to be able to go back to work. Most of the cases Dr. Nicholson's research team treated were US armed forces personnel who can only return to work if they are in perfect health.

The chief characteristic of mycoplasma appears to be that they reside in intracellular space where they attack the mitochondria, thereby impairing the Krebs cycle and disturbing the energy production of the body. They feed on the lipids inside the cell and thus reduce the ability of the body to detoxify toxic chemicals, a process done primarily by lipids.

These findings are so solid, that an editorial in the *Journal of the American Medical Association* as far back as 1997 by Cassell (vol. 278 p. 2051ff) opined that it is nothing less than malpractice not to look for these infections in such patients. [29]

The implications of these findings are very disturbing: here is the very real possibility of a new epidemic—another AIDS or SARS, only fed continuously by chemicals found in the environment everywhere. Containment through old, tried and true methods of quarantine or the promotion of safe sex habits would be quite useless as more and more people become hypersensitized to a chemicalized environment. Transmission of the mycoplasma-mediated environmental illness could take place through anything from a blood transfusion to traditional exchange of body fluids or be transmitted to a fetus through its mother. MCS in all its forms is not readily controllable through behavior modifications such as ceasing to smoke or using condoms. MCS in all its forms will only stop when the environment in which we live is restored to a state in which an organism, with an immune system evolved over some 100 million years can actually survive.

The fourth item was not presented by me at our meeting and is here added because of its profound relevance to all considerations about MCS and its family of illnesses. Following my attendance at your department I had the opportunity to interview Dr. Albert Donnay and speak to him about my meeting with you in Ottawa. His position as research coordinator of the *Johns Hopkins Multi-Centre Study of MCS Immunology* places him in the position of having access to the latest information on MCS issues. The appendix attached to this report contains the information pertaining to the newly recognized fact that "9 out of 10 MCS cases are actually carbon monoxide poisoning cases", as Donnay put it. The entire subsequently observed cascade of symptoms develops out of that. When asked what the trigger for the remaining one · out of ten cases would be, he said, "Mostly solvents." The interesting point is that carbon monoxide poisoning is a well-understood traditional problem with a new symptomatology. Thus, a simple, traditional test which involves comparing the blood gases in a person as found in venous and arterial blood establishes with certainty whether an oxygen deficit exists. The implications for diagnosis and therapy are equally important, as early intervention is possible, treatment is relatively cheap, rehabilitation is highly likely, and a huge saving of money and suffering is within reach.

The sources of low-level carbon monoxide poisoning are many indeed in our society which totally relies upon fossil fuels and natural gas products. The mechanism of poisoning is also well-understood: carbon monoxide acts as a facilitating neurotransmitter in the body. Indeed, this interview prompted my husband to quip : "The solution clearly is to return to the horse and buggy since horse manure is healthier than gasoline." The serious fact behind the joking remark is, of course, the historical fact, that the industrial age has brought about exposures to steady concentrations of substances for which our biological evolution did not prepare us.

In conclusion, it can be said that medical science is learning that new patterns of disease do evolve, formerly harmless bacteria are able to become nasty when given new opportunities, and old poisons can create new responses. All of which pose new demands for social assistance upon governments and the helping professions.

SUGGESTIONS TO THE DEPARTMENT
OF HUMAN RESOURCES

MCS is a disease caused by chemicals toxic to many organs and bodily systems. It has been researched by medical science with increasing intensity since the mid-1990s. MCS and its related, or overlapping illnesses, Chronic Fatigue Syndrome, Fibromyalgia and Gulf War Syndrome afflicts *severely* some 10 million people in the United States and about 1 million in Canada. The information currently available indicates that in Canada about 50 to 60 individuals annually seek some assistance because they are *seriously* disabled. The most immediate concern for the Department is to develop assessment criteria when a Canadian citizen presents with a diagnosis that specifically identifies MCS as the cause of the disability.

Below is a list of sources which contain *diagnostic criteria* developed by experts in the treatment of MCS. As I am a medical science writer and not a practicing doctor, it is not appropriate for me to inform you how to diagnose MCS. Nor can I authoritatively suggest to you which biomarkers you ought to look for in an applicant's file and which tests you can trust as definitive. Given the fact that you wish to develop assessment criteria, your Department and the Canadian public are best served if doctors trained in this area are consulted. The best source would be Dr. L. Marshall whose letter to the Minister is included in this appendix. Also helpful might be the following whose material is also included in the appendix: [30]

1. Dr. A. Lieberman of the *American Academy of Environmental Medicine* presented at the 1999 annual international conference of that organization a summary of diagnostic and tools including tests that identify specific biomarkers.

2. The *Canadian Medical Association*'s recent series on health and environment issues commenced with an article entitled "Identifying and managing adverse environmental health effects: 1. Taking an exposure history." The authors of this series work at various Canadian universities and would no doubt be helpful to your Department.

3. Dr. G. Heuser summarized in an article published in 2000 in the *International Perspectives in Public Health*, vol. 13, the diagnostic protocol for MCS in its various forms.

4. Dr. Albert Donnay's material included in the appendix is invaluable, as it provides the latest information available with regard to biomarkers and applicable tests.

5. A helpful published source for both diagnostic and therapeutic procedures is the *Laboratory Evaluations in Molecular Medicine: Nutrients, Toxicants and Cell Regulators*, by J. A. Bralley and R.S. Lord, published by the Institute for Advances in Molecular medicine, 2001

My suggestion for the Department are as follows:

- To consider calling a meeting with Canadian doctors trained in environmental medicine who work with MCS patients on a regular basis by consulting Dr. L. Marshall whose position as research director for the environmental health clinic at Sunnybrook and Women's College Hospital in Toronto allows for access to whatever information the Department would be seeking. Furthermore, Ottawa happens to have an unusual concentration of doctors trained in this field. To my knowledge, all are graduates of the AAEM: Dr. Jenny Armstrong, Dr. John Molot, Dr. Ross Michealson are all located in downtown Ottawa. Dr. J. Krop in Mississauga, whose primer in environmental medicine I published and gave you copies of, is a Fellow of the AAEM and annually teaches courses on diagnosis and treatment of MCS. He is one of the researchers and clinicians who signed the 1999 international consensus statement on MCS. His input would undoubtedly be most valuable to this exercise.
- A consultation with representatives of patient advocacy groups, such as you have now had with RAINET already, would probably also be most helpful. The Ottawa-based *Environmental Illness Society of Canada* comes to mind, of course, as does the *Environmental Hypersensitivity Association of Ontario*.
- Forming a committee, or working through an existing one, with Health Canada for the purpose of following up on the recommendation made in May 2000 by the Standing Committee on Environment and Sustainable Development: *"The Committee recommends that Health Canada take the necessary steps to bring about legal recognition of multiple chemical sensitivity syndrome."* (p.55) The object of this interdepartmental discussion would be the recognition of MCS, the coverage of its treatment by Medicare, and the initiation of a program for MCS patients that provide them with financial assistance while helping them to get cured (if possible) or to recover sufficiently to become functional and financially independent in a safe environment. MCS is more than a disease: it is an education.

MCS is a disability unlike any other. While it is the duty of your department to assist those Canadian citizens who are usually permanently disabled, a pro-active interface with Health Canada and, if at all possible, with the Ministry of Industry and Technology, would be most urgently indicated. People afflicted with MCS acts as the proverbial canaries in the mine. An economically viable technology, a wealth-creating industry, and a healthy population are not only possible but more likely if the lessons learned from MCS are incorporated into government policy. No country can afford a growing population of chronically ill people, nor can we afford more epidemics like AIDS or outbreaks like SARS. In conclusion, it is instructive to consider the experience of other, industrialized nation 's with MCS:

The German government funded a pilot project in 1994 and opened a hospital exclusively for environmental illness patients in the North near the Danish border in the town of Bredstett. The clinical director, Dr. Eberhard Schwarz, trained at the Environmental Health Clinic in Dallas, Texas. After the first 5 years the medical school of the University of Leibzig was asked to do an evaluation of the project measuring such scores as cost of treatments compared to conventional symptom-control oriented interventions, ability to return to work and stay in the work force, money saved on disability payments, impact on the integrity of the family, etc. The results were so impressive, the German government announced in 1999 it would open four more such hospitals throughout the country. Also, between 1990 and 2000 all German medical schools funded chairs for environmental medicine.

In the UK a similar project was undertaken at Breakespear Hospital in Hamel Hampstead. The endorsement of the Royal Family was of great help to the project. However, the fact that the Countess of Mar of the House of Lords was cured of MCS (developed through chronic exposure to sheep-dip on her sheep farm), which had disabled her completely and had become life-threatening, resulted in a tremendous impetus to research, legal reforms and increased medical acceptance.

The impressive results obtained by Dr. Garth Nicholson, mentioned earlier, should be emphasized again. His unique combination of traditional medicine (e.g. antibiotics and the classic knowledge of infectious disease etiology) with the new insights into toxicology has resulted in helping people with the most severely disabling traditional diseases (Multiple sclerosis, Amyotrophic lateral sclerosis, Systemic lupus erythematosus etc.) as well as MCS victims back to work. Encouraging are especially the positive implications for reduced costs involving health care and disability and increased economic productivity.

Helke Ferrie
KOS Publishing
1997 Beechgrove Road, Alton, Ontario, L0N 1A0,
Tel. 519-927-1049 e-mail: **Helke@inetsonic.com**

Note: *This report was prepared on the basis of personal experience, attendance at various medical conferences, interviews with physicians and MCS patients, and available medical literature sources. The information in this report does not* *pretend to be complete or even comprehensive and is likely to contain some errors of interpretation which are entirely my responsibility and will be corrected if I am made aware of them.*

Notice to MCS Victims

Below is an e-mail sent to me by one of the most active people in the fight for global recognition of MCS. Diana Buckland has been the moving force behind the current campaign to get the Australian government to recognize this condition which would lead not only to medical help becoming more readily available, but especially to preventive measures to be made law, so this increase in MCS stops. The information in this e-mail is of great value because all those links allow you to access the scientific in formation, find out about clinics and doctors who work with such patients, and the kind of political activism that you may be able to become involved in.

This is a global disease because chemicals do not know national borders. This information needs to be shared among MCS victims everywhere, so use it! RAINET and I are doing our small part to help get MCS recognized in Canada, and the chances of success are getting better, especially since the Canadian government's Standing Committee on Environment (see first article in Section 1 of this book) has already recommended such recognition. But it won't happen unless you help, too:

- write to your MPs,
- approach your Senators,
- demand action on this issue from the Canadian Medical Association,
- join or start a patient group,
- write to your local paper and ask for an article on MCS,
- suggest to your doctor to take the appropriate training at the *American Academy of Environmental Medicine,*
- write to the World Health Organization and ask what they are doing about MCS

  raise Hell, politely and determinedly in any way you can.

Feel free to contact me as well. You may download my MCS report from my website and use it: **www.kospublishing.com**

Resources

Date: Sat Mar 27, 2004 12:01:11 PM Canada/Eastern
I HAVE BEEN DOING THIS FOR SIX MONTHS STRAIGHT…SEARCHING THE
INTERNET FINDING ALL THESE KINDS OF PLACES (Environmental clinics,
websites etc.) TO SEND MY EMAIL REGARDING GLOBAL RECOGNITION CAM-
PAIGN FOR MCS AND THE AUSTRALIAN GOVERNMENT ENQUIRY.
MAY I BE SO BOLD TO ASK YOU ALL TO HELP ME BY FORWARDING TO ANY OF
THESE BRILLIANT PLACES YOU DISCOVER, MY EMAIL REGARDING THE GLOBAL
RECOGNITION CAMPAIGN AND AUSTRALIAN GOVERNMENT ENQUIRY.
Thank you—this is for the benefit of us all—I have left all my links here so you all have
access to all the info. Thanks.

Kind Regards,
Diana Buckland
4 Mia Street Kallangur, 4503 Queensland Australia
email: dbucklan@bigpond.net.au
Representative of Australian Chemical Trauma Alliance

http://members.ozemail.com.au/~actall/
Global Recognition Campaign / Multiple Chemical Sensitivity
http://www.wtv-zone.com/infchoice/mcs_australia.html
http://www.wtv-zone.com/infchoice/mcsawareness.html
http://www.wtv-zone.com/infchoice/our_garden.html
http://www.wtv-zone.com/infchoice/mcs/crippling.html
www.ehponline.org/press (Environmental Health Perspectives—more than 12% of population reports extreme sensitivity to common chemicals)
http://www.abqtrib.com/archives/opinions04/030904_opinions_mckee.shtml
http://www.universityofhealth.net/PR/3304PRUSNOMHearing.htm (Mercury warning)
http://www.dragonfleye.org/envir.htm (School Environmental Health Policy)
http://www.acaengineering.com.au (Steam Weed Control Equipment)
http://mozzierid.com.au/home.html (Mosquito Magnet) March 27, 2004 3:11 PM

ENDNOTES

[1] N.Ashford & C. Miller, *Chemical Exposures: Low Levels and High Stakes*, 2nd ed.,Van
Nostrand, 1998, p. 172

[2] A. Hoffer, *Putting It All Together: The New Orthomolecular Nutrition*, Keats, 1996, p. 163

[3] T. G. Randolph, MD, *Environmental Medicine—Beginnings and Bibliographies of Clinical
Ecology*, Clinical Ecology Publications 1987. Dr. Randolph, a professor of medicine at the
University of Chicago in the 1940s and 50s is generally credited with being the first
medical researcher to identify chemical-induced illness and to have initiated the research
into that field. Later, both Rachel Carson and Linus Pauling built on his work. P. Radetsky,
Allergic to the Twentieth Century, Little Brown & Co., 1997, is possibly the best history of
environmental illness from the 1950s to the late 1990s for the general reader.

[4] T. Kerns, *Environmentally Induced Illness: Ethics, Risk Assessment and Human Rights*, McFarland & Co., 2001, p. 13-15 summarizes EPA reports on chemical production, release and safety up to 1995, the last year for which data were available; it also contains international legal information on toxic chemicals.

[5] "Multiple Chemical Sensitivity: a 1999 consensus", in *Archives of Environmental Medicine*, Vol. 54 (3), 1999, pp. 147-49. This paper is part of RAINET's submission documents.

[6] To get an appreciation of what is involved in clinical practice, the British textbook on environmental medicine for doctors is highly recommended: H. Anthony et al, *Environmental Medicine In Clinical Practice*, BSAENM Publications 1997. The majority of the original basic science involved in MCS studies, which led to the 1999 Consensus Statement, is contained in one of the first US textbooks on the subject edited by A.B. Tarcher et al, *Principles and Practice of Environmental Medicine*, Plenum, 1992; its authors are primarily from the EPA, many US universities and several European medical schools. A current summary of what to look for in environmental illness in general is in the *Canadian Medical Association's Journal* (CMAJ) series from April 16 to June 25, 2002. The two international journals devoted to environmental medicine, including occupational medicine, are *Archives of Environmental Health* (published by the US National Institutes of Health) and *Environmental Health Perspectives* (published by the Harvard School of public Health).

[7] D.L. Davis, *When Smoke Ran Like Water: Tales of Environmental Deception and the Battle Against Pollution*, Basic Books, 2002. Professor Devra Lee Davis, a Scholar in Residence at the US National Academy of Sciences, teaches at the Carnegie Mellon University and is a Senior Advisor to the World Resources Institute in Washington DC and the World Health Organization. She has been one of my most reliable sources for the research in MCS over the past 4 years, ever since I interviewed her in 1999.

[8] S. Steingraber, *Living Downstream—An Ecologist Looks at Cancer*, Wesley, 2nd ed., 1999

[9] See proceedings of "Everyday Carcinogens: Stopping cancer before it starts". Workshop on Primary Cancer Prevention 1999, McMaster University, Hamilton, Ontario, on **www.stop-cancer.org**. The most current revised mortality statistics for cancer are in the *Journal of the American Cancer Institute*, No. 94, 2003: the over-all annual trend of increase is stated as being 2-4%, depending on the type of cancer.

[10] *Environmental Health Perspectives* vol. 110 (7), July 2002

[11] French Canadian MCS researcher, Dr. Albert Donnay, who is the research coordinator of the Johns Hopkins Multi-Center Study of MCS Immunology, in personal conversation during a medical conference in 1998 in Baltimore, Maryland, told me that the first cases of Myasthenia gravis were described by the Romans about 2,000 years ago after the city of Rome built its first city-wide sanitation system using lead pipes, a potent neurotoxin, cytotoxin and endocrine disruptor. The illness was re-discovered in 19th century Baltimore, named Neurasthenia. Sir William Osler suspected that the cause was the newly introduced gas lighting and heating. Osler he did not know that it is the carbon monoxide and nitrous dioxide released in small, steady amounts that acts as a most potent neurotoxin. In the 1960s Dr. Theron Randolph reported some 800 cases of neurological illnesses cured through the simple removal of gas appliances. Osler advised one of his patients diagnosed with "neurasthenia", to leave Baltimore and live in her New England country estate instead, where she was free from all symptoms. This patient, Mary Garrett, was the fabulously wealthy daughter of a railroad baron. She provided **all** of the seed money for the building of Johns Hopkins hospital and medical school, attaching only the condition that

women should be allowed to study medicine, a condition vigorously supported by Dr. Osler. See, M. Bright, *Sir William Osler—A Life in Medicine,* Toronto, 1999, pp.199-205,.

[12] T. Randolph, 1987, pp. 73-6. During the 1998 AAEM international conference I asked about 300 of the attending doctors why they became environmental physicians. The answer in **each and every case** was the same: he or she or a spouse had become ill with MCS and their medical training left them unprepared to deal with MCS; so they sought training in this field

[13] One example of WHO endorsement is found in a summary report published in *Scientific American*, April 2002, in an article entitled "Drink Your Shots".

[14] MCS precipitated by neurotoxic substances of the **solvent** variety is generally irreversible and causes the most serious damage; those victims are the most likely ones to apply for assistance to this Department.

[15] M. Cullen, "The Worker with Multiple Chemical Sensitivities: An Overview" in M. Cullen (ed.), *Occupational Medicine: State of the Art Reviews,* Hanley & Belfus, 1987

[16] The hundreds of individuals who eventually were forced to seek WCB, a process that lasted until 2002, were subject to the most vicious campaign by industry lobbyists to discredit their MCS diagnosis (made in many cases at Johns Hopkins Medical School and based on internationally recognized test). However, MCS expert Albert Donnay organized an information campaign for the WCB panelists who threw out the insurance industry "experts reports", investigated and judged as false their alleged "scientific" material and the applications were handled properly.

[17] A detailed history of the understanding of MCS is in N . Ashford and C. Miller, *Chemical Exposures: Low Levels and High Risks,* Van Nostrand & Reinhold, 2nd ed. 1998, chapter 7.

[18] Kilburn proved that asbestos *causes* lung cancer, the first cancer thus proven to be caused by an agent in the environment, which opened up the research into carcinogens; today 96% of all cancers are accepted as being environmentally based, and only 4% are considered genetically anchored; see S. Steingraber, *Living Downstream: An Ecologist Looks At Cancer,* 2nd ed., Wiley, 1999. The most recent landmark study involving 90,000 identical twins, showed that the polluted environment is the principal cause of cancer: *New England Journal of Medicine,* July 13, 2000.

[19] K. Kilburn, "Measuring the effects of chemicals on the brain", *Archives of Environmental Health,* No. 54 (3), p. 150 ff

[20] C.M. Ryan et al, "Cacosmia and neurobehavioral dysfunction associated with occupational exposure to mixtures of organic solvents", *American Journal of Psychiatry* No. 145: 11, Nov. 1988, pp. 1442-1445

[21] The PET and SPECT research results were presented by N. Ashford and G. Heuser at a conference held in Ottawa, May 2001, hosted by the *Environmental Illness Society of Canada.* Heuser's research is published in G. Heuser and J.C. Wu, "Deep Subcortical (including limbic) Hypermetabolism in Patients with Chemical Intolerance: Human PET Studies", *Annals of the New York Academy of Sciences,* vol. 933, 2001

[22] Among some of the best sources for this type of information on systemic conflicts of interest see Dr. Theron Randolph's history of clinical ecology, the already noted chapter 7 of Ashford & Miller's famous book), Linus Pauling in *How To Live Longer and Feel Better,* Avon, 1986, Dr. James P. Carter, *Racketeering in Medicine,* Hampton Roads Press, 1993, US Congressman D. Haley (US Congressman), *Politics in Healing,* Potomac Valley Press, 2000, J. Lisa, *The Assault on Medical Freedom,* Hampton Roads Publishing Co., 1997, the Globe

& Mail report of February 6, 2002, the editorial in the *Canadian Medical Association Journal*, Feb. 19, 2002, the Canadian Association of University Teachers' *Olivieri Report*, Toronto, 2002, and my own website which contains the *Glasnost Report* prepared by 3 medical organizations (including some OMA Sections) and several patient advocacy groups (including RAINET) **www.collegeofphysicianswatchdog.com**. A book on this subject by me, entitled *Malice in Medicine*, is in preparation for publication next year.

[23] This information is based on RAINET files, the web site of Albert Donnay, and my own attempt to become a member of ESRI: I was turned down because I was not a corporation.

[24] It occurred to me that this proposed explanation provides a parallel to the already well-known and biologically well-understood phenomenon of "bio-magnification" which occurs when a toxic substance becomes even more toxic by being passed on through the food-chain. An excellent discussion of this phenomenon and its health impacts on Canada's population is found in the Canadian government report, *Pesticides: Making The Right Choice for the Protection of Health and the Environment*, Report of the Standing committee on Environment and Sustainable Development, May 2000

[25] Sources: **wsunews@wsu.edu** and **phmartin@xtra.co.nz**

[26] Source: **www.apps.niehs.nih.gov/odconfer/gxe/home.htm** This research is in press.

[27] See chapter 10 in R.N. Proctor, *Cancer Wars*, Basic Books, 1995, for the story of this research.

[28] In the documentary film *"Exposure: Environmental Links to Breast Cancer"* produced by Women's Healthy Environments Network (WHEN) available worldwide in seven languages. It won Best Health Documentary at the International Independent Film Festival in 2001 and its producer, Dorothy Goldin Rosenberg was awarded the Governor General's Award of Canada. Contact **when@web.ca** or visit **www.whenvironments.ca**.

[29] For Dr. Nicholson's research visit the rather enormous web site **www.immed.org**
Only two of his many publications are suggested reading for the purposes of this report: G. L. Nicholson, "Diagnosis and Treatment of Mycoplasmal Infections in Persian Gulf War Illness—CFIDS Patients" in *International Journal of Occupational Medicine, Immunology and Toxicology* vol. 5, no. 1, 1996. G. L. Nicholson, "Considerations when undergoing treatment for Gulf War Illness/CFS/FMS/Rheumatoid Arthritis" in *International Journal of Medicine* 1998 Vol. 1 p. 123 ff .

[30] Our meeting in June ended with a delightful and informal brain-storming during which I was asked what I would do to assess MCS applicants. I replied that the government should avoid expensive confirmatory tests; there is no need for MRIs, SPECT's and PET scans as these are among the universally recognized tools used in *research*. The reliable and most helpful tests that were cost-effective (done in excellent Canadian laboratories) in my own and my son's case were a set of *standard blood, urine, hormone, saliva, and intracellular tests* as well as *hair analysis* and *screening tests for chemical intolerances* with which all environmental physicians are familiar. As Albert Donnay has pointed out, the blood gas tests are probably essential, as carbon monoxide poisoning is involved in 9 out of 10 MCS cases. All these are also employed in standard medicine where the doctor orders the lab to look for different markers. In an MCS patient, these tests usually confirm the history and make sense of the specific reported disability for the simple reason, that toxicology is generally accepted as an *exact* science.

8

Reform

Dr. Shiv Chopra of Health Canada and Ontario's MPP M. Kwinter: Heroes of Health Care

Vitality Magazine February 2001

Two remarkable victories for freedom of choice in health care have been achieved, which should cause champagne bottles to be uncorked across the country. A national victory came on September 5, 2000 in the Federal Court in Ottawa; and an Ontario victory occurred on December 14, 2000, in the provincial legislature.

York Centre MPP Monte Kwinter's bill is possibly the first private member's bill to become law in Ontario history. This new law, which effectively decriminalizes alternative medicine (as of Dec. 14), puts freedom of choice back in the hands of the patient, and frees up doctors to use alternative and new methods without fear of losing their medical licence.

The Kwinter Bill has taken a medical clause from the international human rights treaty, the *Helsinki Accord* (signed by Canada in 1989) and re-formulated it to decriminalizing medical innovation. It states that a doctor "shall not be found guilty of professional misconduct, or of incompetence... solely on the basis that (he or she) practices a therapy that is non-traditional or that departs from the prevailing medical practice, unless there is evidence that proves that the therapy poses a greater risk to the patient's health than the traditional or prevailing practice."

The need for the Kwinter Bill arose out of the righteous anger of thousands of patients who lost their doctors to the kangaroo courts of the CPSO (College of Physicians & Surgeons of Ontario) which uses the disciplinary process to remove from practice doctors using drug-free medicine, as well as those MDs who anger insurance companies by taking chronic pain seriously.

Kwinter became aware of the need for such legislation when learning of Dr. Gerry Green's loss of licence for using nutritional protocols alongside standard cancer treatment. Throughout the 1990s, several hundred Ontario physicians were also prosecuted unjustly, among the most prominent being environmental medicine expert Dr. Jozef Krop. What all these doctors have in common is the use of non-pharmaceutical treatments (which cannot be patented); they also provided scientific proof for the reality of diseases that are a threat to Big Business, e.g. chemical sensitivity, sick building syndrome, fibromyalgia etc. These doctors also provided objective, scientific proof of the reality of chronic pain and disabilities caused by environmental toxins (resulting in contested insurances having to be paid).

Kwinter sponsored this bill in 1997 and piloted it through four years of stormy medical politics assisted by the dogged determination of Citizens for Choice in Health Care, Voices on Health Care Concerns, Consumers Health Organization of Canada, and many patient and physician groups. The 4-year battle involved Liberals, the NDP and Conservatives, who managed to transcend their political differences—only to be opposed by the College of Physicians and Surgeons of Ontario (CPSO) who insisted that medicine would never be the same again if this bill became law.

Very true! It puts a brake on their bullying of environmental, holistic, homeopathic, naturopathic and chelation therapy doctors. Literally until the last day—December 11, when the committee hearings took place prior to third and final reading of the bill—the CPSO tried to scuttle it. They went on record stating that such legislation would allow doctors to "wrap babies in cabbage leaves to treat pneumonia". This nonsense backfired and helped increase support for the bill.

(When an identical bill was introduced by Roy Bressard in the Alberta legislature, and passed unanimously 1997, it was vigorously opposed by the Alberta Pharmaceutical Association who objected on the grounds that it "creates the possibility that a physician cannot be prosecuted for practicing non-traditional medicine"—impacting on revenues from patent medicines!)

In Ontario, mainstream physicians joined forces with alternative doctors supporting Kwinter individually as well as in groups: two Ontario Medical Association sections (on complementary medicine, chaired by Dr. Linda Rapson and on chronic pain, chaired by Dr. Peter Rothbart) supported the Canadian Society for Environmental Medicine, Gatekeepers of Health, and others in endorsing Kwinter's bill.

On December 14, during third reading, Kwinter read parts of Dr. Rothbart's submission into the legislature's *Hansard* record: "This [bill's] core notion is that the needs of the patient are central to medical practice, that patient outcomes matter most, that alleviating suffering is what medicine is all about... I urge you to pass Bill 2 in the name of medicine."

During the December 11 committee hearings on the Kwinter Bill, MPP Richard Patton of Ottawa provided unexpected human drama by adding to his supportive statements that having recently been diagnosed with cancer himself, "my perspective changed quite dramatically". He had found "that our so-called western conventional medical model is a very, very narrow model". He was deeply impressed by the help he received from naturopaths, saying, "I see the need, obviously, for a more holistic approach." The government, led by Premier Mike Harris, created some real Christmas magic when on December 14, Kwinter's amendment to the *Medicine Act* was finally passed with unanimous consent; it received royal assent on December 21 and is expected to be proclaimed formally by the end of this month.

Over the past decade, as the CPSO prosecutions of some of Ontario's finest and most highly trained doctors escalated, it became clear that a major house-cleaning is needed at the CPSO. OMA Pain Section's Dr. Peter Rothbart was joined by many doctors at a press conference held on November 15, 2000, at Queen's Park, demanding the resignation of the Deputy Registrar of the CPSO, Dr. John Carlisle, who for the past decade has masterminded these unjustified prosecutions against innovative doctors. Last year, criminal lawyer, Michael Code, formerly with the Ontario Attorney General's department, concluded that those doctors' cases, which he spent a year examining, show clear evidence of "abuse of power" and, in one case, even "criminal obstruction of justice".

The medical and citizens' groups, which helped to get the Kwinter bill passed, have since approached the Ontario government asking that the CPSO be radically reformed (requiring Dr. Carlisle's resignation to start with), that all current disciplinary cases be reviewed independently, and doctors' cases unjustly prosecuted be reopened with the view to restore those licenses.

The fact that the government pushed a private member's bill through and rushed it to royal assent is sending a strong message to the CPSO that the government knows that the practice of medicine cannot continue to be hijacked by an old boys' club and their corporate friends. After all, Canadian health care is in crisis, cancer and chronic illness are at epidemic levels, and regardless of one's political philosophy, health care must somehow be made to work. And, of course, nothing evaporates differing political philosophies as fast as personal experience with sickness. As Kwinter told me, "Just about all of us [parliamentarians] take vitamins, and many consult complementary medical practitioners."

Alaska was the first jurisdiction to pass a Kwinter Bill-type law. Licensing authorities in any province or state, where an Alaska Clause type bill is now law, face a new situation: the onus of proof of harm is on the licensing authority with respect to any new diagnostic technique or treatment method: it must prove that they are more harmful than currently used methods. Alaska Clause/Kwinter Bill-type legislation is a powerful tool for achieving health freedom because it puts the patients' choice as well as patient-outcome at the centre of medical practice. The licensing authorities must familiarize themselves to the satisfaction of legal proof with whatever they wish to condemn. They can no longer pre-judge. Now Alberta, Nova Scotia and Ontario have this health freedom legislation, as do many U.S. states.

This changes the climate radically. As a result, this summer, California repealed the law that had made chemotherapy, surgery and radiation the only mandatory cancer treatments. The U.S. National Cancer Institute joined forces with the National Institutes of Health and the FDA in initiating large-scale, formal evaluations of nutritional cancer therapy—headed by nutritional experts, so it is not a rigged exercise.

The second remarkable court victory occurred on Sept. 5, 2000 in Ottawa, when Federal Justice D. Tremblay-Lamer ruled that Health Canada had no business placing a gag order on two of their chief scientists, Dr. Shiv Chopra and Dr. Margaret Haydon. As a result, Health Canada no longer has any legal means by which to prevent its own scientists from informing the public directly if they believe they are being pressured by industry or government to approve a food or drug that is unsafe.

The issue originally ended up in court because these scientists had stated on CBC's Canada AM radio program (June 11, 1998) that our food supply is unsafe, because Health Protection Branch scientists are often pressured to approve drugs for animal and human consumption even though they are known carcinogens and immune system disruptors. During the court case against Health Canada, all 200 Health Canada scientists supported Drs. Chopra and Haydon, as did the 36,000-member Canadian civil service union! As a result, a bovine growth hormone was not approved, and Senator Eugene Whelan's 1998 public inquiry exposed the high level corruption involving Health Canada and life-sciences corporations like Monsanto.

In May last year the defense for the gagged scientists was handled by constitutional lawyer Andrew Raven. The court's resulting decision stated that "where a matter is of legitimate public concern requiring public debate, the [civil servant's] duty of loyalty cannot be absolute to the extent of preventing public disclosure by a government official [the Minister of Health]". After citing famous whistle blowers like Daniel Ellsberg (who exposed the illegality of the Vietnam War) and Karen Silkwood (who was murdered for exposing the crimes of the nuclear power industry) Justice Tremblay-Lamer stated: "I am of the opinion, that preventing [the scientists] from going to the media, in cases of legitimate safety or health concerns regarding policies within Health Canada, is unreasonable." In other words, the gag on the scientists had been lifted. The federal government, threatened by whistle blowers in virtually every department, scrambled to find a way to appeal this decision. After intense debate, the lawyers for the government admitted that nothing in Canada's legal history or statutes supported an appeal—and so the September 5 decision stands unchallenged.

Shortly before Christmas, the pharmaceutical giant Hoechst approached Dr. Chopra and his colleagues regarding approval of a new hormone that increases muscle bulk in bovines and sheep. The hormone is a known cancer trigger and a tumour growth promoter, i.e. a so-called "complete carcinogen". This fact was fully known to both Hoechst and Dr. Chopra. One such carcinogenic hormone is already in Canada's meat supply and was one reason why Drs. Chopra and Haydon went public back in 1998. Dr. Chopra told Hoechst that they could, of course, try once again to bypass the Health Protection Branch, as often in the past, and attempt to get ministerial approval without mandatory scientific safety assessment. However, he added that the Federal Court ruling of December 5 had leveled the playing field and there was nothing to stop him from getting public debate involved! Hoechst backed off.

So whether you prefer champagne or herbal tea, it's time to raise a toast to our public heroes: Ontario's MPP Kwinter and Health Canada's Shiv Chopra and Margaret Haydon, for the remarkable victories they have achieved on behalf of all Canadians.

Sources

Ontario Government *Hansard* for December 11 and 14th, 2000, regarding the amendment to the *Medicine Act*, Bill 2 available at website:
www.ontl/session1/committees/gengov/G040

Justice Tremblay-Lamer's decision of September 5, 2000, is obtainable at the Federal Court, Trial Division, tel. 613-992-4238 or through www.fct-cf.gc.ca, look for the decision of that date.

Update October 2004: *It looks like bovine growth hormone is disappearing from the market at last. Read about it on* **ttp://www.notmilk.com/pelican. html.** *Dr. Chopra won several more actions against Health Canada and was fired in June 2004. A case for wrongful dismissal is now in the courts and supported by the civil service union.*

A Tale of Three Conferences

Vitality Magazine September 2001

In the late 1800s the writer and physician Oliver Wendell Holmes observed: "The mind, once stretched, never regains its original dimensions." The three medical conferences reported here will irrevocably stretch many minds. In May the 30th Annual Conference on Nutritional Medicine was held in Toronto by the International Society for Orthomolecular Medicine which also celebrated the 100th birthday of Linus Pauling, its founder. Later that month, the First International Environmental Illness Conference took place in Ottawa, held by the Environmental Illness Society of Canada and the University of Calgary. In June the University of Toronto had its Complementary Medicine 2001 conference. A grand medical chorus, they proclaimed truth, provided help, and raised profoundly disturbing questions.

The most startling conclusion was that we know the causes of most diseases, how to prevent virtually all of those, and can effectively treat, arrest, ease and even cure them. So, what's going on?

The consensus was that mind and body are an indivisible unity made sick by an increasingly dead and toxic diet, a poisoned environment, and psychological trauma. Astonishingly, body and soul appear to have a near infinite capacity to heal, if treated with the respect Nature deserves. Esther Sternberg is the Chief of the Neuroendocrine Immunology Section of the US National Institutes of Health and the author of the beautiful exposition of the science which connects health and emotions, *The Balance Within* (2000). At the U of T conference she presented a magisterial overview of the communication between the central nervous system and the immune system in the process of illness-causing physical and emotional stress. She said, that while the variability in resistance to stress is genetically set at 35%, "the other 65% is entirely environmentally determined" and thus open to intelligent control or reckless disregard. "We need to change our physical environment to meet the body's demands," she said. She told of the Volvo company replacing the assembly line with small worker groups in charge of the entire car building process, installing openable windows, live plants and brightly painted socializing areas in all their factories, thereby reducing stress everywhere and—naturally—increasing productivity. Management did this when learning of the high incidence of heart disease, hypertension, stroke and depression among workers in traditional car plants.

Providing historical context, Dr. E. Leyton pointed to the dramatic dietary and environmental changes our bodies must handle, mostly in the last 50 years. This is 0.003% of the last two million years of human evolution. It is hardly surprising, that not only our metabolism is in shock, but our very genetic code is under stress, as it tries to build cells and tissues from flawed or missing raw materials. Providing US government research data, Dr. Leyton showed how our depleted soils, pre-ripe harvesting, transportation and processing methods all conspire to deplete our food of all those essential nutrients we have taken for granted for the past few million years. A hunter-gatherer in Australia and Africa enjoys the nutrient and fiber density, enormous vitamin C intake, and basic exercise our culture no longer provides. It is well documented that those "primitives" don't develop cancer and chronic illness until they switch to the Western life style. Nutrition expert, Dr. T. Barnard supported these observations from his own work adding a quote from a medical researcher (speaking about our fast dead-food culture), "When you pass through those Golden Arches, you are on your way to the Pearly Gates."

The obstacles blocking health are (1) an outdated medical model desperately in need of systems and complexity thinking, (2) an economy based on the notion that greed is good, and (3) the body's tendency to defend against physical and mental assaults by adapting temporarily through addiction until it can no longer hold off the collapse into disease.

The obvious solution to these three interlinked obstacles is zero tolerance for poisons, the precautionary principle as a universal social value, the acknowledged human right of patient freedom of choice in medicine, and legal protection from harassment for innovative doctors. These conferences contributed greatly towards focusing on this vision, the creation of a map for action, and the establishment of solid facts—all prerequisite for such an achievement, even if it takes another century to be realized.

The Politics of Health

At the U of T conference, MPP Monte Kwinter told the story of the passage of his private member's bill which he piloted through a formidable political obstacle course until it became law last December with unanimous parliamentary and immense public support. The greatest opposition came from the College of Physicians and Surgeons, Ontario's medical licensing body, which warned the Premier babies would be wrapped in cabbage leaves to treat pneumonia and that sexual assault by psychiatrists would be condoned as a novel treatment. The fact is, however, that the Kwinter Bill was designed to stop the harassment of innovative doctors through CPSO disciplinary action in the absence of patient complaints.

Two such victimized doctors spoke at these conferences: environmental medicine physician Dr. Jozef Krop (12 years in disciplinary harassment) and nutritional and geriatric medicine specialist Dr. Tom Barnard (recently accused by the CPSO of suggesting patients eat healthier foods). MPP Kwinter observed, "The CPSO does things that require some sort of surveillance because they are doing things that make no sense." Indeed! In spite of the Kwinter Bill being law, international pain expert Dr. Frank Adams of Kingston was prosecuted without patient mishap or complaint and in the face of immense public protest. He was forced to leave Canada in March. Last month, Dr. S. Kooner of Windsor, "guilty" of extraordinary success in the treatment of asthma mostly without using drugs, was declared to have fallen below the standard of medical practice. The CPSO wants to revoke his license—yet, no patient was harmed or complained. Both doctors have huge public support. Their cases will now necessitate testing the Kwinter Bill in court. (*See details in Section 5 of this book.*)

Dr. Heather Boon, a U of T pharmacology faculty member and co-author of a textbook on medicinal herbs, described in her presentation on the safety and efficacy of neuroactive herbs (e.g. St. John's Wort, Ginko Biloba etc.), how mainstream research all too frequently alters protocols and dosages (in plain English: cheats) and then misrepresents their effects by inappropriately interpreting the results in a linear fashion. Of course, herbs are not patentable.

Internationally renowned researcher, Dr. Garth Nicholson, Director of the California based Institute of Molecular Medicine, told how military hospital labs deliberately employed destructive techniques to his Gulf War veteran patient samples. They knew that the biologically active substances they would otherwise have found were actually US patented biological warfare bugs—a secret more important to protect than to assist in the cure of their afflicted citizens.

It is now generally acknowledged that pesticides cause cancer and Parkinson's disease. Back in 1979 a US presidential committee advised against their widespread use because bugs and people share the same nervous system enzymes—but industry won out. Autism researcher Dr. B. Rimland, reported how every effort was made by mainstream medicine to downplay and even falsify the facts showing that the triple vaccine for mumps, measles and rubella, introduced in 1978, triggered the horrendous increase in childhood autism. Prior to the MMR vaccine 4-5 children per 10,000 births were autistic; now it is 1 in 150 kids, a 1,000% increase. The FDA knowingly allowed the industry to use up its mercury-contaminated stocks. A huge class action suit has begun and is fought by the same lawyers who brought down Big Tobacco.

Even though detection methods have vastly improved, the cancer rate has steadily increased, mortality has remained the same, and the 5-year post-diagnosis survival rate has remained unchanged. Yet, the non-toxic treatment methods with nutritional and orthomolecular protocols developed by Drs. Gonzales, Gerson, Hoffer, Pauling, Clark, Issels and others have been attacked for decades as quackery. Dr. Gonzales almost got kicked out of medical school for publishing a paper in the Journal of Orthomolecular Medicine.

Dr. B. Berkson, an expert on Alpha Lipoic Acid was asked to monitor the death of some liver cancer patients while still an intern in the 60s. He contacted the National Institutes of Health and learned that in Czechoslovakia and the former USSR, liver cancer was often being cured with Alpha Lipoic Acid. He had it flown in, gave it to the dying patients, and they went home healthy two weeks later. When the next liver-diseased patient came up, he was specifically told by his chief not to use Alpha Lipoic Acid! He did anyway and cured him and nearly got fired. His internationally published research is mostly supported and advanced by European universities. He provided breath-taking case histories of successful treatments also of macular degeneration, diabetes, heart disease, and stroke. In Russia, Alpha Lipoic Acid is used as first-line treatment in hospitals for strokes and heart attacks. His book is highly recommended.

One of the U of T conference organizers, Dr. Linda Rapson, is among the early pioneers who brought acupuncture to Canada almost three decades ago. She developed worldwide-accepted protocols for its spectacularly successful use in pain management in spinal chord injury victims at the Lyndhurst Center in Toronto. At the conference, she observed that progress in medicine can only occur when the patient is in control and doctors and patient work as a team. Amen!

New Vision

Born at the cost of immense human suffering, truth is ultimately indestructible. The non-toxic treatments for cancer are now being seriously studied at the National Institute of Health (NIH) in the US; preliminary results indicate that protocols involving coffee enemas, nutritional and mega vitamin therapy have the leading edge over chemotherapy. Dr. Rapson and her colleagues were recently able to persuade Health Canada to include research of complementary and alternative medicine in the mandate of the new research institutes patterned after the NIH.

Dr.Lynn Marshall, Director of the Environmental Health Clinic at Toronto's Women's College Hospital (WCH), and her colleagues formulated detailed and up-to-date guidelines on how to diagnose and treat environmentally induced illness for the College of Family Physicians. Dr. R. Bray, also at WCH, pulled no punches when calling for the full and proper labeling of water. She advised following the lead of other countries and ban neurotoxic artificial sweeteners, institute zero tolerance on thyroid damaging food colorings, asthma triggering sulfites, neurotoxic MSG, and heavy metals.

Dr. J. Molot, President of the Canadian Society for Environmental Medicine, provided the details on the development of the North American 1999 Consensus Definition in conjunction with Johns Hopkins Medical School, now internationally accepted and published in the Archives of Environmental Health (May 1999 vol 54/3). This is no empty gesture: at the NIH environmental illness expert Dr. Claudia Miller has been put in charge of an entire new division mandated to research this field. It's no longer all in your head, but becoming part of the medical textbooks—and not of the psychiatric ones either.

Dr. G. Heuser of UCLA provided the PET scan evidence for environmental illness showing how toxic chemicals and correct treatment effect the brain. His research into the pathophysiology of environmental illness and practical help are accessible through on **www.toxgun.com**.

The Ottawa conference hosted several of these internationally respected experts who had a few days earlier been invited to address the National Defense Department of Canada on environmental illness. Since the military establishments of the world are among the worst polluters, this was amazing. The big brass sat and listened, no questions or comments were allowed. Time will tell what effect this will have.

Professor D. Davis of U of T outlined the way complementary medicine is now being integrated into the teaching of medical students, starting in the undergraduate years. We are catching up with the Renaissance, Dr. Sternberg observes: four hundred years ago over the entrance of Padua's famous university was written "Universa Universit Patavina Libertas" (Here in Padua all are free to study all).

How pressingly important such measures have become is brought home by the study on the socio-economic impact of our toxic environment commissioned by the EI Society of Canada. One in 8 Canadian adults is affected; one in 50 can't work because of environmental illness. This causes an annual loss of $10 billion in productivity and $ 1 billion in taxes. Of those affected about 60% become homeless or end in suicide, thereby causing an additional burden on social services.

In the State of Utah the legal system has caught on that juvenile delinquency has a lot to do with toxins in food, air and water, Dr. J. Ross reported in Ottawa. Judges now regularly offer repeat offenders the choice between jail or medical detoxification while placed under probation. The results have been so dramatic that judges have started to order detoxification even for first time offenders.

Hard Truths

The clinical case material presented at all three conferences was of such excellence, practical value, and encyclopedic knowledge, that my advice is to purchase the tapes on these presentations listed at the end. Hand a copy to your family doctor: a new era of patient-doctor collaboration is at hand.

Dr. Barnard's lecture provided important information on essential fatty acids, enzymes, nutrition, and prevention of disease. Gynecologist Dr. A. Pettle's immense knowledge of the interaction between hormones, diet, and psyche may put you at last on the path to recovery from migraines, PMS, depression, and obesity. Having suffered much from clueless gynecologists until I discovered their alternatives, I muttered passionately, "Yes! Right on!" as I listened to him. Equally excellent was Dr. B. Bronson's presentation on her research into the brain chemistry of women and the importance of understanding why pharmaceutical hormone products are so dangerous and natural products preferable.

For those battling with Gulf War Syndrome, and some of the terrible autoimmune diseases, great news is found in the presentation by Dr. Nicolson. Dr. J. Krop showed a fantastic, non-simulated movie tracking the actual destruction of nerves by mercury vapor as it arises from dental fillings. It is available on the internet through the University of Calgary. He provided the details on the protocol for mercury amalgam removal.

A most exciting section of the U of T conference dealt with the interface of spirituality, near-death experiences, and the biology and treatment of post-traumatic stress (PTSD). Dr. A. Newberg, who researches the biology of religious experience, and Dr. Y. Kason, a near-death experience researcher, announced that in the latest Diagnostic and Statistical Manual of the American Psychiatric Association, religious experience is no longer listed as a disease! The spontaneous image this brought to mind was a huge, uproarious chorus of laughter arising from Jesus, Buddha, Mohammed, Chunag Tzu and all the saints of history.

The presentation and workshop by Dr. J. Young on EMDR in treatment of PTSD provided me with the deep satisfaction a writer sometimes is granted: Dr. Young became an EMDR therapist after reading an article on it written by my EMDR practicing physician husband and me in 1997.

What is Complementary?

A big mystery remains. After considering all these mind-stretching facts, what on earth is all this supposed to be complementary to? What is "standard", and do we even want to know? Is the car complementary to the horse and buggy? Is the computer complementary to the manual typewriter? Dr. T. Barnard was right when observing this "is fundamental, good medicine."

Sources and Resources

On autism: **www.austismresearchinstitute.com**

On Gulf War Syndrome and some chronic autoimmune diseases; **www.immed.org**

For science based information on vitamins and supplements, nothing beats the Linus Pauling Institute: **www.lpi.orst.edu**

For orthomolecular/nontoxic psychiatry e-mail **centre@orthomed.org**

For herbal medicine subscribe to *The Canadian Journal of Herbalism* 416-536-1509

From *Complementary Medicine 2001* (conference no 010615) through Audio Archives of Canada 905-889-6555: on nutrition and disease Dr. Tom Barnard (050), Drs. Barnard, Burford-Mason, Leyton (170); on healing psychological trauma with EMDR: Dr. J. Young (180/181); on women's health issues: Dr. A. Pettle (190)

From the *Nutritional Medicine Today* (conference no 010503): on autism Dr. B. Rimland (110), on Alpha-Lipoic Acid and insulin resistance Dr. B. Berkson (090), on dysbiosis and all gut problems Dr. A. Bested (080), to learn how fantastic recoveries were achieved through orthomolecular medicine: the FORUM panel tapes with Margot Kidder and friends (050 & 055)

From the *Environmental Illness* conference call Conference Tape at 613-824-2583 for the tapes of Dr. G.H. Ross on Environmental Medicine, Dr. G. Nicholson on Mycoplasma, and Dr. J. Krop on mercury amalgam.

B. Berkson, *The Alpha Lipoic Acid Breakthrough,* 1998

P. Breggin, *Toxic Psychiatry,* 1994

Dossey, L. *Healing Words: The Power of Prayer and the Practice of Medicine,* 1997

M. Gershon, *The Second Brain,* 1994

J. Glenmullen, *Prozac Backlash,* 2000

Y. Kason, *Farther Shores,* 1994

Newberg, *Why God Won't Go Away,* 2001

U. Reiss, *Natural Hormone Balance for Women,* 2001

E. Sternberg, *The Balance Within: The Science Connecting Health and Emotions,* 2000

When Two Worlds of Medicine Clash...the World of Orthomolecular Medicine Comes Up a Winner

Vitality Magazine June 2003

Early in April, at the height of the SARS scare, among the many events can-celled in Toronto was the conference of the international society of cancer researchers (15,000 registered to attend) because they feared contracting or taking home the SARS virus. The 32nd annual conference of the Interna-tional Society for Orthomolecular Medicine (ISOM) never even considered canceling. In his welcoming address Dr. Gert Schuitemaker remarked, "We have no fear of contracting or passing on SARS. We just increase our daily doses of vitamin C, Selenium and Zinc and we know we are just fine." The contrast between two utterly different worlds of modern medicine is astounding: the high-tech crowd is scared and admits helplessness. The low-tech crowd fears nothing, because their medicine is founded on an insight that confers ultimate personal and scientific security, best summed up in the words of the 18th century scientist Francis Bacon who observed, "We control Nature by obeying her."

Two Medical Paradigms

The assumptions informing the SARS scare are similar to ancient fears of angry, arbitrary gods who need to be understood (sequence the virus' genome) and propitiated with their very own ritual to be observed in perpe-tuity (develop a vaccine) which is very lucrative for the high priests (phar-maceutical companies). By contrast, understanding disease in terms of orthomolecular medicine places physicians and patients into an intelligent dialogue with Nature's healing powers.

Not surprising to an orthomolecular doctor is the fact that SARS mortal-ity (326 dead worldwide by May) involved only people immune-compro-mised through bad nutrition or pre-existing health conditions (*Lancet*, May 3, 2003). SARS patients develop viral pneumonia, potentially fatal due to the destruction of the oxygen-carrying alveoli in the lungs. An inflammation-producing protein, known as tumor necrosis factor, is overproduced as the immune system goes into hyper-alarm. Standard medicine combats that with steroids and anti-viral drugs, which can cause dangerous anemia and suppress the immune system—that system which sounded its alarm in the first place because it was already too weak to fight.

Compared to orthomolecular medicine, this standard medical reasoning strikes one as terrifyingly prehistoric. What a SARS patient really needs is a *boost* to the immune system, not its suppression. Paradoxically, standard medicine agrees that recovery depends entirely on the immune system eventually mounting a successful defence against the virus. The only substances, which enable such a defense, are vitamins C and E, the minerals selenium and zinc, and bioflavonoids like quercetin and myricetin (found in organically grown red onions, apple peel, berries, tea, wine and certain vegetables). Why standard medicine doesn't read the mainstream journals, such as the *Journal of Medical Virology* is a mystery, for there the information is found on how these substances in mega-doses kill both RNA and DNA viruses by boosting the immune system into appropriate responses. Basic biochemistry fortunately informs the Beijing zookeepers: they are feeding their animals huge amounts of vitamins to ensure they don't catch SARS (*New York Times*, May 10, 2003).

Not only did the ill-prepared immune systems of some people over-react dangerously, but so did the whole world, according to virus expert and Nobel laureate David Baltimore, Stephen Lewis of the UN's AIDS program, and the relief organization *Doctors Without Borders*. They pointed out that over the last six months, a North American had a 10,000 times greater chance of dying from ordinary flu than from SARS (every day 55 people die of regular flu).

SARS Mystery

SARS may be more than another nasty virus. One of the key SARS researchers, Dr. Frank Plummer of Canada's National Microbiology Laboratory disagreed with the World Health Organization's assertion that SARS is caused by a specific corona virus, because only 40% of SARS patients tested were found to have it. Corona viruses mutate often in hours, but strangely this one didn't change in seven weeks. Really "weird" said Dr. Plummer, is the fact that the samples taken from people all over the world were genetically identical—a unique finding for a virus which adapts rapidly to local conditions and ought to have been different in every sample. Furthermore, some people, who recovered from this virus, became ill again: same-strain coronavirus infections were totally unknown, until now.

Fundamentally unnatural is the fact that this virus is a hybrid: one side is like a virus that causes respiratory disease, the other looks like one that causes hepatitis and pneumonia (*New Scientist* April 26, 2003). Nature does not go in for genetic recombinant technology. Are 60% of cases just regular viral pneumonia patients? And are the remaining 40% "real" SARS cases the result of an experiment gone wrong, as speculated in the international journal *Virology* (No. 77, 2003)?

Indeed Canada's University of Western Ontario virologist and anti-GMO activist Prof. Joe Cummins wondered why the "large body of reports on the genetic manipulation of corona viruses" is ignored and suggests that the SARS virus might well be a "a unique virus that arose as a laboratory accident or purposeful experiment." (From interview with Bill Sardi) The biotech companies Prodigene and Monsanto used coronaviruses to make an oral live-stock vaccine (projected market: US $ 140 billion by 2020). Indeed, it is vaccines that all biotech companies are now pinning their hopes on, as reported in *Nature* (April 24, 2003) as the "industry is battling for survival". Its stocks fell by 50% in the past two years because of waning investor confidence and increasing worldwide rejection of GMO foods. However, China granted permits for those vaccine experiments and China's Guangdong province is the epicenter of classic SARS from where it spread across the world.

A Sane Medicine that Works

The late great chemist Linus Pauling (two time Nobel prize winner) coined the term orthomolecular in 1968, meaning "right molecule": "Treatment of disease is a matter of varying the concentration of substances (right molecules) normally present in the body." Orthomolecular medicine is based on two principles: First, illness is seen as a biochemical alarm reaction caused by inadequately nourished cells unable to support bodily systems. Specific vitamins, amino acids, minerals, coenzymes etc. need replenishing to restore function. Inadequate nutrition comes from processed foods and pesticides which kill essential nutrients, a repetitive mono-diet lacking sufficient organic fresh fruits and vegetables, and acquired addictions to sugar, alcohol, tobacco, and other toxic substances such as artificial sweeteners and anti-depressant drugs.

Second, it is acknowledged that everybody is biochemically different due to variation in the personal history of biological and emotional stress, nutrition, genetic endowment, and cultural habits. Orthomolecular medicine has broad therapeutic guidelines, which are then fine-tuned to individual needs. Even hereditary diseases are seen as indications that this person has unusual requirements for a specific nutrient. Treatment involves nutrients because drugs (temporarily useful in an emergency) are *designed to interfere* with the body's dynamics, i.e. its enzyme system, while nutrients always and unfailingly work as constructive helpers for those enzymes.

This year's Orthomolecular conference was dedicated to the memory of David Horrobin who sadly died in his 50s on April 1. He lived long enough to see his life's work on the diseases caused by essential fatty acid (EFAs) deficiencies replicated and accepted by mainstream medicine. His research was the largest and most successful assault on poisons like Ritalin and antidepressants. Harvard University and Johns Hopkins Medical school confirmed that EFAs are the central players in a family of conditions ranging from hyperactivity to schizophrenia and include diabetes, thyroid diseases, asthma and allergies (*Medical Post* April 29, 2003). Horrobin began his research career after being fired as medical director from a New York psychiatric hospital in the 1970s because his dietary interventions cured even the most chronic mental patients so rapidly that hospital profits were threatened.

This conference always begins with the FORUM at which patients speak of their experiences with orthomolecular medicine. The FORUM has been organized for years by Robert Sealey, a chartered accountant whose mind and life were saved by Dr. Hoffer after escaping the living hell of standard psychiatry. His books now offer practical help and guidance for victims of mental disorders. He is of special help to people, whose manic-depression wrecked their finances, as he can show them the road back to financial and mental balance.

The testimonies included a Princeton University theologian who suffered a cortisone-induced psychosis after contact with poison oak. Misdiagnosed for years and drugged out of whatever mind remained, she finally was rescued and now rescues others from the same possible fate. A young musician and his mother described the descent into florid insanity (and the painstaking, dramatic stages of complete recovery) following exposure to street drugs, allergy-inducing foods and an especially high sensitivity to the toxicity of tobacco. The film by Hollywood star Margot Kidder (of "Superman"), "Masks of Madness", was also shown. It is impossible to attend a FORUM meeting and not be profoundly shaken and overwhelmingly grateful that doctors like Abraham Hoffer exist in this world.

The scientific presentations, in addition to Dr. Hoffer's marvelous overview of the history of orthomolecular medicine, included presentations on new discoveries about Vitamin B3 by Dr. Jonathan Prousky, Vitamin D by Dr. Reinhold Vieth, and addiction research into curing alcoholism, street drugs and antidepressants by Dr. Joan Mathews Larson. These presentations were so outstanding, the reader is urged to order the tapes and organize their own orthomolecular conference at home for family and friends.

Dr. Hoffer told, how in the 1950s he realized one day that the chemical structure of mescaline, LSD, and certain proteins our bodies produce under stress are all hallucinogens. Testing his psychiatric patients confirmed this insight, which eventually led to the understanding that such stress-based imbalances were mediated through the lack of EFAs, as Dr. Horrobin later proved.

Dr. Prousky reported of his successful new uses of vitamin B3 (niacin) for classic migraine, for example. The flush-producing pure B3 opens the constricted blood supply within minutes. In severe allergic reactions B3 works quickly and dramatically because it causes T cells to release the body's healing histamine.

Dr. Vieth, a Canadian researcher and world expert on Vitamin D reported on the new RDA's based on his work, namely a minimum of 1,000 units daily. His research explores this vitamin's effect on preventing osteoporosis, cancer and chronic disease.

Dr. Larson is internationally famous for her work with alcoholism treated as a nutritional deficiency response. While AA can claim only a success rate of 40% (followed up for 7 years), her treatment boasts a success rate of 75% followed up over 20 years. Her work now has expanded to include curing victims of food-mediated and anti-depressant-induced addictions. The case histories she reported from her institute were jaw-droppers. An extraordinary experience in childhood eventually guided her towards orthomolecular medicine: her family had invited a blind child for a summer vacation and, along with the other children in the house, she had been given cod liver oil daily. By the end of the summer the child's sight was fully restored.

The conference also celebrated Dr. Hoffer's 85th birthday. Having spent his life showing how processed, sugar-laden foods cause mental and physical illness, it comes as sweet vindication that the World Health Organization published its report, "Diet, Nutrition and the Prevention of Chronic Disease" on April 23. In it the WHO tells the food and soft drink industry to reduce sugar to 10% of caloric intake from 25%, and remove vending machines from schools. As reported in *The Medical Post May* 13, 2003, the Sugar Association's president Andrew Briscoe wrote to the WHO Director-General that he would see to it that the US would stop its financial contribution to the WHO if the report were not withdrawn. The WHO made the threat public and stood firm.

Are intimations of a Golden Age of Medicine coming into focus, promising that medicine will serve humanity once again instead of Big Business? History has given us some intimations of the epidemiology of good nutrition: During World War I Denmark suffered a severe drought as well as the Allied food blockade. The government slaughtered 80% of the country's livestock and fed the grain (mostly vitamin- and mineral-rich rye and wheat bran) to its citizens instead. Mortality from all causes fell by 17% and when the great pandemic influenza of 1918 struck (killing 40 million people worldwide in one year), Denmark was virtually spared completely.

In England during World War II refined flour became unavailable: the population was healthier after the war than before. In addition to the need for healthy food, a real "war on drugs" is needed—those mostly symptom-controlling and nutrient-depleting pharmaceutical phantoms on which our government spends annually $ 2 billion more than on medical services (*Medical Post* May 13, 2003). Those and the genetically engineered freaks the food industry tries to force us to eat are, however, most successfully combated by consumer resistance and conscious engagement with "the right molecules". An orthomolecular way of life offers the way to health.

Sources and Resources

J.M. Larson, *Seven Weeks To Sobriety*, Ballantine, 1997

J.M. Larson, *Depression-Free Naturally*, Ballantine, 2001

Hoffer, M.D., *Orthomolecular Medicine for Physicians*, Keats, 1989

Hoffer, M.D., *Vitamin C & Cancer: Discovery, Recovery, Controversy*, Quarry Books, 2000

Hoffer, M.D., *Hoffer's Laws of Natural Nutrition*, Quarry, 2001

Hoffer, M.D., *Vitamin B 3 and Schizophrenia*, Quarry, 1998

Hoffer, M.D., *Putting It All Together: The New Orthomolecular Nutrition*, Keats, 1996

D. Horrobin ed., *Phospholipid Spectrum Disorders in Psychiatry*, Marius, UK, 1999 (this is the definitive text on the relationship between essential fatty acids and the brain)

R.P. Huemer ed., *The Roots of Molecular Medicine: A Tribute to Linus Pauling*, Freeman, 1986

M. Lyon, M.D., *Healing The Hyperactive Brain*, Focused Publishing, 2000

R. Sealey, *Finding Care for Depression*, Sear Publications, 2002

S. Simmie & J. Nunes, *The Last Taboo*, McClelland & Stewart, 2002

R. J. Williams MD et al, *A Physician's Handbook on Orthomolecular Medicine*, Keats, 1979

R.J. Williams, *Biochemical Individuality*, Keats, 1998

The conference presentations are available on tape from Audio Archives 905-889-6555

Finding orthomolecular medical practitioners

International Society for Orthomolecular Medicine (chapters in 17 countries); in Toronto: 416-733-2117, e-mail: **centre@orthomed.org**

The Naturopathic Medical Research Clinic, Toronto 416-944-8824, **www.nmrc.ca**,, e-mail: **info@nmr.ca**

Clinic for Optimal Health, Toronto, President: Dr. V. DeMarco

Canadian College of Naturopathic Medicine, Toronto

Joan M. Larson's *Health Recovery Centre*, Minneapolis, MN, USA, offers intensive treatment for recovery from alcoholism, suicidal depression, addiction to anti-depressants 1-800-554-9155 or 612-827-7800

Mood Disorder Association of Ontario, 416-486-8049, **www.mooddisorders.on.ca**

For a comprehensive overview of SARS and systemic biases blinkering medicine see Bill Sardi's May 2003 report on the Knowledge of Health website. For full information on how to treat and prevent SARS, and any other viral disease, see Dr. Jozeph Puleo's website, the founder of the *World Natural Health Organization:* **www.wnho.net**. In Canada see **www.HealthyWorldDistributing.com** or 1-888-508-4787 or **john@cureforsars.net** (1-800-336-9266). Other recommended and reliable sources are **www.drhui.com** and **www.garynull.com** and **www.orthomed.com**

Postcards from the Road Less Travelled

Vitality Magazine February 2004

"Two roads diverged in a yellow wood,
And sorry I could not travel both
And be one traveler, long I stood
And looked down one as far as I could
To where it bent in the undergrowth ....

I shall be telling this with a sigh
Somewhere ages and ages hence:
Two roads diverged in a wood, and I –
I took the one less traveled by,
And that has made all the difference."

Robert Frost 1916

Frost's famous poem is cited usually in support of decisions made in opposition to a prevailing worldview and by people who stood their ground against the pressure of conventional wisdom. But this great poem also has the power to illuminate the very darkest corners of the human heart where decisions were made to travel roads once less traveled and which became highways of misery and death for untold numbers of people.

Consider the fact that the wealth of the pharmaceutical industry is based primarily on three classes of drugs: cholesterol lowering drugs to prevent and treat heart disease and stroke, synthetic hormone therapy, and anti-depressants. Furthermore, remember that cancer therapy has become an industry focused on chemotherapy and radiation (with or without surgery). Yet, the historical fact is that there once were two roads. Medicine chose the one we now know as the standard approach to cancer, heart disease, menopause and mental illness. That choice powerfully reinforced assumptions about causes as well. Indeed, the road chosen will inevitably unfold an environment that determines an entire world view. If you always travel in mountains, you cannot imagine the ocean.

Now let us suppose that the other road had been taken instead and had revealed that cholesterol has nothing much at all to do with the causation of heart disease and stroke; that synthetic hormone replacement therapy is a potentially fatal mistake; that treating cancer with toxic drugs and toxic rays stems from a fundamental misunderstanding of the nature of cancer; that anti-depressants do not restore the mind but actually can cause worse depression, suicide and violence as well as cancer, diabetes and irreversible brain damage.

This is a bit like imagining what would have happened if America had never been discovered. Then the tobacco industry would never come into being. While history cannot be switched into reverse like a movie, science can return to a previous bifurcation and start all over again—now full of important knowledge gained from enormous past mistakes. Since the time of the ancient Greeks, Western civilization has held that learning tends to come through suffering, and modern medicine is currently once again on that steep learning curve. This time, the task is not to control infection, find new surgical methods, discover the trick of anesthesia, and invent the concept of public health. This time, medicine needs to recognize how perilously close it is to moral bankruptcy. Only good medicine can undo the damage of bad medicine, and there are some amazingly good doctors out there working to renovate their profession.

The Road to Fame and Fortune

When Dr. Max Gerson provided the proof to US Congressional Committees in the early 1950s that even metastasized cancer can be cured through dietary regimes, alone the American government appears to have been primarily motivated by agonized idealism: they chose to give financial support for the development of radiation therapy, hoping that after the nightmare of Hiroshima there would be something beneficial in radiation for humanity. It took over 40 years before the National Institutes of Health finally was forced to acknowledge that no advance had been made in all that time in prevention, cure, or mortality rates, and serious research into the Gerson therapy is finally starting (see **www.dr-gonzalez.com**.

Turning to look briefly at the standard therapies for depression, cardiovascular disease, menopause, and asthma, we find that here the emperor is not only naked, but armed and dangerous. Two books show us how medicine was led down the garden path some 50 years ago. The first is by Dr. David Healy, the internationally renowned pharmacologist and psychiatrist whose expert testimony in law suits against various drug companies including Eli Lilly, the manufacturer of Prozac, resulted in that drug's dirty laundry finally becoming public knowledge. His book, *Let Them Eat Prozac*, published a few months ago by the Canadian Association of University Teachers and Lorimer, is so spell-binding a medical who-dunit, that it was appropriately reviewed by the master of spy novels, John Le Carre who wrote: "This very important book will demonstrate beyond your worst dreams that the commercial needs of Big Pharma are the natural-born enemy of independent scientific research."

Dr. Healy observes that the development and use of antidepressants followed the same path as that of the cholesterol-lowering drugs both based on a *choice* of assumptions favoring patents, rather than scientific integrity and patient outcome. He writes that: " the net effect of control" over science by business is that "certain aspects of the field (of research) are selected over others. A premium is put on certain data in a manner that builds up bandwagons and skews the field. This process is not confined to psychiatry. The cardiovascular field, for instance, contained in the late 1960s competing views as to what were important factors in preventing heart attacks. One lead suggested that blood homocysteine levels were important, another that blood lipid levels were the critical factor. The homocysteine hypothesis suggested a range of dietary approaches...such as taking folate or B vitamins. The lipid-lowering approach gave rise to a generation of patented drugs" which are "among the most profitable agents ever made. Rival evidence for homocysteine was effectively buried for almost 30 years." (He cites the prestigious journal *The Lancet* No. 354. 1999 and a new textbook published in 2000 which is finally leading us out of the toxic mess of lipid-lowering drugs; their worst property is that they deplete the body of CoEnzyme Q_{10}, the very substance upon which the health of the heart depends, thereby causing heart attacks.)

Dr. Healy's book describes how scientists who came up with evidence showing how dangerous the Selective Serotonin Reuptake Inhibitor (SSRI) class of drugs really might be, were silenced through classic, criminal dirty tricks . They didn't work on him, thank god, for here we have drugs like Paxil, which carry a 750% risk of cancer—compared to a daily pack of cigarettes a 400%. (The older antidepressants "merely" doubled that risk.) Increased risk of suicide, diabetes, irreversible neurological damage, weight gain, loss of sexual libido and homicidal violence are among SSRIs other devastating side-effects. A group of pharmacists decided to publish an entire 600-page compendium on the nutrient depletion of all synthetic drugs, published it in plain language for their victims and with all the biochemistry for the doctors duped into prescribing them.

How does this system work? An internet search under the heading "financial conflicts" locates for the past decade more than 3,000 articles in *The Lancet* alone, with the new *England Journal of Medicine*, the *Journal of the American Medical Association* and the *British Medical Journal* not far behind with about a thousand more between them. These articles focus on profit and deception. Thus, the profit margin on Prozac is 224,973 % per bottle of 240 pills (FDA figures). The deception is found in the fact that less than 50% of all research published is written by the researchers whose names are in the by-line; they are ghost written by industry hacks hired by Big Pharma. Dr. Healy calls this "the slippery slope" that gives a senior researcher an "extensive publication record very little of which he actually produced"; indeed, he or she "may actually get to the point of expressing surprise that people still write their own articles". This is how "control of what is said passes from the clinician to the companies." The result is that "big names become big names in this field [as chosen by the companies] because they are pushed forward by pharmaceutical company support." These big names then also sit on the committees that draft the standards of practice for the doctor treating us (JAMA Feb. 6, 2002).

And the money is good: "The returns for those at the top of this pyramid, including consultancy fees, fees for being principal investigators in trials, speaker's fees, chairman's fees, and other fees, may be substantial", some being "in the range of US $ 800,000 a year." But money is never the only incentive, and companies know that and make all this "personally gratifying. These players will be seen as the opinion leaders in the field…[they] may be too busy to do hands-on scientific work or even see patients, and may never observed the effects of the drug they are talking about, will be the ones informing others about that drug in some exotic location, by delivering a message worked out by the pharmaceutical company beforehand. All that is really required of the big name is to remember the brand name of the drug and to stick to the script."

Speaking about the trail of suicides, Dr. Healy estimates that the SSRI Zoloft increases the risk of suicide 2,000 times, or 1 per every 10 prescriptions. He concludes by observing that "one of the many chilling things about the Prozac story is that a mistake or a conspiracy would probably have cost fewer lives. Instead, a sequence of historical events [a path made into a highway] made a poor drug fashionable…and removed the natural cautions and safeguards…" He wonders, "Could key employees in a company like Eli

Lilly have been expected to appreciate the scale of the public health disaster ahead of them...and that, ultimately more harm than good would be done?"

The similar story can be told about synthetic hormones about which it was known since 1973 that they and those also containing estrogen from pregnant horses are potentially carcinogenic. But menopause had been made into disease like depression, and soon manufacturer made profits of US $ 37 million annually on just Premarin; it seemed not to bothered them that the yellow dye used in the sugar coating was listed as a separate, additional carcinogen by the FDA since the early 1980s. How many doctors read FDA reports? In 2002 the facts finally became public in the *Journal of the American Medical Association.*

Since then, in Canada alone, the use of synthetic estrogens dropped by 65%. Everything we were told turned out to be the opposite: HRT does not appreciably protect against osteoporosis (vitamin D does the job properly), memory loss (natural-source testosterone does that nicely), but it does dramatically increase the risk of cancer, heart attack, stroke and blood clots, and in combination with synthetic progesterone it's even worse. Inevitably, the medical profession will now begin to learn about the natural-source hormones.

Meanwhile, the drug industry is facing litigation on an astronomical scale: Bayer in Germany is currently fighting 11,300 lawsuits worldwide. Monsanto is facing liabilities in the range of US $ 2.3 billion. Merck downsized by thousands of employees last year; international financial institutions consider them poor risks. Finally, the medical profession in 2001 drew up a new international Physicians Charter to revive basic rules of ethical conduct known since Hippocrates. The leading journals now insist that articles must actually be authored by the person submitting them. Last September, the World Health Organization informed Britain's National Institute for Clinical Excellence that they better sever their ties to the drug industry if they wish to remain credible, as did the Canadian Association of University Teachers in 2002 to all our medical schools. That's some progress.

A skullduggery tale of equally tragic scope is found in Dr. Felix Ravikovich's book *The Plot Against Asthma and Allergy Patients* published by my company past November. Coming from the former Soviet Union, where no Big Pharma existed and no highway into Drug Hell was therefore paved, doctors struck out on a different path developing effective and safe low-tech methods for the treatment of asthma and allergy that naturally carry none of the toxic side-effects and growth-stunting properties of cortisone therapy. His book, like Dr. Healy's, reads like a detective story as he takes us through the scientific discoveries made in Europe and North America about the self-healing properties of the body's own histamine which can reverse asthma and allergy when used therapeutically. Yet, this information published in the leading medical journals world-wide remains hidden from patients. Indeed, the very scientists who made these great discoveries, remain mysteriously silent and do nothing to support clinical application, even though the World Health Organization in 2002 declared asthma to be a world-wide epidemic. Every 5th child in Canada suffers from it.

Worse even is the fact that the standards of practice enforced by the regulatory agencies, such as the Ontario College of Physicians and Surgeons, expressly forbade Dr. Ravikovich in 1994 the use of histamine in treating asthma—in spite of the protest of hundreds of patients on a CBC Fifth Estate show in the late 1990s. No patient was harmed, thousands were helped, and his research is found in the leading journals—not good enough for Ontario, it seems. In December, the head of immunology of the Swiss government's medical research institution in Davos, Professor Cezmi Akdis, wrote to Dr. Ravikovich: "Today I received your book and read most of it with great enthusiasm. My congratulations for bringing out such a good book which covers your life-time experience in a very critical area…. It will hopefully awake some clinical allergists."

Dr. Healy's and Dr. Ravikovich's expositions of the dark side of medicine will eventually make a difference. This valuable information is not lost. Dr. Ravikovich is fond of quoting a Russian saying, "If the door is bolted against the truth, it will come in by the window."

Sources and Resources:

Alternative Medicine Guide, Heart Disease, Stroke and High Blood Pressure, Future Medicine Publishing 1998

Dr. E.M. Cranton, *Bypassing Bypass Surgery,* Hampton Roads 2001M.

Dr. M. Gerson, *A Cancer Therapy,* 6th ed., (1958) Gerson Institute, 1999

Dr. G. N. Grob, *The Deadly Truth: A History of Disease in America,* Harvard University Press, 2002

Dr. D. Healy, *Let Them Eat Prozac,* Lorimer, 2003

Dr. J.M. Larson, *Depression-Free Naturally,* Ballantine, 1999

Dr. J.R. Lee, *What Your Doctor May Not Tell You About Breast Cancer,* Warner Books, 2002

R. Pelton et al, *The Nutritional Cost of Prescription Drugs,* Morton Publishing, 2000 (edition for non-medical readers) and/or *Drug-Induced Nutrient Depletion Handbook,* Lexi-Comp & American Pharmaceutical Association, 2001, ISBN 1-930598-45-9 (for doctors and health care professionals)

Dr. F. Ravikovich, *The Plot Against Asthma and Allergy Patients,* Kos, Dr. U. Reiss, *Natural Hormone Balance for Women,* Pocket Books, 2001

Dr. J. Whitaker, *Reversing Heart Disease,* Warner Books, 2002

Final Comments

I placed this article at the end of this book because the information in it illustrates that the world of medicine we have at the moment is not in any way absolute or even remotely approaching completion, but medicine is a work in progress—"painful progress", as one of the characters in that great play *Angels in America* puts it at the end, in reference to all humanity in general. Many diverging paths are open to us all, whether we are doctors or patients, and we can chose to explore different ones. If one believes in *absolute* authority of any kind, that science has figured something out once and for all, that there is one truth and we must obey its dictates, one becomes a statistic of that path which one chose.

Some paths are better than others, and that also shows in their statistics! But all paths lead to new diverging options in the course of history. Orthomolecular and environmental medicine and nutritional cancer therapies have the best statistics for survival and recovery, but they, too, are constantly searching for improvement, and basic science is bringing out more and more information on how to work *with* the body, how to understand what Nature wants.

One of Canada's great scientists and activists, Ursula Franklin, observed in the Massey Lectures of 1990: "Whenever suggestions for political action are placed before the government of Canada, the first consideration always seems to be, 'What about the Americans. They may not like it. They may let their displeasure be seen and felt. They may retaliate!' And what about nature? Obviously nature is not taking kindly to what is going on in the real world of technology. Nature *is* retaliating, and we had better understand why and how this is happening. I would therefore suggest to you that, in all processes of planning, nature should be considered as a strong and independent power. Ask, 'What will nature do?'" (p.86) This applies to all issues of environment and health because there can be no health without the recognition that the environment is the basis of all health.

Humanity is young. We survived as bi-pedal creatures with rapidly growing brains for some 3 million years and are physically and emotionally a hardy lot. We are, after causing much damage, likely to wake up from our nightmare of greed and sloth and stop working against the environment that sustains us. Our explorations of health and disease and the conscientious correction of our errors in judgment are only beginning, and that beginning is very promising. We understand now, what former University of Toronto environmental studies professor Henry Regier called "new domains of ignorance". Just as the advent of agriculture in the Neolithic period brought with it infectious diseases, and the rise of urbanism some five thousand years ago allowed chronic illnesses to evolve as patterns of disease, our chemical era has presented us challenges we could never have imagined.

So, the following comments by Ursula Franklin on Regier's observation are poignantly pertinent to the dominant position the environment holds for human health and survival, to all developments of therapy, and to drugs in particular: "…with every development new domains of ignorance are discovered which become evident only as the project proceeds. The emergence of domains of ignorance is basically quite inevitable. Some of the side effects of technical processes could not have been known…but the existence of domains of ignorance is quite predictable. That means, that it is necessary to proceed with great caution when moving into the unknown and the unknowable." (p. 128)

Finally, in addition to considering nature's dominant position, and learning humility in the face of the only barely predictable dynamics of nature, we also need to understand that it matters profoundly what we imagine health to be, what we imagine about the prognosis of our condition, what we imagine to be the correct approach, whether we are doctors or patients, and that fatalistically accepting the verdict of some authority is the end of our creative involvement with life. In medicine especially, the great observation of the Buddha applies to patient and physician alike: "All that we are is the result of what we have thought—it is founded on our thoughts, it is made up of our thoughts. With our thoughts we make the world."

Source

U. Franklin, *The Real World of Technology* (Massey Lectures 1990), revised edition, Anansi, 1999

Books of Interest

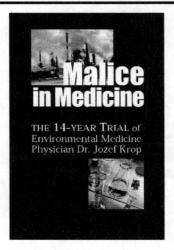

THE 14-YEAR TRIAL of Environmental Medicine Physician Dr. Jozef Krop

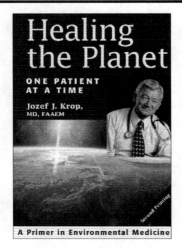

A Primer in Environmental Medicine

From 1988 to 2002 Dr. Jozef Krop fought for the legal right to practice state-of-the-art environmental medicine. Without patient complaint, the prosecuting College of Physicians and Surgeons of Ontario (mandated to control doctors' licenses) maintained that environmentally induced illness is at best a psychiatric disorder and ignored international medical consensus on Multiple Chemical Sensitivity, Sick Building Syndrome and related medical conditions. Dr. Krop's battle was supported by a stellar international panel of medical experts and by thousands of patients made ill by industrial chemicals and pesticides; legal costs exceeded 1 million dollars, all paid by public donations. This book tells the dramatic story of a physician's successful challenge of corruption in the medical regulatory system.

6" × 9" | 400 pages | PB | $25.00
November 2005

The general reader learns from his book to:
• identify health hazards in the home and work-place environments and what to do about them
• find help through a comprehensive resource section covering everything from pesticides to food allergies, electromagnetic fields, holistic dentistry, safe building materials, how to become a practitioner in environmental medicine and much more
• recognize warning signs that indicate probable environmental illness and how to find medically reliable help

Readers who are health professionals may use this book
• to find the references from the mainstream medical literature covering the field of environmental toxins and the treatment of environmental illness
• basic treatment and detoxification protocols for patients with environmental illness

ISBN 0-9731945-0-2
6" × 9" | 368 pages | PB | $25.00 | 2003

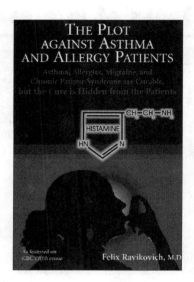

DR. FELIX RAVIKOVICH obtained his medical degree and specialized in Internal Medicine in the former Soviet Union. Since 1985, he has practiced in Toronto specializing in allergy and asthma. His presentations at international conferences on the effective treatment with histamine were published in leading medical journals. This is his first book for the general public and medical colleagues.

Dr. Ravikovich describes his clinical experience with histamine—a synthetic version of the body's substance that stimulates the body to heal itself. His histamine therapy freed hundreds of asthma, allergy and migraine sufferers from drugs that have disastrous effects on the patients' health and the course of the diseases for which these drugs are prescribed.

Unlike other books that concentrate on triggers, this book spells out the primary cellular and genetic defects in patients with allergies, asthma and related diseases and shows how to repair these defects. The author substantiates this through the theoretical works of the world's leading scientists.

Dr. Ravikovich undertook an extensive detective search of literature in molecular biology, immunopharmacology, genetics, and clinical medicine that led him to unprecedented revelations. The scientific foundation for the treatment that could save millions from suffering and dying has been concealed by the medical elite to enable the pharmaceutical industry to develop only those drugs that do not cure and ensure indefinite patient dependence.

Dr. Ravikovich tells the story of his own battle with the medical regulatory authorities which work actively to suppress good, scientifically grounded medicine and protect—not patients— but corporate interests.

ISBN 0-9731945-1-0 | **2003**
6" × 9" | **432 pages** | **PB** | **$25.00**

Books of Interest

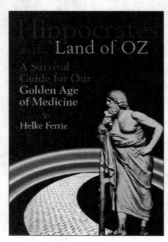

"There are no magic bullets. But miracles occur daily—if we accept illness as a teacher. The first doctor to be consulted is the one living in our hearts. Trusting that inner physician's advice is a political act of liberation for yourself and others."

"Why eat organic? The single most important health decision you can ever make is to protect your body from the witches' brew of money-science. Regaining the Garden of Eden is a task to be accomplished and we have the knowledge to re-create that garden."

"The requirements of human biology cannot be made to harmonize with the priorities of a world economy in which pesticides are of central importance."

"We have choices our ancestors never dreamed of. It takes an open mind and a fearless curiosity to benefit from what is available in medicine and the determination to protect that freedom of choice."

"Exploring how to have healthy children is a worthy meditation. They are not only our future, they are also the very incarnation of God's unfolding imagination. Paradoxically, it is up to us to protect and nurture this mystery."

ISBN 0-9731945-2-9
6" × 9" | 400 pages | PB | $25.00
February 2005

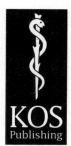

Order form

KOS can be contacted at the address given below to obtain more information or to place an order for any of our publications.

KOS PUBLISHING INC.
1997 Beechgrove Road
Alton, Ontario Canada L0N 1A0   **www.kospublishing.com**
Tel: (519) 927-1049 • Fax: (519) 927-9542
Email: helke@inetsonic.com • info@kospublishing.com

Name:_____   Date: _____

Address: _____   Payment: ○ Cheque ○ Visa

City: _____   ○ Master Card

Prov./State:_____   Name on Card: _____

Postal/Zip Code:_____   Card #: _____

Telephone: _____   Expiry Date: _____

Email:_____   Signature: _____

ISBN	TITLE	QTY.	PRICE	TOTAL
0-9731945-0-2	*Healing the Planet*		$28.95	
0-9731945-1-0	*The Plot Against Asthma and Allergy Patients*		$25.00	
0-9731945-3-7	*Dispatches from the War Zone of Environmental Health*		$25.00	
0-9731945-2-9	*Hippocrates in the Land of Oz*		$20.00	
	Malice in Medicine		$25.00	
			SUB-TOTAL	
			TAXES	
			TOTAL	

About the Author

HELKE FERRIE is a medical science writer with a master's degree in anthropology and prehistoric archaeology. Her special area of interest is human evolutionary biology and the anthropology of disease. She started writing on issues of medicine and environment as a result of a serious illness caused by mercury and pesticide poisoning in the mid-1990s. Having raised a family of 12 adopted and 3 biological children, she and her physician husband of over 30 years now live with various cats and dogs north of Toronto. Her better half practices psychotherapy (EMDR) and she runs KOS Publishing Inc. dedicated to books on "medicine that works." She writes monthly for Toronto's *Vitality Magazine* and frequently for *Alive* and US-based publications.